Manual of

I.V.

Therapeutics

Manual of

I.V.

Therapeutics

Lynn Dianne Phillips, RN, MSN, CRNI
Instructor of Nursing
Butte Community College
Oroville, California

 F. A. DAVIS COMPANY • Philadelphia

F. A. Davis Company
1915 Arch Street
Philadelphia, PA 19103

Printed in the United States of America

Last digit indicates print number: 10 9 8 7 6 5

Publisher, Nursing: Robert G. Martone
Nursing Acquisitions Editor: Evan R. Schnittman
Production Editor: Crystal S. McNichol
Cover design by: Steven R. Morrone

As new scientific information becomes available through basic and clinical research, recommended treatments and drug therapies undergo changes. The author(s) and publisher have done everything possible to make this book accurate, up to date, and in accord with accepted standards at the time of publication. The authors, editors, and publisher are not responsible for errors or omissions or for consequences from application of the book, and make no warranty, expressed or implied, in regard to the contents of the book. Any practice described in this book should be applied by the reader in accordance with professional standards of care used in regard to the unique circumstances that may apply in each situation. The reader is advised always to check product information (package inserts) for changes and new information regarding dose and contraindications before administering any drug. Caution is especially urged when using new or infrequently ordered drugs.

Library of Congress Cataloging-in-Publication Data

Phillips, Lynn Dianne, 1947–
    Manual of I.V. therapeutics / Lynn Dianne Phillips.
       p. cm.
    Includes bibliographical references and index.
    ISBN 0-8036-6911-9 (soft : alk. paper)
    1. Intravenous therapy. I. Title.
    [DNLM: 1. Blood Transfusion—methods—nurses' instruction.
    2. Drug Administration Routes—nurses' instruction. 3. Fluid
    Therapy—methods—nurses' instruction. 4. Infusions, Intravenous—
    methods—nurses' instruction. WD 220 P561m]
    RM170.P48 1993
    615'.6—dc20
    DNLM/DLC   92-48825
    for Library of Congress   CIP

TO MY FAMILY

My husband, Don, for your support and encouragement during this project.

My children, Christa and Timothy.

My parents, Larry and Margie Schuetz, for always believing in your children.

TO ALL MY STUDENTS:

This is for you!

PREFACE

I.V.-related skills, according to an American Journal of Nursing 1991 Survey, are performed by 85 percent of the nurses in the acute setting. During many years of educating nurses about techniques in I.V. therapy, I have heard this question asked over and over again: "Why don't we have more of this information in nursing school?" Another common question is "Why doesn't our staff development department have more classes so that we can keep up our skills in I.V.-related therapy?" Lack of time is the response. Using time as a valued resource, this manual can be used by student and novice nurses in the hospital or alternate setting where I.V. therapy skills are necessary or as a resource for expert practitioners.

My search for a self-paced comprehensive text for students and educators, along with my quest for a research book for practitioners, has resulted in the modular-experiential approach to learning I.V. therapy skills presented in this text. *Manual of I.V. Therapeutics* provides a text from which instruction builds from simple to complex, incorporating theory into clinical application. The skills of recall, assessment, and nursing diagnosis, along with summaries, provide the foundation to produce a knowledgeable therapist. The psychomotor skills associated with I.V. therapy are presented in step-by-step procedures based on standards of practice. The effective behavior of valuing standards of practice for safe delivery of patient care is presented in the form of an Activity Journal at the end of each chapter that focuses on the reader's own area of practice.

This book uniquely combines a workbook, text, and pocket guide. Each chapter in Units Two and Three has accompanying objectives, defined glossary terms, a pre-test and a post-test, worksheets, an Activity Journal, and a Quality Assessment Model. Nursing assessment and nursing diagnoses are threaded throughout the manual. Standards of practice are emphasized using Intravenous Nursing Society 1990 Revised Standards of Practice and Occupational Safety and Health Administration (OSHA) guidelines.

This manual is divided into three units: Unit One lays the foundation for practice, Unit Two covers basic I.V. therapy, and Unit Three covers advanced practice. Unit One provides two chapters designed to introduce the reader to the legal responsibilities, risks, and steps of quality assurance using assessment. The history includes past, present, and future trends that contribute to the changing clinical picture of I.V. therapy.

Unit Two provides the essential foundation for I.V. therapy practice, which includes techniques for venipuncture using a 15-step format, fluids and electrolyte balance, parenteral fluids, and special problems of the pediatric and geriatric patient. Unit Two also emphasizes a modular approach. Assessment is a key concept in Units Two and Three, along with the focus on nursing diagnosis.

Unit Three includes four chapters covering content specific to transfusion therapy, I.V. medication administration, central lines, and nutritional support.

The appendices include reference charts for physical and chemical compatibility, normal reference laboratory values, and the guidelines for personnel dealing with cytotoxic agents. Dilution rates for I.V. drugs and the NANDA 10th National Conference nursing diagnoses list and definitions are included for reference. Due to the changing role of the Licensed Practical Nurse/Licensed Vocational Nurse (LPN/LVN), a list of states that have expanded the role of I.V. therapy in the LPN/LVN practice is provided.

I hope this working manual provides you, whether a practicing health care provider or nursing student, valuable insight into safe I.V. practice and a reference for the rapidly advancing field of I.V. therapy.

ACKNOWLEDGMENTS

The author would like to acknowledge the following:

My I.V. therapy students at Butte College from 1990 to 1992 for your valuable input and enthusiasm for this manual.

The nurses in the specialty practice of I.V. therapy, who are angels.

Christie Boggs, Lead Secretary, Area III Butte Community College, for the computer assistance, corrections, and help in presenting this material to the publishers in a readable form.

The nursing department at Butte Community College for all their support and encouragement during this project.

Robert G. Martone, Publisher, Nursing, whose foresight brought the project to F.A. Davis.

Evan R. Schnittman, Nursing Acquisitions Editor at F.A. Davis, who assisted in the final development of this manual.

Ruth DeGeorge, Executive Editorial Secretary, who kept track of the manuscript and always greeted me with a warm, friendly voice.

Crystal McNichol, Production Editor, for finalizing galley and page proofs and laughing with me.

Herbert Powell, Director of Production, for guiding my manuscript through the production process.

The author would also like to thank the following reviewers, whose constructive criticisms helped to bring this manual to completion.

Barbara Brown, RN, MN, CCRN
Community College of Allegheny County — North
Pittsburgh, Pennsylvania

Suzanne M. Davis, RN, MSN
Greenville Technical College
Greenville, South Carolina

Jane Freeman, PhD
Jacksonville State University
Jacksonville, Alabama

Rosalie Graveline, RN, MEd
River College
St. Joseph's School of Nursing
Nashua, New Hampshire

Carol O. Long, RN, MSN
Arizona State University
Tempe, Arizona

Patricia Murray, RN
Amarillo College
Department of Nursing
Amarillo, Texas

Beverly Reno, RN, MSN
Northern Kentucky University
Highland Heights, Kentucky

Lorna Schumann, RN, PhD
Intercollegiate Center for Nursing Education
Spokane, Washington

CONTRIBUTING AUTHOR

Leslie Baranowski, BSN, CRNI
Clinical Manager I.V. Therapy Services
Roseville Hospital
Roseville, California

CONSULTANTS

Maxine Acevedo, CRNI, MPA
Manager of I.V. Therapy
University of California-Davis Medical Center
Sacramento, California

Leslie Baranowski, BSN, CRNI
Clinical Manager I.V. Therapy Services
Roseville Hospital
Roseville, California

Laylee Charlang, BSN, OCN
Quality Assurance Coordinator
OptionCare Inc.
Chico, California

Carol Jorgensen Huston, RN, MSN
Professor of Nursing
California State University
Chico, California

Edie Jonas, BSN, CRNI
Assistant Director I.V. Services
Roseville Hospital
Roseville, California

Joan Lotti, CRNI
Nutritional Support Consultant
Staff Nurse
Enloe Hospital
Chico, California

Bessie Marquis, RN, CNAA, MSN
Professor of Nursing
California State University
Chico, California

Mary Mirch, BSN, MS
Assistant Professor of
Allied Health and Nursing
Glendale Community College
Glendale, California

CONTENTS

UNIT THREE:
Advanced Practice

TABLES

INTRODUCTION TO THE PRACTICE OF INTRAVENOUS THERAPY

CHAPTER 1

Intravenous Therapy: Past, Present, and Future Trends

The foundation for intravenous (I.V.) therapy began slowly with contributions from chemists, physicians, and architects. The specialty practice of I.V. therapy as we know it today has many heroes and heroines who have made an imprint on this area of medicine. The history of I.V. therapy is woven with individuals aided by advances in technical development. Five hundred years have elapsed from the discovery of the circulation of blood to today's state-of-the-art tunneled catheters, implanted ports, and blood component therapy. A review of the roots of I.V. therapy precedes the study of the theoretic and practical applications of I.V. therapy.

RENAISSANCE ERA (1438 to 1660)

The history of I.V. therapy began with the discovery by Sir William Harvey of the circulation of blood. Until the late Renaissance period it was known that the arteries and veins both contained blood, but it was believed that the blood ebbed and flowed "like the human breath." The essential parts of the circulatory system and the capillary networks were unknown, and for centuries this fundamental error was accepted as truth. Harvey was the first to discover that the heart is both a muscle and a pump, and he lectured extensively in Europe to educate other physicians.

Sir Christopher Wren, the famous architect of St. Paul's Cathedral in London, worked with a chemist and produced the first hypodermic needle. Wren inserted a hollow pipe in the blood vessel of dogs and injected wine, ale, opium, scammony, liver of antimony, and other substances directly into the bloodstream and studied their effect. He was thus credited for using a quill and bladder to inject the first I.V. substance.

A German physician, Johann Majors, was the first to use Sir Christopher Wren's discovery of the hypodermic needle and injected unpurified compounds into humans. The disastrous consequences of this early experimental work were compounded by the fact that infections occurred at the site of injection, resulting in death.

In 1667, the first well-documented transfusion from an animal to a human

Table 1 – 1   □   **SUMMARY OF KEY HISTORIC ADVANCES IN THE RENAISSANCE ERA**

Year	Key Perspectives
1543	Andreas Vesalius published written account of his work on anatomy and surgery based on dissections.
1616	Sir William Harvey discovered circulation of blood.
1628	Sir William Harvey published theories on circulation, considered to be the beginning of modern I.V. therapy.
1660	Sir Christopher Wren invented the first hypodermic needle.
1662	German physician Johann Majors injected compounds into human, using Wren's needle.
1667	First well-documented transfusion from animal to human performed in Paris by John Denis. This led to the edict from the church and parliament prohibiting all further work on transfusion therapy.

was performed. The Parisian physician John Baptiste Denis infused lamb's blood directly into the circulation of a 15-year-old boy. The boy died quickly. This early experiment was not well received, and in 1687, by edict of the church and parliament, animal-to-human transfusions were prohibited in Europe (Schmidt, 1959, pp 59 – 62). Because of this edict, 150 years passed before injecting substances into the circulation again became of interest, in the 19th century. Table 1 – 1 summarizes the key historic advances before the 19th century.

THE 19th CENTURY

In 1831, the Anatomy Act was designed to regulate human dissection; Florence Nightingale was 8 years old and Joseph Lister, 4; and an outbreak of cholera, the second pandemic, was spreading across Asia and Europe from India. Dr. William Brooke O'Shaughnessy, a recent Edinburgh graduate, age 22, wrote his first paper on cholera. He became engrossed in the cause and cure of cholera. O'Shaughnessy described cholera and studied the blood drawn from patients with the disease. He wrote to *The Lancet* on February 4, 1832:

> The blood drawn in the worst cases . . . is unchanged in its anatomical or globular structure. . . . It has lost a large proportion of its water . . . . It has lost also a great proportion of its neutral saline ingredients . . . . Of the free alkali contained in healthy serum, not a particle is present.
> Cited in Cosnett, 1989

The first practical application of O'Shaughnessy's observations was by Dr. Thomas Latta, who used infusions of saline to treat the intractable diarrhea of cholera. He published his results in *The Lancet* on June 2, 1832. However, no previous records existed of water and salts being given deliberately to restore constituents of the blood. Of the first 25 reported cases treated by saline, eight survived. Because there was severe criticism of this method of treatment, when the pandemic spread to America from 1852 to 1863, the use of I.V. saline was not accepted (van Heyningen, 1983). During this same period, James Blundell, an English obstetrician, revived the idea of injecting blood into humans. In 1834 he proved that animal blood was unfit to inject into humans, and instead used human blood to save many women threatened by hemorrhage during childbirth.

During the latter part of the 19th century advances were made in medicine. Accelerated knowledge regarding bacteriology, pathology, and pharmacology revealed new approaches to problems of medicine. Horace Wells demonstrated the use of nitrous oxide and ether as a form of anesthesia. A chemist, Charles Jackson, assisted W. T. G. Morton in his first surgical operation with ether at Massachusetts General Hospital in Boston on October 16, 1846. This method of anesthesia spread quickly throughout America and Europe, but chloroform soon came to be preferred to ether.

In 1847, a Viennese obstetrician, Ignaz Semmelweis, noted that physicians moving from autopsies to the maternity unit were passing highly pathogenic substances to the obstetric patients. He was the first to require that physicians wash their hands in a solution of chlorine before examining an obstetric patient. Through this simple procedure of cleanliness, the death rate in the maternity wards was reduced by more than 90 percent between 1846 and 1848.

Louis Pasteur, a chemist, later demonstrated the scientific basis for Semmelweis' theory, proving bacteria were living microorganisms. However, Pasteur's ideas were challenged and it was not until Lister's work in 1867 that the germ theory was accepted and the war won. Lister's work focused on sterility in the operating room and led to the practice of asepsis. His aseptic technique came to replace older antiseptic methods, and was universally accepted. Later William Halsted introduced the use of rubber gloves (Kalisch & Kalisch, 1986, pp 130–136) (Table 1–2).

The primitive state of medical knowledge and practice in the 1880s had an influence on the morbidity or mortality of infants and young children of the time. Infant mortality rate during this time varied from 250 to 500 of 1000 live births. The high morbidity and mortality rates of the late 19th century accounted for the average lifespan of 35 to 38 years. Enteric disorders, malnutrition, and common respiratory and contagious diseases constituted the major causes of death during the 19th century. Table 1–3 lists the life expectancies from the 1600s to the present.

Medications during the turn of the century were limited primarily to the coal tar products, which were used to treat febrile illnesses and influenza. The following is a list of the 10 most commonly administered compounds during the 19th century (Kalisch & Kalisch, 1986, p 127):

1. Ether
2. Morphine
3. Digitalis
4. Diphtheria antitoxin
5. Smallpox vaccine
6. Iron
7. Quinine
8. Iodine
9. Alcohol
10. Mercury

Table 1–2 □ SUMMARY OF KEY HISTORIC EVENTS OF THE 19th CENTURY

Year	Key Perspectives
1818	English obstetrician James Blundell revived the idea of transfusions for hemorrhage during childbirth. He proved that animal blood was unfit to inject into humans and that only human blood was safe.
1831	The Anatomy Act, designed to regulate human dissection, was debated. An outbreak of cholera, the second pandemic, spread across Asia and Europe from India.
Dec 1831	Dr. William Brooke O'Shaughnessy wrote a paper on cholera and applied chemistry to its cure. He cited detailed descriptions of blood from cholera patients. He recommended restoring blood to natural specific gravity and restoring saline matter of blood.
June 1832	Dr. Thomas Latta of Scotland successfully used I.V. saline on cholera patients, based on Dr. O'Shaughnessy's work on cholera.
1852–1863	Despite further pandemics I.V. saline was not widely used.
1845	Horace Wells demonstrated the use of nitrous oxide and ether for anesthesia.
1846	W. T. G. Morton, with assistance from chemist, used ether in first surgical operation with this agent at Massachusetts General Hospital in Boston.
1847	Dr. Ignaz Semmelweis noted that infection was transferred from postmortem patients to obstetric patients. He was first to require physicians to wash hands in solution of chlorine before the examination of maternity patients.
1857	Dr. Pasteur demonstrated scientific basis for Semmelweis' theory.
1867	Lord Lister achieved success with meticulous attention to sterility during surgical procedures.
Late 1800s	Dr. Edward Robinson Squibb founded pharmaceutical company and manufactured products including talcum and ether anesthesia in tins.

THE 20th CENTURY

In 1900, Dr. Karl Landsteiner proved that not all human blood was alike with the discovery of three of the four main blood groups. This led the way to compatible blood transfusions and the development of blood banks. Until 1914,

Table 1–3 □ LIFE EXPECTANCY FROM 1600s TO THE PRESENT

Year	Age (years)
1600s	21
1700s	25
1800s	35–38
1901	48
1920s	54
1940s	65
1982	Women 78; men 70
2000	Women 81; men 73

with no way to prevent the coagulation of blood, every transfusion was performed via the direct method, recipient to donor; however, with the discovery of sodium citrate, blood could be stored and blood banking began.

Until Dr. Florence Seibert discovered pyrogen substances in distilled water, many problems existed related to pyrogens (proteins foreign to the blood) within solutions. Researchers worked to eliminate those pyrogens, and the administration of parenteral solutions became safer. Before 1925, the most frequently used parenteral solution was normal saline solution because of its isotonic relationship to blood. After 1925, dextrose was used extensively to provide a source of calories. I.V. solutions, however, were used only in the critically ill patient.

The first I.V.-hydrolyzed protein and fat were administered to animals during the early 20th century, leading the way for today's nutritional support solutions. In 1937, Dr. W. C. Rose identified amino acids essential for growth in rats, which led to the development of protein hydrolysates for infusion into humans.

In 1940 Dr's Karl Landsteiner and Alexander Wiener discovered the Rhesus system which moved transfusion therapy ahead by leaps and bounds. Along with changes in blood groupings, great strides were made at Massachusetts General Hospital, where nurses were first assigned to be I.V. nurses. The services of the I.V. nurse consisted of administering I.V. solutions and transfusions, cleaning infusion sets, and cleaning and sharpening needles. The role of the nurse changed primarily because of the shortage of physicians during World War II. Nurses took over jobs that physicians had always done: administering injections, suturing wounds, taking blood pressure readings, drawing blood, as well as providing I.V. infusion therapy. Nurses were trained in I.V. therapy by the anesthesiologist in the operating room.

In 1950, the Rochester needle was introduced. This device consisted of a resinous catheter on the outside of a steel needle; the catheter was slipped off the needle and into the vein and the needle removed. The first change in the steel needle appeared in 1957, when McGaw Laboratories introduced small vein sets with foldable wings as grips. In 1958, the Intracath (Deseret Pharmaceutical Co.), a plastic catheter lying within the lumen of the needle, was introduced in individual sterile packaging. This type of catheter reduced the need for surgical cutdown for placement of the 1940s catheter (Plumer & Cosentino, 1987, p 5).

In the mid-1950s I.V. therapy was used for two main purposes: major surgery and dehydration. Solutions of 5% dextrose and water or normal saline for surgical patients were infused over 3 to 4 hours and discontinued at night (Millam, 1987).

Less than 20 percent of hospital patients received I.V. therapy in the mid-1950s. The site most frequently used by nurses during this period was the antecubital vein. A 16- to 18-gauge steel reusable needle was used and stabilized with leather restraints. Disposable plastic sets became available and replaced reusable rubber tubing, and frequent infiltrations with metal needles led to the development of the flexible plastic catheter for insertion by the cutdown method (Crossley & Matsen, 1972).

Medications were not routinely administered by the I.V. route, but rather were given intramuscularly. For seriously ill patients with diseases like meningitis, penicillin or chloromycetin was given by continuous I.V. drip. When patients required medication added to their infusions, an intern carried out this procedure, often using medication that had been unrefrigerated for long periods of time. When blood was needed, the patient received whole blood in a glass bottle, administered by the intern with assistance from the nursing staff.

The momentum for change in the I.V. therapy field occurred during the 1960s. A variety of solutions were marketed, expanding the choice to approximately 200. Piggyback medications were used, and filters and electronic infusion devices flooded the market.

In 1960 peripherally inserted central catheters (PICCs) became common on critical care units. Recently they have become popular alternatives for central venous access (Viall, 1990). In 1963 at the Harrison Department of Surgical Research at the University of Pennsylvania, a young surgical resident, Stanley Dudrick, conducted the first experiment to determine definitely whether or not long-term total I.V. nutrition was feasible. Dudrick's experiments quickly were applied to starving adult patients who would probably not have survived without total parenteral nutrition (Dudrick & Rhoads, 1972).

In 1967, the first hyperalimentation was given to patients at Children's Hospital in Philadelphia. In 1968, RhoGAM was manufactured and available to the physician for Rh-negative mothers to prevent hemolytic disease of the newborn.

In 1970, blood components and the prescribing of selected components for individual situations, such as packed cells for the anemic patient, were instituted. In 1976, a fat emulsion, Intralipid (Abbott Pharmaceuticals), was instituted as an adjunct to nutritional support. Cutdowns continued to be used until the mid-1970s for severely ill patients, to prevent the complication of infiltration. Catheter sites were changed only when the catheters were not functioning. It was not until the early 1970s that the Centers for Disease Control (CDC) developed recommendations for infection control related to I.V. therapy. In the 1970s there was a scarcity of I.V. information in nursing journals and, of course, I.V. therapy journals were nonexistent until the late 1970s. Nursing schools presented I.V. therapy in a limited manner, with more theory than practical management. In 1975, tunneled catheters such as Hickman-Broviac and Groshong were introduced and have increased in popularity for long-term access.

The past 10 years have been the fastest growing for the I.V. therapy field. The National Intravenous Therapy Association (NITA) published recommendations for practices in 1980. The US House of Representatives on October 1, 1980, recognized and nationalized I.V. Nurse Day throughout the country. It was

> resolved, that I.V. Nurse Day be nationally celebrated in honor of the National Intravenous Therapy Association Inc. on January 25 of each year. . .

according to the proclamation presented by the Honorable Edward J. Mackey from the Fifth Congressional District of Massachusetts (Gardner, 1985). The NITA first national Certification Examination for Intravenous Nurses was offered in March 1985. In 1987, NITA changed its name to Intravenous Nurses Society (INS) (Table 1-4). In 1987 the CDC developed its system of "universal precautions," primarily to reduce the risk of transmitting HIV, the virus that causes AIDS and hepatitis B (HBV), to health care workers. The Body-Substance Isolation System, developed by nurses and their colleagues working in

8

Table 1–4 □ **SUMMARY OF KEY ADVANCES IN THE 20th CENTURY**

Year	Key Perspectives
1900	Karl Landsteiner discovered three of four main blood groups.
1914	Sodium citrate used to preserve blood. Hydrolyzed protein and fats given intravenously to animals.
1923	Dr. Florence Seibert discovered pathogens in distilled water. Sterilization practices for infusion therapy changed.
1937	W. C. Rose identified amino acids essential for growth in rats; this led to development of protein hydrolysates for infusion.
1940	Drs. Landsteiner and Wiener discovered Rhesus (Rh) factor.
1940	Work by Tocantins and O'Neil led to use of intraosseous infusions.
1945	Development of flexible plastic I.V. catheter inserted by cutdown method.
1950	Rochester needle introduced.
1957	McGraw Laboratories introduced a steel needle with foldable wings as grips.
1958	Deseret Pharmaceuticals introduced the Intracath.
1960	First hyperalimentation experiment on animals began. Peripherally inserted central lines used in critical care units.
1963	Research by Stanley Dudrick at University of Pennsylvania involved first experiment to determine whether long-term total I.V. nutritional support was feasible.
1968	RhoGAM used to treat Rh hemolytic disease.
1970	Blood components made available for use in specific situations. CDC guidelines for I.V. therapy published.
1972	Concept of accessing an implantable port introduced.
1975	First central venous tunneled catheter developed. Broviac right atrial catheter designed and introduced.
1976	Fat emulsions used for nutritional support.
1977	National Cancer Institute testing of intraperitoneal chemotherapy began in selected patients.
1980	NITA published recommended practices for therapy. US House of Representatives recognized I.V. Nurse Day.
1982	Implantable ports developed for long-term access.
1983	Resurgence of interest in intraosseous infusions in children.
1986	Resurgence of interest in PICCs for adults.
1987	CDC developed system of "universal precautions."

large hospitals, reduces the risks to patients and health care workers (Jackson & Lynch, 1990).

Tunneled catheters such as Hickman-Broviac and Groshong have provided a means of central venous access for delivery of hyperalimentation and cytoxic therapy. In the past 5 years, totally implanted access devices consisting of subcutaneous reservoir connected to a catheter positioned in the central circulation provided alternatives for patients requiring long-term access. The changes in management of patients needing long-term I.V. therapy with permanent central venous lines have expanded the field of I.V. therapy. The role of the nurse has changed along with advanced technical innovations. Today, 80 percent of all hospitalized patients receive I.V. therapy, and many receive home I.V. therapy. A 1990 *American Journal of Nursing* survey found that 81 percent of nurses performed I.V. skills more than 75 percent of the time (Griffith, Thomas, & Griffith, 1991). The role of the nurse has also changed in home care settings with patients requiring home care monitoring of I.V. therapy.

FUTURE TRENDS

Looking ahead to the 21st century, it is inconceivable that nurses will be limited to the responsibilities they hold today. By the turn of the century nurses will be assuming more and more health care responsibilities. Changes in expenditures for health care, the hospital costs, and the seriously ill patients will all have an impact on the nursing profession. Patients in the hospitals of the year 2000 will be those needing highly intensive and sophisticated treatment.

Technology will continue to evolve in health care. Patients will find treatment in noninstitutional settings such as outpatient centers, diagnostic centers, self-care centers, and health-related shopping centers. It is projected that patients will be better able to match the nature of their disease or illness with the appropriate care setting and will have more autonomy in the prevention and treatment of their illness. Satellite telemedicine and video network hookups will be in common use. Nurses will routinely provide services outside hospitals, addressing patients' relatively minor problems in noninstitutional ways (Kalisch & Kalisch, 1986, p 751). Nurses will be case managers of catastrophic cases and work through insurance agencies as independent practitioners.

The growth or expansion of the nurse's role is both necessary and desirable. The changing role of the nurse leads to the development of many new programs designed to prepare the nurse to use new skills and assume new responsibilities. New roles are emerging, with nurses developing an interdependent, collaborative, and peer relationship with physicians. I.V. therapy is just one of those interdependent roles needing a sound foundation in basic as well as advanced theory (Grippando, 1986, p 257).

The role of the registered nurse is well defined in the initiation, maintenance, and therapeutic modalities as identified in each state's nursing practice act. Standards of practice established by the INS and CDC have set guidelines for the role of the registered nurse in all aspects of I.V. therapy and nutritional support.

Because of the shortage of licensed personnel in many settings, the role of the licensed practical/vocational nurse (LPN/LVN) as an integral part of the I.V. therapy team is in the process of evaluation. The role of the LPN/LVN has been expanded in 20 states to encompass the initiation, maintenance, and delivery of solutions, antibiotics, blood components, and peripheral nutritional support. Each of the 20 states has established the expanded role of the LPN/LVN with clear guidelines for practice. Another 26 states delegate the role of I.V. therapy to the institution in which the LPN/LVN is practicing. Four states have elected to deny I.V. therapy in the scope of LPN/LVN duties. Refer to Appendix I for the survey on the expanded role of the LPN/LVN.

At present the INS has recognized that the LPN/LVN has a place in the scope of I.V. nursing and is preparing a credentialing examination for the LPN/LVN.

TRENDS OF THE 21st CENTURY
✓ Bionics of artificial limbs and organs will continue to evolve.
✓ Artificial hearts and kidneys will prolong lives of people for many years.
✓ Nurses in ambulatory care facilities will provide the majority of health services.

✓ Robots, within the average hospital budget, will be used for retrieving supplies.

✓ Computers will proliferate for concise record keeping.

✓ Diagnosis and care plans will be computer generated, based on prospective payment system.

✓ Computer-assisted educational programs will replace classroom work in hospitals.

✓ Computer-based patient information systems will be available, using plastic cards with health record on a microchip. Computers will be used in the home for self-care and patient education of the chronically ill or disabled.

✓ Medical centers will be known as tertiary centers and will serve as information resources.

✓ Health care conglomerates will monopolize the industry, using nurses and doctors in management, administration, and consultation.

✓ Nonprofit institutions will be rare.

✓ Fees for services will disappear.

✓ Nursing service corporations will offer services to individuals and corporations on a contractual basis. Hospitals will contract for entire nursing departments.

(Spitzer, 1987; Kalisch & Kalisch, 1986, p 749)

References

Cosnett, J.E. (1989). Before our time: The origins of intravenous fluid therapy. *Lancet*, (4), 768–771.

Crossley, K., & Matsen, M. (1972). The scalp vein needle. *J.A.M.A., 220*, 985.

Dudrick, S.J., & Rhoads, J.E. (1972). Total intravenous feeding. *Science American, 226*, 73–80.

Gardner, C. (1985). United States House of Representatives honors the National Intravenous Therapy Association. *National Intravenous Therapy Association, 14*(1), 5.

Griffith, Thomas, & Griffith. (1991). LPN's widen their role, disagreement grows. Controversies in care. *American Journal of Nursing, 90*(2), 16–17.

Grippando, G.M. (1986). *Nursing perspectives and issues* (3rd ed.) New York: Delmar.

Jackson, M.M., & Lynch, P. (1990). Infection control: In search of a rational approach. *American Journal of Nursing, 90*(10), 65–73.

Kalisch, P.A., & Kalisch, B.J. (1986). *The advance of American nursing* (2nd ed.) Boston: Little, Brown.

Millam, D.A. (1987). I.V. therapy 30 years ago. *National Intravenous Therapy Association, 10*, 118–121.

Plumer, A.L., & Cosentino, F. (1987). *Principles and practices of intravenous therapy* (4th ed.) Boston: Little, Brown.

Schmidt, J.E. (1959). *Medical discoveries who and when*. Springfield, IL: Charles C Thomas

Spitzer, R. (1987). Catch the wave of nursing in the '90s. *Nursing 87* (Career Suppl.), 8–10.

Viall, C.D. (1990). Your complete guide to central venous catheters. *Nursing 90, 2*, 34–41.

van Heyningen, W.E., & Seal, J.R. (1983). *Cholera: The American scientific experience 1947–1980*. Boulder: Westview Press.

CHAPTER 2

Risk Management and Quality Assurance

CHAPTER CONTENTS

Glossary

CDC: Centers for Disease Control

Civil law: Law that affects the legal rights of a private person or a corporation

Criminal law: Offense against the general public, affecting the welfare of society as a whole

Corrective action: A defined plan to eliminate deficiencies

Documentation: A written or printed recording of original, official, or legal information

INS: Intravenous Nurses Society

JCAHO: Joint Commission on Accreditation of Healthcare Organizations

Liable: Legally responsible for damages; answerable

Malpractice: Negligent conduct of a professional person

OSHA: Occupational Safety and Health Administration

Outcome: Element in quality assessment denoting the effects of care on the health status of patients

Process: Actual performance and observation of performance based on compliance with policy and procedure and professional standards of practice —a key element in quality assessment

Quality assurance (QA): An ongoing systematic process for monitoring, evaluating, and problem solving

Risk management: Process that centers on identification, analysis, treatment, and evaluation of real and potential hazards

Statutes: Written laws enacted by the legislature

Structure: Element in quality assessment reflecting resources available

Tort: Private wrong, by act or omission, which can result in a civil action by the harmed person

LEARNING OBJECTIVES

Upon completion of this chapter, the reader will be able to:

☐ Define the terminology related to risk management and quality assurance.

☐ Identify the sources of laws.

☐ Summarize the evolution of standards of care.

☐ Identify the three types of standards in nursing.

☐ Identify the areas of breach of duty in intravenous nursing.

☐ State the key points in an incident report.

☐ State the definition of quality assurance.

☐ State the three components of the quality assurance model.

☐ Identify the nursing responsibilities of an intravenous therapy team.

RISK MANAGEMENT

In the 1930s, nurses were required to follow almost blindly every physician's order without question. By the 1960s, the courts began to recognize that nurses were exercising more independent judgment in caring for patients and, therefore, should accept legal responsibility for their own actions. The 1980s launched the formation of new health care delivery options. These changes have led to increased specificity of clinical standards for all types of health care providers.

Risk management concepts (Table 2–1) include the concerns an organization faces with exposure to losses. The chances of loss or risks are treated in an organization by financing, purchase of insurance, or through practicing loss control. Loss control is preventive and protective activities that are performed before, during, and after losses are incurred. Prevention of patient injury and employee injury, reduction of losses, and survival of the organization are the key concepts supporting risk management (Goldman, 1991). To understand risk management, one must understand the sources of laws and standards of care guiding practice.

Sources of Law

In the United States there are four primary sources of law: (1) the Constitution, (2) statutes, (3) administrative law, and (4) common law. The Constitution is the basic framework on which our government is built. The Constitution, however, has little direct involvement in the area of **malpractice**.

Statutes are laws enacted by the legislature and are passed by the House of Representatives and the Senate as basic rules for society. There were a minimal number of statutes dealing with malpractice before the malpractice crisis of the mid-1970s. Today there are only a few federal statutes dealing with malpractice; however, there are many such state statutes.

Administrative law is a form of law made by administrative agencies. Examples of administrative agencies that make laws are the National Labor Relations Board and Interstate Commerce Commission. The administrative agencies have limited effect on malpractice.

The final source of the law is common law. This is court-made law. Most law in the area of malpractice is court-made law. The courts are responsible for interpreting the statutes. Most malpractice law is not addressed by statute but is established by the courts (Fiesta, 1988, pp 3–5).

Legal terms that nurses should become familiar with are (1) criminal law,

Table 2–1 □ **STRATEGIES FOR RISK MANAGEMENT**

Establishment of nursing standards of practice
Incident reports
Informed consent
Documentation
Identification of occupational risks

(2) civil law, (3) tort, (4) malpractice, and (5) rule of personal liability. **Criminal law** relates to an offense against the general public because of its harmful effect on society as a whole. Criminal actions are prosecuted by a government authority, and punishment includes imprisonment, fine, or both. The administration of intravenous (I.V.) therapy, if performed in an unlawful manner, can involve the nurse in a criminal offense. Violation of the Nurse Practice Act or the Medical Practice Act by a licensed person is considered a criminal offense.

Civil law affects the legal right of a private person or corporation. When harm occurs, the guilty party may be required to pay damages to the injured person.

A private wrong, by act or omission, is referred to as a **tort**. This can result in civil action by a harmed person. Common torts related to nursing practice include negligence, assault and battery, false imprisonment, slander, libel, and invasion of privacy. When dealing with a rational patient who refuses treatment, it is best to explain the treatment, verbally reassure the patient, and then notify the physician of refusal.

✎ **Note:** Coercion of a rational adult patient in order to place an I.V. cannula device constitutes assault and battery.

Negligent conduct occurs when a nurse does not act in a reasonable and prudent manner, with resultant damage to a person or that person's property. Malpractice is the negligent conduct of professional persons. However, carelessness is not synonymous with negligence. Medical malpractice is generally defined as "a departure from the accepted standards of practice which the average qualified health care provider of the same or similar specialty as the defendant would deliver at the time and under the circumstances with consideration for the resources available and advances in medical science" (Lumsden, 1990).

✎ **Note:** If an act of malpractice does not create harm, legal action cannot be initiated.

The rule of personal liability is "every person is liable for his own tortuous conduct" (his or her own wrongdoing [Bernzweig, 1981, p 68]. A physician cannot protect the nurse from an act of negligence by bypassing this rule with verbal assurance. Nurses are **liable** for their own wrongdoings in carrying out physicians' orders. This rule is relevant to nurses in the areas of medication errors (the most common cause of malpractice claims) and administration of I.V. fluids. Nurses have a legal and professional responsibility to be knowledgeable regarding the I.V. fluids and medications that are administered (Plumer & Cosentino, 1987, pp 11–12).

Standards of Care

Evolution of Standards

In 1912 the Third Clinical Congress of Surgeons of North America resolved that "some system of standardization of hospital equipment and hospital work should be developed. Institutions having the highest ideals may have proper recognition before the profession, and those of inferior standards should be stimulated to raise the quality of their work. In this way patients will receive the

15

best type of treatment, and the public will have some means of recognizing those institutions devoted to the highest ideals of medicine." From 1919 to 1970 the adopted standards referred to the minimum level "considered essential to proper care and treatment of patients in the hospital" (Roberts, Coale, & Redman, 1989).

At the national level, the standards of nursing practice are established by the American Nurses Association (ANA) and the Joint Commission for Accreditation of Healthcare Organizations (**JCAHO**), along with various specialty organizations. At the state level, the various Nurse Practice Acts regulate nursing practice. At the local level, specific standards are set forth in the hospital or agency procedure manual (Creighton, 1987) (Table 2–2).

A nursing standard is a specific statement about the quality of some facet of nursing care. This statement contains the criteria by which the effectiveness of that facet can be evaluated. Standards are the criteria for measuring performance against the optimal achievable degree of clinical excellence. Standards are formulated to communicate expectations of nursing practice.

The Food and Drug Administration (FDA) regulates products in the United States, including over-the-counter and prescription drugs and pharmaceutic agents, food, cosmetics, veterinary products, biologic agents, and medical devices. Nurses use many medical devices and usually are the primary reporters of device problems.

Table 2–2 □ **AGENCIES INFLUENCING STANDARDS OF PRACTICE**

Year	Association	Ruling
1970	Joint Commission on Accreditation of Hospitals (JCAH)	Revised its focus and published a manual for hospitals that defined optimum achievable standards.
1974	ANA	Published generic and specialty standards for nursing care.
1978	CDC	Set standards for infection control practice regarding infusion therapy.
1980	National Intravenous Therapy Association (NITA)	Set standards of practice for I.V. therapy
1987	JCAHO (formerly JCAH)	Mailed "Agenda for Change," which changed the commission's focus from evaluating a health care organization's capability of delivering quality care to helping institutions provide quality health care.
1987	Omnibus Budget Reconciliation Act. (P.L. 100–203)	Set standards for accreditation of home care.
1989	JCAHO	Issued standards regarding what constitutes high-quality home care services.
1990	INS (formerly NITA)	Published revised Standards of Practice for I.V. therapy.

In 1976, the Medical Device Amendment to the federal Food, Drug and Cosmetic Act of 1938 clearly placed the responsibility for ensuring that medical devices in domestic commercial distribution are safe and effective for their intended purposes. The nurse is the best judge of product integrity by inspection of equipment before use. Examples of medical device problems related to the I.V. therapy practice are:

1. Loose or leaking catheter hubs
2. Occluded cannulas
3. Defective infusion pump tubing
4. Contaminated infusates
5. Misleading labeling
6. Inadequate packaging
7. Cracked or leaking I.V. solution bag

✎ **Note:** It is the health care professional's responsibility to report medical device problems (Scott, 1990).

Nursing Standards

Standards of nursing care reflect the mission, values, and philosophy of the agency. Nursing process, professional accountability, fiscal responsibility, and other areas of care are included within these standards. Standards should reflect the type of care that the patient will receive on a given unit or within a given service. These are called performance standards and should (1) include the minimum acceptable behavior for the nurse, congruent with department standards and standards of practice; (2) define performance in observable, measurable behaviors; (3) be specific to the staff nurse role and job description; (4) include all aspects of the nurse's role, including leadership and organizational expectations; (5) serve as the basis for employee selection decisions and performance appraisal system (Porter, 1988).

There are three types of standards in nursing:

1. Standards of structure, which consider organizational framework
2. Standards of process, which encompass patient procedures in health care setting
3. Standards of outcome, which consider the objectives or goals of patient care

All three types of standards must be given equal weight and scrutinized with the same degree of diligence to ensure quality of care (Meisenheimer, 1985, p 53).

✎ **Note:** The Intravenous Nursing Society **(INS)** has set standards of practice for I.V. therapy. Standards of practice must be met in all settings in which I.V. therapy is delivered (INS, S17).

The Nurse's Role as an Expert Witness

Studies indicate that 70 to 80 percent of all civil litigation involves medical and scientific evidence and the testimony of experts (Wecht, 1979). In the profession of nursing, especially the specialty of I.V. therapy, the likelihood of being involved in some legal matter, directly or indirectly, is great (Weinstein, 1984).

In every negligence or malpractice proceeding, the injured party or plaintiff must prove that the defendant did not act as a reasonable, prudent professional would have acted in the same or similar circumstance. An expert is required to explain the appropriate standard of care and to indicate the deviation from standard care (Fiesta, 1991b).

The role of the expert is *not* to establish standards of care. Rather, the expert is present to educate the judge and jury regarding the standards already established by the profession. Expert nursing testimony increases with the technical complexity of a case. An expert witness is usually selected from the same area of experience as that of the defendant nurse. Additional expertise, such as national I.V. certification or research experience, is also important (Fiesta, 1991).

✏ **Note:** The specialty area of I.V. therapy is a high-risk technical area.

Breach of Duty

Once the standard of care has been established and legal duty shown in negligence cases, the injured party must prove breach of duty has occurred. In negligence cases, breach of duty often involves the matter of foreseeability. Forseeability is the legal requirement that the case must be judged on the unique facts as they were at the time of the occurrence because it is always easier to state what should have been done in retrospect. Certain events may foreseeably cause a specific result. The following is a list of breach of duties related to I.V. therapy nursing:

1. Delay in administration of medication
2. Unfamiliarity with drug
3. Inappropriate route of administration
4. Failure to qualify orders
5. Negligence in patient teaching

Also, the nurse must be aware at all times that failure to observe, failure to intervene, and verbal rather than written orders are potential risks for all nursing areas. Nurses must assess the patient and formulate a nursing diagnosis to meet the patient's needs. Courts have not extended the concept of nursing diagnosis to the liability of the nurse's practice at this time.

Malpractice cases are most frequently based on negligence in physical care. Many documented cases of malpractice exist related to all procedures performed on patients. Sometimes the breach of duty occurs because a nurse fails to perform a procedure according to proper standards of care.

✏ **Note:** Because of the risk of malpractice, policy and procedure manuals are vitally important in all aspects of physical nursing care. Practicing and performing specific physical care based on the policies and procedures ensures quality care.

The practice of verbal rather than written orders potentially places the nurse at higher liability risks. Most states require that verbal orders be countersigned by the physician within 24 hours (Fiesta, 1988, pp 51–79).

18

Incident Reports (Occurrence Situation)

Incident reports, which should be filed every time something unusual occurs, are considered an internal recording mechanism for quality assurance. Incident reports are simply records of an event. The incident must be objectively charted, but reference to an incident report should not appear in the legal patient record. Incident reports should contain the following 10 key points:

1. Patient's admitting diagnosis
2. Date incident occurred
3. Patient's room number
4. Age of patient
5. Location of incident
6. Type of incident
7. Nature of occurrence (committing medication error, mislabeling, misreading, not following policy and procedure, overlooking order on chart, not checking patient identification); must be noted (on incident report) if a physician's order was needed after occurrence
8. Factual description of incident
9. Patient condition before occurrence
10. Results of occurrence or injury

✎ **Note:** Incident reports are meant to be nonjudgmental, factual reports of the problem and its consequences (Gardner, 1987). Because the term "incident report" acquired many threatening commonalities, the terminology has been replaced with "occurrence situation or event" (Fiesta, 1991a).

Incident reports are useful for identification of patterns of I.V. medication errors or potentially dangerous situations. Trend analysis monitors patterns of occurrences. Nursing staff must feel free to file reports; an incident report is not an admission of negligence. These reports have the potential for saving lives by identifying unsafe practices. Table 2–3 presents risk management screens for I.V. therapy.

Informed Consent

One of the most effective proactive strategies taken in risk management is the informed consent. The purpose of informed consent is to provide patients with enough information to enable them to decide rationally whether or not to undergo treatment. The focus is on the patient's understanding the procedure rather than simply signing a consent to have a procedure performed (Goldman, 1991).

In order for a consent to be valid, according to Hogue (1986), three conditions must be met: (1) the patient must be capable of giving consent; (2) the patient must receive the necessary information to make an informed decision; and (3) the patient's consent must not be coerced. Getting the consent form signed may be the nurse's responsibility, as defined by policy. If the patient does not give informed consent, there may be grounds for liability. The consent form is actually a **risk management** tool designed to avoid charges of malpractice, along with protecting the consumer. Table 2–4 identifies the necessary components of informed consent.

19

Table 2–3 ☐ I.V. THERAPY RISK MANAGEMENT SCREENS

Incident reports are written for any of the following occurrences. The incident should be reported to the supervisor or quality assurance director or risk manager.

1. Medication error
2. I.V. fluid error
3. Anaphylaxis or severe allergic reaction
4. Severe irritation or breakdown at site
5. Site infection
6. Phlebitis stage +2 or +3 (INS standards)
7. Needle stick to patient, family member, or health care personnel
8. Neurologic deficit, sign, or symptom not present before I.V. therapy
9. Patient withdraws consent for treatment or refuses treatment
10. Equipment failure or malfunction with potential impact on patient care
11. Patient complaint related to I.V. therapy
12. Other adverse or unexpected event (specify)
13. Break in policy or procedure (specify)
14. Particulate or other observable contaminant of I.V. fluid or medication
15. Severe infiltration or extravasation of vesicant agent

For home infusion services, add the following screening for risk management:

1. Diarrhea, fever, arrhythmia, sudden weight loss or gain, and infections other than site infections
2. Questioned safety of home environment for continued home I.V. therapy
3. Rehospitalization for I.V. therapy

Source: From "Occurrence Screens: A Risk and Quality Control Tool for Intravenous Nurses" by M.W. Tan, 1990, *Journal of Intravenous Therapy, 13*, p. 308–311. Adapted by permission.

Table 2–4 ☐ KEY COMPONENTS OF INFORMED CONSENT

Process

1. Accurate and complete information
2. Including an understanding of:
   Risks
   Benefits
   Alternative
3. Understanding of:
   Language idioms
   Intelligence
   Hearing loss
4. Opportunity for dialogue

Consent

1. After consideration of all options
2. Agreed in verbal and written word
3. Documentation of consent obtained

Source: Courtesy of Kathleen Sazama, M.D., J.D. Associate Medical Director, Center for Blood Research, Sacramento, California.

✎ **Note:** The consent form helps establish a good relationship with the patient, as well as helping to protect everyone—the nurse, the doctor, the hospital, and the patient.

Documentation

Documentation by nurses and other health care providers is another strategy for risk management. All charting should accurately describe the care rendered the patient. Documentation should be objective and free of criticism or complaints. Charting should be legible and include only standard abbreviations. Documentation should contain no vacant lines, and every entry should be signed. Completion of documentation should be prompt. Charting must be timely, complete, and accurate to provide a true account of actual care.

✎ **Note:** If you are working in a clinic, in an office, or in home care, be sure to chart dates of return visits, canceled or failed appointments, all telephone conversations, and all follow-up instructions (Creighton, 1987).

Occupational Risks

There are occupational risks associated with I.V. therapy. The two key types of risks are physical hazards and exposure to infectious organisms.

Physical Hazards

Physical hazards associated with I.V. therapy include, but are not limited to, accidents, abrasions, contusions, and chemical exposure.

Accidents

Needle-stick injuries are associated with recapping the needle, improper discarding of needle in container, accidental needle sticks while performing tasks, and carelessness. Accidental needle-stick injuries can lead to exposure to hepatitis B, human immunodeficiency virus (HIV), malaria, varicella zoster, and Rocky Mountain spotted fever (McCray, 1986).

✎ **Note:** According to INS *Standards of Practice* (1990), the recapping of needles and stylets increases potential risk to the practitioner. Therefore, needles and stylets should not be recapped, broken, or bent. They must be disposed of in rigid, puncture-resistant, nonpermeable, tamper- and leakproof containers that will eventually be incinerated or autoclaved (S41).

Abrasions and Contusions

Abrasions and contusions can be caused by needle sticks and by contact with broken glass, sharp container edges, or any other jagged-edged item. Small or undetected skin abrasions can be potential portals for microorganisms such as *Staphylococcus aureus*, herpes simplex, and HIV.

✎ **Note:** Use caution when assembling and manipulating I.V. equipment. Excellent handwashing practices prevent the invasion of microorganisms. Needleless and protected needle systems are now available.

21

Chemical Exposure

Handling of cytotoxic (antineoplastic) drugs can be hazardous. Although little research has been done on the long-term risks at the levels of exposure encountered by unprotected health care workers, cytotoxic drugs have been associated with human cancers at therapeutic levels of exposure and are known carcinogens and teratogens in many animal species.

Cytotoxic drugs can cause chromosome breakage in circulating lymphocytes and mutagenic activity in urine, as well as skin necrosis (after surface contact with abraded skin) and damage to normal skin. Nurses preparing cytotoxic drugs should wear surgical latex gloves (double gloves if this does not interfere with technique) and wear a protective disposable gown made of lint-free, low-permeability fabric with closed front, long sleeves, and elastic or knit-closed cuffs. Because surgical masks do not protect against the breathing of aerosols, a biologic safety cabinet or air-purifying respirator should be used when preparing the drug. A plastic face shield or splash goggles should be worn if a biologic safety cabinet is not used (OSHA, 1986). Refer to Appendix D for the Occupational Safety and Health Organization (OSHA) complete guide to personnel dealing with cytotoxic drugs.

Exposure to Infectious Organisms

Intravenous therapy nurses are constantly exposed to patient's secretions and excretions. Nurses should follow standards established by OSHA with regard to gloving and excellent handwashing practices (OSHA, 1991).

✎ **Note:** All patient body secretions can be potentially infectious; therefore, strict guidelines must be adhered to by all personnel having contact with patients.

Handwashing is a routine infection control practice to decrease the potential risk of contamination and cross-infection.

Occupational Safety and Health Administration's Occupational Exposure to Bloodborne Pathogens: Final Rule*

OSHA has stiffened the bloodborne rules enforcing new regulations regarding universal precautions. OSHA's new standard makes universal precautions fully enforceable for the first time and spells out what inspectors will look for. Health care workers should be aware of how the rules are observed in each agency.

Health care employees face a significant risk as the result of occupational exposure to materials that may contain bloodborne pathogens, including hepatitis B virus (HBV), which causes Hepatitis B, a serious liver disease and HIV, which causes AIDS. The exposure can be minimized or eliminated using a

---

*For further rules and a text of the standard write OSHA Publications, Room N 3101, 200 Constitution Avenue, NW, Washington, DC 20210.

combination of engineering and work practice controls, personal protective clothing and equipment, training, medical surveillance, hepatitis B vaccination, signs and labels, and other provisions (OSHA, 1991).

The following list is a summary of some of the rules to be observed in the workplace.

Hepatitis B Vaccine. The vaccine must be offered at no charge to the employee "at a reasonable time and place" and "within 10 working days of initial assignment."

Universal Precautions. It is now a legal requirement to observe this concept, in which "all human blood and certain human body fluids are treated as if known to be infectious for HIV, HBV, and other bloodborne pathogens."

Sharps and Waste Disposal. Reusable contaminated sharps have to be placed in puncture resistant, leakproof, and labeled or color-coded containers that are "easily accessible . . . . maintained upright, and placed routinely."

Protective Equipment. The whole range of equipment must be available wherever blood or other infectious materials might reach an employee's clothes, skin, eyes, mouth, or other mucous membranes.

Gloves. Gloves must be worn when hand contact with infectious materials can be reasonably anticipated. Utility gloves must be discarded if cracked, peeling, torn, or punctured. Hypoallergenic gloves must be provided to those allergic to other gloves.

Laundry. Contaminated laundry has to be handled "with a minimum of agitation" and moved in labeled or color-coded bags or containers. Wet laundry requires leakproof containers. Laundry workers must wear gloves.

Communicating Hazards. Orange-red or fluorescent orange warning labels must be affixed to containers of "regulated" waste, refrigerators and freezers containing infectious materials, and containers used to transport them. Labels must include the official BIOHAZARD legend. (OSHA, 1991)

QUALITY ASSURANCE

Quality assurance (QA) is a systematic process to ensure desired patient outcomes. A QA program should be established that objectively identifies, evaluates, and solves problems associated with I.V. patient treatment modalities. A QA program for I.V. therapy should be ongoing and include structure, process, outcome, **corrective action**, and reevaluation (INS, 1990, S19).

Risk management handles errors, whereas QA seeks perfection. Both are mutually compatible and interdependent. QA works at preventing malpractice claims and promotes better patient outcomes. All hospital departments are involved in both QA and risk management activities (Fiesta, 1991).

Initially QA monitoring and evaluation activities focused on capacity for providing care according to established standards and tracked retrospectively through audits. Current QA programs concentrate on monitoring outcomes of care as close to the scene and time of care delivery as is feasible.

Beginning in the 1980s, health care consumers, third-party payers, and health care providers began looking at positive patient outcomes as a measure of quality. JCAHO was the driving force in this movement, along with peer review organizations (PROs), Medicare/Medicaid reimbursement regulations, federal and state laws, court interpretations of liability, and private health insurers' standards (Cassidy & Friesen, 1990). In the early 1980s, guidelines initiated by JCAHO were formed to provide a Nursing QA committee. This committee recognized that QA had to be ongoing to ensure high-quality patient care. The committee in each facility should include management, chief nursing officers, and members of staff (O'Brien, 1988). Nursing QA focuses on two endeavors: checking achievement of standards and solving patient care problems.

Approaches to Quality Assurance Using Assessment

Assessing the achievement of nursing care standards involves measuring quality of care provided. This is part of the nursing process: observing care delivered, assessing patient satisfaction, documenting care received, and evaluating outcomes based on short- and long-term goals. Involving staff in quality assessments can increase their awareness of standards, as well as enhancing their assessment skills (New & New, 1989).

I.V. therapy quality assurance includes compliance with policy and procedure manuals, documentation of I.V. therapy – related complications, equipment evaluation, and chart documentation. The QA process may be performed by lengthy studies, short-term sampling, or problem solving with documentation and reporting (Plumer & Cosentino, 1987, p 37). Three categories are used to create a model for QA. Each category is linked as a measurement of quality patient care. These three components are:

- Structure
- Process
- Outcome standards (Donabedian, 1988).

Structure

Structure denotes the attributes of the setting in which care occurs. This is defined as evaluation of resources: material and human. Material resources are classified as facilities, equipment, or financial budget. Equipment is the chief material resource in I.V. therapy quality assurance. Human resources include the number and qualifications of nurses performing I.V.-related procedures.

STRUCTURE RESOURCES

Material Resources	Human Resources
1. Facilities	1. Number of nurses
2. Equipment	2. Qualifications of nurses performing I.V. nursing duties
3. Financial budget	

Process

Process denotes what is actually done in giving and receiving care. It includes the patient's activities in seeking care and the practitioner's activities in making a nursing diagnosis, along with evaluation of actual performance of procedures. This link sets the standards by which evaluation can take place.

PROCESS BASED ON STANDARDS OF PRACTICE

Patient Activities	Nurse Activities
1. Patient knowledge	1. Assessments related to standards of practice
	2. Intervention and establishment of short- and long-term goals

Outcome Standards

Outcome denotes the effect of care on the health status of patients. Improvement in the patient's knowledge and changes in patient health status are components of outcome criteria. The assessment of outcomes is a method for establishing quality of care. Outcome in the practice of I.V. therapy should reflect final results of the therapy, including patient recovery and rates of complications. Table 2–5 is the QA model used throughout this book.

Table 2–5 □ **QUALITY ASSESSMENT MODEL**

Structure
(Resources that affect outcome) Resource: Human Material
▼
Process (Standards)
(Actual giving and receiving of care based on standards of practice) Activities: Patient Nurse
▼
Outcome Standards
Effects of care by Patient contribution Nursing evaluation

25

Helpful guidelines (Delaney & Lauer, 1988, p 322) for evaluation of quality include the following:

1. Centers for Disease Control (**CDC**): *Guidelines for Prevention of Intravascular Infections*
2. Intravenous Nursing Standards of Practice, 1990.
3. Joint Commission on Accreditation of Healthcare Organizations (JCAHO) Performance Standards for I.V. Therapy
4. American Association of Blood Banks (AABB)

OUTCOME

Patient Knowledge	Evaluation of Care
1. Patient participation in care and verbal understanding of procedures	1. Evaluation of nursing compliance to institutional policy 2. Evaluation of standards of care

In summary, the goals of QA assessment are to (1) prevent complications, (2) decrease morbidity and mortality, (3) decrease cost, (4) shorten hospital stay, (5) increase patient comfort; and (6) increase patient knowledge.

This model can be used as a basis for research, to set up standards of quality control, and to educate staff members regarding the practice of measurable quality nursing care based on assessment.

INTRAVENOUS THERAPY NURSING TEAMS

According to the INS (S17), "Intravenous teams provide clinical expertise, cost effective care and decrease the risk of complications related to intravenous therapy. Intravenous nursing teams provide desired patient outcomes and decrease morbidity and mortality associated with this therapy."

The responsibilities of the I.V. team should be set according to the policies and procedures of each institution. These responsibilities include, but are not limited to, the following:

1. Inserting I.V. cannulas
2. Administering prescribed I.V. solutions and medications and blood products
3. Monitoring and maintaining I.V. sites and systems
4. Evaluating the patient's response to prescribed therapy
5. Teaching patient and family and evaluating their comprehension
6. Documenting pertinent information on the patient's record.
7. Compiling statistics to qualify and quantify I.V. services.

I.V. therapy nurses should also be active on committees relevant to the specialty practice of I.V. nursing, such as:

Pharmacy and therapeutics
Infection control
Nutritional support
Transfusion therapy
Quality assurance and risk management

SUMMARY OF CHAPTER 2

MANAGEMENT AND QUALITY ASSURANCE

Risk Management

Sources of Laws

United States has four primary sources of law:

Constitution
Statutes
Administrative law
Common law

Legal terms are:

Criminal law
Civil law
Tort
Malpractice
Rule of personal liability

Common torts in the nursing practice include negligence, assault and battery, false imprisonment, slander, libel, and invasion of privacy.

Coercion of a rational adult patient in order to place an I.V. cannula device constitutes assault and battery.

Standards of Care

National level: Standards of nursing practice established by the ANA and JCAHO
State level: Nurse Practice Act
Local level: Hospital/agency policy and procedure manuals

Nursing standards reflect the mission, values, and philosophy of the agency. There are three types of standards in nursing:

1. Standards of structure, which consider organizational framework
2. Standards of process, which encompass patient procedure in health care setting
3. Standards of outcome, which consider the objectives or goals of patient care

INS has set the following standards of practice for I.V. therapy:

Breach of Duty

Breach of duty related to I.V. therapy includes:

1. Delay in administration of medication
2. Unfamiliarity with drug
3. Inappropriate route of administration

27

4. Failure to qualify orders
5. Negligence in patient teaching

Incident Reports

Incident reports should be filed every time there is an unusual occurrence. An incident reports is simply a record of an event.

Informed Consent

In order for a consent to be valid, three conditions must be met:

1. Patients must be capable of giving consent.
2. Patients must receive the necessary information to make an intelligent decision.
3. Consent must not be coerced.

The consent form is actually a risk management tool designed to avoid charges of malpractice.

Documentation

All charting should accurately describe the care rendered the patient, and should be written objectively. Charting must be timely, complete, and accurate to help the patient secure a better quality of care and to help protect nurses, physicians, and hospitals.

Occupational Risks

Physical hazards

- Accidents, including needle-stick injuries
- Abrasions and contusions
- Chemical exposure

Exposure to infectious organisms

Quality Assurance

1. Quality assurance works at preventing malpractice claims and promotes better patient outcomes.
2. Assessment is a key ingredient in ensuring quality of care.
3. The three components of quality assurance are structure, process, and outcome standards.

   Structure: Denotes the attributes of the setting — material (equipment) or human (nurses, qualifications).

   Process: Standards of practice; denotes what is actually done in giving and receiving care. Patient activities such as knowledge and nursing activities such as assessments related to standards of practice, interventions, and establishing short- and long-term goals are included in this category.

Outcome standards: Denotes the effect of care on the health status of the patient. Patient knowledge as manifest by the patient's contribution to his or her own care and evaluation of nursing care are included.

Goals of QA

Prevent complications
Decrease morbidity and mortality
Decrease cost
Shorten hospital stay
Increase patient comfort
Increase patient knowledge

References

Bernzweig, E.P. (1981). *Nurse's liability for malpractice* (3rd ed.) New York: McGraw-Hill.

Cassidy, D.A., & Friesen, M.A. (1990). QA: Applying JCAHO's generic model. *Nursing Management, 21*(6), 22–27.

Creighton, H. (1987a). Legal significance of charting Part II. *Nursing Management, 18*(10), 14–15.

Creighton, H. (1987b). Legal importance of policy and procedures Part I. *Nursing Management, 18*(4), 22–28. Delaney, C.W., & Lauer, M.L. (1988). *Intravenous therapy, a guide to quality care.* Philadelphia: J.B. Lippincott.

Donabedian, A. (1988). The quality of care. How can it be assessed? *JAMA, 260*(12), 1743–1748.

Fiesta, J. (1988). *The law and liability: A guide for nurses* (2nd ed.) New York: Wiley.

Fiesta, J. (1991a). QA and risk management reducing liability exposure. *Nursing Management, 22*(2), 14–15.

Fiesta, J. (1991b). Nurse's role as an expert witness. *Nursing Management, 22* (3), 28–29.

Gardner, C. (1987). Risk management of medication errors. *National Intravenous Therapy Association, 10*(1), 266–278.

Goldman, T.A. (1991). Risk management concepts and strategies. *Journal of Intravenous Nursing, 14*(3), 199–204.

Hogue, E. (1986). What you should know about informed consent. *Nursing 86, 6,* 47–48.

Intravenous Nurses Society (1990). *Standards of practice.* Philadelphia: Lippincott.

Lumsden, D.J. (1990). Legal risks in a changing practice environment. *Journal of Intravenous Nursing, 13*(1), 59–67.

McCray, E. (1986). Occupational risk of acquired immunodeficiency syndrome among health care workers. *New England Journal of Medicine, 314*(17), 1127.

Meisenheimer, C.G. (1985). *Quality assurance: A complete guide to effective programs.* Rockville, MD: Aspen.

New, N.A., & New, J.R. (1989). QA that works. *Nursing Management, 20*(6), 21–24.

O'Brien, B. (1988). QA: A commitment to excellence. *Nursing Management, 19*(11), 33–40.

OSHA (1986). OSHA work-practice for personnel dealing with cytotoxic (antineoplastic) drugs. *American Journal of Hospital Pharmacy, 43,* 1193.

OSHA (1991). Occupational safe exposure to bloodborne pathogens: Final rule. Department of Labor Docket No. H-370, Dec 6, 1991.

Plumer, A., & Cosentino, F. (1987). *Principles and practices of intravenous therapy*. Boston: Little, Brown.

Porter, A.L. (1988). Assuring quality through staff nurse performance. *Nursing Clinics of North America, 23*(3), 649–655.

Roberts, J.S., Coale, J.G., & Redman, R.R. (1989). A history of the Joint Commission on Accreditation of Hospitals. *JAMA, 238*, 936–940.

Scott, W.L. (1990). Medical-device complications. Reporting a quality assurance mechanism. *Journal of Intravenous Nursing, 13*(3), 178–182.

Tan, M.W. (1990). Occurrence screens: A risk and quality control tool for I.V. nursing. *Journal of Intravenous Nursing, 13*(5), 308–311.

Wecht, C.H. (1979). Medical expert testimony: Every doctor's concern. *Legal Aspects of Medical Practice, 2*.

Weinstein, S.M. (1984). Expert testimony: The I.V. nurse's responsibility. *National Intravenous Therapy Association, 7*, 423–424.

Bibliography

Baker, D.L. (1990). Measuring outcome criteria. *Journal of Intravenous Nursing, 13*(4), 253–258.

Beyers, M. (1988). Quality: The banner of the 1980's. *Nursing Clinics of North America, 23*(3), 617–623.

Creighton, H. (1987c). Legal importance of policy and procedures Part II. *Nursing Management, 18*(5), 14–15.

Harris, S.H., Kreger, S.M., & Davis M.Z. (1989). A problem-focused QA program. *Nursing Management, 20*(2), 54–60.

Hughes, F.Y. (1987). Quality assurance in home care services. *Nursing Management, 18*(12), 33–36.

Macklin, D.C. (1990). The evolution of standards. *Journal of Intravenous Nursing, 13*(4), 249–252.

Micheletti, J.A., & Shlala, T.J. (1990). Evolving QA initiative in home healthcare. *Nursing Management, 20*(8), 24–28.

Nacker, J.G., & Brubakker, K.M. (1990). Accuracy of infusing I.V. fluids: A QA approach. *Journal of Intravenous Therapy, 13*(1), 23–26.

Schroeder, P. (1988). Directions and dilemmas in nursing QA. *Nursing clinics of North America, 23*(3), 657–664.

Sumner, W. (1985). Needlecaps to prevent needlestick injuries. *Infection Control, 6*(12), 495.

Watson, C.A., Bulechek, G.M., & McCloskey, J.C. (1987). QAMR: A quality assurance model using research. *Journal of Nursing Quality Assurance, 2*(1), 21–27.

UNIT TWO

THE BASICS: FOUNDATION FOR PRACTICE

CHAPTER 3

Fundamentals of Fluid Balance

CHAPTER CONTENTS

Glossary

Active transport: Passage of a substance across a cell membrane by an energy-consuming process that permits diffusion to take place

Antidiuretic hormone (ADH): A hormone secreted from the pituitary gland that causes the kidney to conserve water; sometimes referred to as the "water-conserving hormone"

Diffusion: The passage of molecules of one substance between the molecules of another to form a mixture of the two substances

Extracellular fluid (ECF): Body fluid located outside the cells

Filtration: The process of passing of fluid through a filter using pressure

Homeostasis: The ability to restore equilibrium under stress

Hypertonic: Having an osmotic pressure higher than 375 mOsm/liter

Hypotonic: Having an osmotic pressure less than 250 mOsm/liter

Insensible loss: Output that is difficult to measure, such as perspiration

Interstitial fluid: Fluid between the cells

Intracellular fluid (ICF): Fluid inside the cells

Intravascular fluid: The fluid portion of blood (plasma)

Isotonic: Having an osmotic pressure equal to that of blood; equivalent osmotic pressure

Osmolarity: A measure of solute concentration; refers to the number of osmoles per liter of solution. It is measured in mOsm/liter

Osmosis: The movement of water from a lower concentration to a higher concentration across a semipermeable membrane

SIADH: Syndrome of inappropriate antidiuretic hormone, a condition in which excessive antidiuretic hormone is secreted, resulting in hyponatremia

Sensible loss: Output that is measurable

Solute: The substance that is dissolved in a liquid to form a solution

---

LEARNING OBJECTIVES

Upon completion of this chapter, the reader will be able to:

☐ Define terminology related to fluids and electrolytes.
☐ Identify the three fluid compartments within the body.
☐ Identify the mechanisms of daily intake and daily output.
☐ State the functions of body fluid.
☐ List the four fluid transport systems.
☐ Define the concept of osmosis and delineate examples of this concept.
☐ State the average insensible loss for 24 hours.

☐ Recall the homeostatic organs.
☐ Contrast the movement of water in hypotonic, hypertonic, and isotonic solutions.
☐ Summarize the major fluid balance disorders.
☐ List the six major body systems assessed for fluid balance disturbances.
☐ Identify the patient with fluid volume deficit and fluid volume excess, using the nurses' quick assessment guide.
☐ Determine nursing diagnosis appropriate for the care of a patient experiencing fluid balance disturbance.

Pre-test, Chapter 3

Instructions: The pre-test is to review prior knowledge of the theory content of fluid balance. Each question in the pre-test is based on the learning objectives of the chapter. Match the definition in column 2 to the correct term in column 1.

Column 1	Column 2
1. _____ Extracellular	A. Ability to restore equilibrium
2. _____ Intravascular	B. Body fluid outside the cell
3. _____ Intracellular	C. A measure of solute concentration
4. _____ Osmolarity	D. The fluid portion of blood (plasma)
5. _____ Homeostasis	E. Body fluid inside the cell

6. What are the three fluid compartments related to body fluid?
   A. Intracellular, interstitial, intravascular
   B. Transcellular, intraorbital, intraspinal
   C. Extracellular, extravascular, interstitial

7. What are the functions of body fluid?
   A. Maintain blood volume
   B. Transport material to and from cells
   C. Assist digestion of food through hydrolysis
   D. Regulate body temperature
   E. All of the above

8. How is *fluid* primarily passively transported within the body?
   A. Osmosis
   B. Adenosine triphosphate (ATP) in cell membrane
   C. Diffusion
   D. The sodium-potassium pump

9. Which of the following is the range of milliosmoles (mOsm/liter) for an isotonic solution?
   A. 150 to 250
   B. 250 to 375
   C. 320 to 460
   D. 350 to 550

10. Which of the following may be signs and symptoms of fluid volume deficit?
    A. Bounding pulse, decreased blood pressure, and moist rales
    B. Increased respiratory rate, warm moist skin, and decreased temperature
    C. Decreased pulse, decreased blood pressure, and poor skin turgor
    D. Dyspnea, jugular vein distention, and sternum fingerprinting

11. A patient has the following signs and symptoms: moist rales, increased respiratory rate, dyspnea, and 3+ edema of the ankles. What is the appropriate nursing diagnosis?
    A. Fluid volume deficit
    B. Fluid volume excess
    C. Tissue integrity impaired
    D. Tissue perfusion altered, renal

12. What is the average insensible loss in an adult?
    A. 200 to 400 mL per day
    B. 400 to 600 mL per day
    C. 500 to 1000 mL per day
    D. 800 to 1200 mL per day

13. Diffusion is a passive process in which molecules move from:
    A. An area of low concentration to one of high concentration
    B. An area of high concentration to one of low concentration
    C. A region of low pressure to one of high pressure, using hydrostatic pressure

True-False

14. **T F** Hypertonic solutions have a range of 250 to 350 mOsm/liter.

15. **T F** The area that can be used to assess for skin turgor in an adult is the sternum.

ANSWERS TO PRE-TEST, Chapter 3

1. B   2. D   3. E   4. C   5. A   6. A   7. E   8. A   9. B

10. C   11. B   12. C   13. B   14. F   15. T

 The purpose of this chapter is to introduce the reader to fundamental concepts of fluid balance and the physical assessment of patients with fluid volume deficit and fluid volume excess.

> When they went ashore the animals that took up a land life carried with them a part of the sea in their bodies, a heritage which they passed on to their children and which even today links each land animal with its origin in the ancient sea.
>
>   Carson, 1961, p 28

BODY FLUID COMPOSITION

Body fluid refers to body water in which electrolytes are dissolved. Water is the largest single constituent of the body. Body water, the medium in which cellular reactions take place, constitutes approximately 60 percent of total body weight (TBW) in young male adults and 50 to 55 percent in female adults. Refer to Table 3–1 for values of total body fluids in relation to age and sex. Fat

35

Table 3–1 □ PERCENTAGES OF TOTAL BODY FLUID IN RELATION TO AGE AND SEX

Age	% of Water = Body Weight
Full-term newborn infant	70–80
1-year-old	64
Puberty to 39 years	Men: 60
	Women: 55
40–60 years	Men: 55
	Women: 47
>60 years	Men: 52
	Women: 46

Source: From *Fluid and Electrolyte Balance: Nursing Considerations* (p. 5) by N. M. Metheny, 1987, Philadelphia. J.B. Lippincott Company. Copyright 1987 by J.B. Lippincott Company. Reprinted by permission.

tissue contains little water, and the percentage of total body water will vary considerably, based on the amount of body fat present. In addition, total body water progressively decreases with age, comprising about 50 percent of body weight in the elderly (Goldberger, 1986).

FLUID DISTRIBUTION

Total body fluid (water and electrolytes) in adults, as well as children, is distributed within the cell, referred to as **intracellular fluid (ICF)**, and outside the cell referred to as **extracellular fluid (ECF)**. The water and electrolytes distributed in the intracellular compartment comprise 40 percent of the total body fluid. Fluid distributed in the extracellular compartments comprises 20 percent of the total body fluid. The extracellular compartment is further subdivided into the **interstitial** (fluid lying between the cells, or tissue fluid) and the **intravascular** (plasma) compartments, with 15 percent in the tissue (interstitial) space and 5 percent in the plasma space. Figure 3–1 is a diagrammatic representation of body fluid distribution.

✎ **Note:** Lymph and cerebrospinal fluids, although highly specialized, are usually regarded as interstitial.

An exchange of fluid continuously occurs among the intracellular, plasma, and interstitial compartments. Of these three spaces, only the plasma is directly influenced by the intake or elimination of fluid from the body. Changes in the intracellular and interstitial fluid compartments occur in response to changes in the volume or concentration of the plasma.

The internal environment needs to remain in **homeostasis**; therefore, the intake and output of fluid must be relatively equal, as in healthy individuals. In illness this balance is frequently upset, with intake of fluid becoming diminished or even ceasing. Output of fluid may vary according to the influences of increased temperature, increased respirations, draining wounds, or gastric suction.

Normal sources of water per day include liquids, water-containing foods, and metabolic activity. In healthy adults the intake of fluids varies from 1000 to

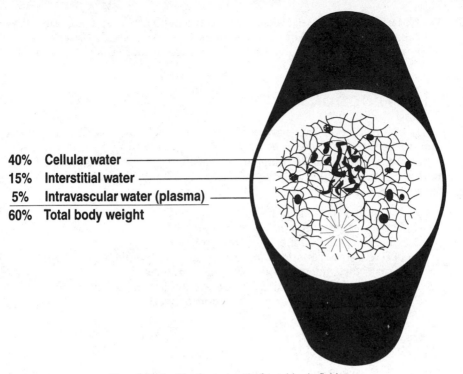

40% **Cellular water**
15% **Interstitial water**
5% **Intravascular water (plasma)**
60% **Total body weight**

Figure 3–1 ☐ Percentages of total body fluid.

3000 mL/day, and 200 to 300 mL are produced from oxidation (Chenevey, 1987).

The elimination of fluid is considered **sensible** (measurable) **loss** or **insensible** (not measurable) **loss**. Water is eliminated from the body by the skin, kidneys, bowels, and respirations. Approximately 300 to 500 mL are eliminated via the lungs every 24 hours, and approximately 500 mL per day are eliminated by the skin as perspiration. The amount of insensible loss in an adult is considered to be 500 to 1000 mL/day. Losses through the gastrointestinal tract are only about 100 to 200 mL/day owing to the reabsorption of most of the fluid in the small intestines (Table 3–2). Increased losses of gastrointestinal fluids can occur because of diarrhea or intestinal fistulas (Metheny, 1987, p 7).

Table 3–2 ☐ **WATER BALANCE: INTAKE AND OUTPUT**

Intake (mL)		Output	
Liquids	1200	Breathing	500
Food intake	1000	Perspiration	500
Oxidation	300	Urine	1400
Total	2500	Feces	100
		Total	2500

✎ **Note:** Significant sweat losses occur if the patient's body temperature exceeds 101°F (38.3°C) or if room temperature exceeds 90°F. Insensible loss is also increased if respirations are increased to more than 20 per minute (Metheny, 1990).

FLUID FUNCTION

Fluids within the body have several important functions. The ECF transports nutrients to the cells and carries waste products away from the cells by means of the capillary bed. Body fluids are in constant motion, maintaining living conditions for body cells (Metheny, 1987, p 6). The fluid within the body also has the following functions:

1. Maintains blood volume
2. Regulates body temperature
3. Transports material to and from cells
4. Serves as aqueous medium for cellular metabolism
5. Assists digestion of food through hydrolysis
6. Acts as solvent in which solutes are available for cell function
7. Serves as medium for the excretion of waste

FLUID TRANSPORT

Movement of particles through the cell membrane occurs via four transport mechanisms: diffusion, osmosis, filtration, and active transport. Materials are transported between the ICF and ECF compartments by these four mechanisms (Table 3–3).

Passive Transport

Diffusion

Diffusion is the passive movement of molecules or ions from a region of high concentration to one of low concentration. Diffusion occurs through semipermeable membranes by either passing through pores, if small enough, or dis-

Table 3–3 ☐ **MECHANISMS OF TRANSPORT**

Passive Transport
Diffusion
Osmosis
Filtration

Active Transport
ATP by cell membrane
Sodium-potassium pump

solving in the lipid matrix of the membrane wall. If there is no force opposing diffusion, particles will distribute themselves evenly. Many substances can diffuse through the cell membrane, and these substances diffuse in both directions.

Influencing factors in the diffusion process are concentration differences, electrical potential, and pressure differences across the pores. The greater the concentration, the greater the rate of diffusion. Increase in the pressure on one side of the membrane increases the molecular forces striking the pores, thus creating a pressure gradient.

Osmosis

Osmosis is the passage of water from an area of lower concentration of particles toward a higher concentration of particles across a semipermeable membrane. The most important factor that determines rate of diffusion of a substance is the concentration difference of the substance crossing the cell membrane.

The concentration of a solution containing more solute particles increases the collisions, creating a greater osmotic pressure. Osmotic pressure is measured in mOsm. Osmolality refers to the total number of osmotically active particles per liter of solution, whereas **osmolarity** is the concentration of a solute in a volume of solution. The two terms are very similar and are often used interchangeably. The term osmolarity will be used within this text. The normal osmolarity of body fluids is 290 mOsm/kg and the osmolarity of ICF and ECF is always equal. The terms *tonicity* and *osmolarity* are used interchangeably (Chenevey, 1987). Tonicity reflects the concept and effects of hypotonic, hypertonic, and isotonic solutions on body cells. Figure 3–2 is a diagrammatic representation of the movement of water by osmosis in hypotonic, isotonic, and hypertonic solutions.

Isotonic solutions, such as 0.9% sodium chloride (NaCl) and 5% dextrose and water, have the same osmolarity as normal body fluids. Solutions that have an osmolarity of 250 to 375 mOsm/liter are considered isotonic solutions and will have no effect on the volume of fluid within the cell; these solutions will remain within the ECF space. Isotonic solutions are used to expand the ECF compartment.

Hypotonic solutions are solutions that contain less salt than the ICF space, and when infused, have an osmolarity below 250 mOsm/liter and move water into the cell, causing the cell to swell and possibly burst. By lowering the serum osmolarity, fluids shift out of the blood vessels into the interstitial tissue and cells. Hypotonic solutions hydrate cells and can deplete the circulatory system. An example of a hypotonic solution is 2-1/2% dextrose and water.

Hypertonic solutions, conversely, cause the water within the cell to move to the ECF compartment where the concentration of salt is greater, causing the cell to shrink. Hypertonic solutions have an osmolality of 375 mOsm/liter and above. These solutions are used to replace electrolytes. When hypertonic dextrose solutions are used alone, they also are used to shift ECF from interstitial tissue to plasma. Examples of hypertonic solutions would be 5% dextrose/0.9% sodium chloride, 5% dextrose/Normosol M, amino acid solutions, and

HYPOTONIC
Less than body less 250mEq/L

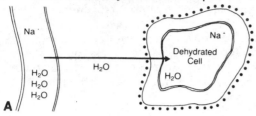

A

ISOTONIC
Equal to body 290 mEq/L

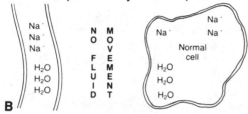

B

HYPERTONIC
More than body greater 375 mEq/L

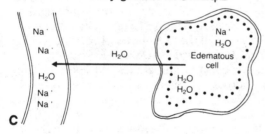

C

Figure 3–2 □ Effects of fluid shifts in isotonic, hypertonic, and hypotonic states. (From *Pharmacotherapeutics: A Nursing Process Approach, second edition* [p. 249.] by Mathewson-Kuhn, 1991, Philadelphia, F.A. Davis Company. Copyright 1991 by F.A. Davis Company. Reprinted by permission.)

5% dextrose/lactated Ringers. Refer to Figure 3–3 for a chart of tonicity (osmolarity) ranges.

Filtration

Filtration is the transfer of water and dissolved substance from a region of high pressure to one of low pressure; the force behind this process is hydrostatic pressure. The pumping heart provides hydrostatic pressure in the movement of water and electrolytes from the arterial capillary bed to the interstitial fluid. The plasma compartment (intravascular space) contains more protein than the other compartments. Plasma protein, composed of albumin, globulin, and fibrinogen, creates an osmotic pressure (colloid osmotic pressure) at the capillary membrane, thus preventing fluid from the plasma from leaking into the interstitial spaces. Osmotic pressure created within the plasma by the presence of protein (mainly albumin) keeps the water in the vascular system (Chenevey, 1987).

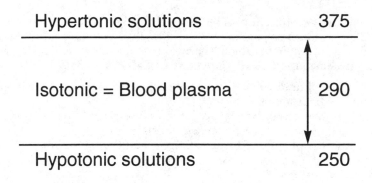

Hypertonic solutions	375
Isotonic = Blood plasma	290
Hypotonic solutions	250

Figure 3–3 ☐ Tonicity/osmolarity ranges of solutions.

Active Transport

Active transport occurs when it is necessary for ions (electrolytes) to move from an area of low concentration to one of high concentration. By definition, active transport implies that energy expenditure must take place for the movement to occur against a concentration gradient. ATP is released from the cell to enable certain substances to acquire the energy needed to pass through the cell membrane. For example, sodium concentration is greater in ECF; therefore, sodium tends to enter by diffusion into the intracellular compartment. This tendency is offset by the sodium-potassium pump located on the cell membrane. In the presence of ATP, the sodium-potassium pump actively moves sodium from the cell into the ECF.

HOMEOSTATIC MECHANISMS

Several homeostatic mechanisms are responsible for the balance of fluid and electrolytes within the body. Those mechanisms involve organs that keep the composition and volume of body fluid within limits of normal: kidneys; heart and blood vessels; lungs; and adrenal, parathyroid, and pituitary glands (Table 3–4).

Table 3–4 ☐ **HOMEOSTATIC ORGANS AND MECHANISMS**

1. Kidneys
2. Heart and blood vessels
3. Lungs
4. Glands
   Adrenal: Aldosterone, cortisol, epinephrine
   Parathyroid: PTH
   Pituitary: ADH

41

Kidneys

The kidneys are vital to control of fluid and electrolyte balance. They normally filter 170 liters of plasma per day in the adult, while excreting only 1.5 liters of urine. They act in response to blood-borne messengers such as aldosterone and **antidiuretic hormone (ADH)**. Functions of kidneys in fluid balance are:

✓ Regulation of fluid volume and osmolarity by selective retention and excretion of body fluids
✓ Regulation of electrolyte levels by selective retention of needed substances and excretion of unneeded substances
✓ Regulation of pH of ECF by excretion or retention of hydrogen (H^+) ions
✓ Excretion of metabolic wastes (primarily acids) and toxic substances (Metheny, 1987, p 8)

✎ **Note:** Renal failure can result in multiple fluid and electrolyte imbalances.

Heart and Blood Vessels

The pumping action of the heart provides circulation of blood through the kidneys under pressure, which allows urine to form; renal perfusion makes renal function possible. Blood vessels permit plasma to reach the kidneys in sufficient volume (20 percent of circulating blood volume) to regulate water and electrolytes.

Lungs

The lungs regulate acid-base balance by regulating the H^+ ion concentration and are important homeostatic organs. Functions of the lungs in body fluid balance are:

✓ Regulation of metabolic alkalosis by compensatory hypoventilation, resulting in carbon dioxide (CO_2) retention and increased acidity of the ECF
✓ Regulation of metabolic acidosis by causing compensatory hyperventilation, resulting in CO_2 excretion, thus decreasing acidity of the ECF
✓ Removal of 300 to 500 mL of water daily through exhalation (insensible water loss)

Glands

The glands responsible for aiding in homeostasis are the adrenal, parathyroid, and pituitary glands. The adrenal cortex is important in fluid and electrolyte homeostasis. The primary adrenocortical hormone influencing the balance of fluid is aldosterone. Aldosterone is responsible for the renal reabsorption of sodium, which results in the retention of chloride and water and the excretion of potassium. Aldosterone also regulates blood volume by regulating sodium retention.

Epinephrine, another adrenal hormone, increases blood pressure, enhances pulmonary ventilation, dilates blood vessels needed for emergencies, and constricts unnecessary vessels. The adrenocortical hormone cortisol, when produced in large quantities, can produce sodium and fluid retention and potassium deficit.

The parathyroid gland, which is embedded in the corners of the thyroid gland, regulates calcium and phosphate balance. The parathyroid gland influences fluid and electrolytes, increases serum calcium levels, and lowers serum phosphate levels. A decrease in parathyroid hormone (PTH) lowers serum calcium levels and increases serum phosphate levels.

The pituitary hormone influencing water balance is the ADH. This hormone, which affects renal reabsorption of water, is also referred to as the "water-conserving hormone." Functions of ADH are to maintain osmotic pressure of the cells by controlling renal water retention or excretion and controlling blood volume.

✎ **Note:** Excessive secretion of ADH results in syndrome of inappropriate antidiuretic hormone **(SIADH)**.

FLUID IMBALANCES: FLUID VOLUME DEFICIT AND EXCESS

Fluid imbalances may reflect an increase or a decrease in total body fluid or an altered distribution of body fluids. Assessment skills of history taking and physical examination, along with an understanding of fluid physiology, are necessary for identification of fluid volume excess and deficit disorders. Along with physical assessment skills, clinical assessment of total body water can be inaccurate unless serial documentation of body weights are performed.

There are two major alterations in ECF balance: fluid volume deficit and fluid volume excess. ECF volume deficit reflects a contracted vascular compartment due either to a significant ECF loss or to an accumulation of fluid in the interstitial space. Gastrointestinal dysfunction is the most common cause of ECF deficit. Other etiologies are listed in Table 3 – 5. Clinically, ECF deficit is characterized by an acute weight loss, altered cardiovascular function (which reflects the underlying ECF volume deficit), and complaints of nausea and vomiting. Symptomatology reflects a dehydrated state with sunken eyeballs, poor skin turgor, and oliguria. Treatment for ECF volume deficit entails fluid replacement (orally or intravenously) until the oliguria is relieved and the cardiovascular and neurologic systems stabilize.

✎ **Note:** Extreme caution must be exercised in fluid replacement therapy, to avoid fluid overload. ECF volume excess causes an expansion of the ECF compartment.

The primary cause of ECF excess is cardiovascular dysfunction. Table 3–5 shows further etiologies of ECF volume excess. Clinically, ECF volume excess has distinct signs and symptoms, such as weight gain of 5 percent of TBW and alterations in cardiovascular function with presence of edema, hypertension, tachycardia, and respiratory dysfunction. Treatment of ECF volume excess is directed toward sodium and fluid restriction, administration of diuretics, and the treatment of the underlying cause (Dolan, 1991, pp 438 – 441).

43

Table 3–5 ☐ **CONTRAST ECF DISORDERS**

	Fluid Volume Deficit	Fluid Volume Excess
Definition, Etiology (Causes)	Hypovolemia Fever with diaphoresis *GI dysfunction* (most common) Fluid and electrolyte loss Diarrhea Overdose of cathartics *Renal* dysfunction *Neurologic* dysfunction Lethargy and coma *Endocrine* dysfunction Diabetes insipidus	Hypervolemia *Cardiovascular* dysfunction CHF, pulmonary edema Too rapid administration of I.V. saline *Renal* dysfunction Serum protein depletion and hyponatremia Cirrhosis with ascites and portal hypertension *Endocrine* dysfunction Hyperaldosteronism
Clinical Picture	Acute weight loss *Neurologic:* Changes in mental status, disorientation, lethargy, convulsions *Cardiovascular:* Postural hypotension, dizziness Syncope, vertigo, pulse weak Absence of neck vein distension Decreased CVP, decreased cardiac output *GI:* Nausea, vomiting, anorexia *Fluid intake versus output:* Increased thirst, decreased urine output, poor skin turgor over sternum and forehead Dry skin and mucous membranes Sunken eyeballs; hyperthermia	Acute weight gain *Neurologic:* Changes in mental status, level of consciousness, seizures *Cardiovascular:* Hypertension, tachycardia, bounding pulse Increased CVP, neck vein distension *Edema:* True pitting edema, taut and shiny skin. *Respiratory:* SOB, tachypnea, dyspnea, cough, rales, pulmonary edema. *Renal:* Urine output is disproportionately less than fluid intake.
Laboratory Data	Electrolyte parameter (by itself) is indicative of fluid deficit *Serum:* Hematocrit: Increased Hemoglobin: Increased	Electrolyte parameter (by itself) is indicative of fluid excess. *Serum:* Hematocrit: Normal to low Hemoglobin: Normal to low

Table 3–5 □ **CONTRAST ECF DISORDERS (*Continued*)**

	Fluid Volume Deficit	Fluid Volume Excess

	Proteins: Increased
	Osmolarity: Normal
	BUN: > 20 mg/100 mL
	Urine:
	Sodium: < 50 mEq/L
	Osmolarity: > 500
	  mOsm/kg
	Specific gravity: 1.030
		Proteins: Normal to low
		Osmolarity: Normal
		BUN: Normal to low
		Urine:
		Sodium: Reduced
		Osmolarity: < 500
		  mOsm/kg
		Specific gravity: < 1.010

Treatment	1. Restore fluid and
	   electrolyte balance
	   using I.V. isotonic
	   saline
	2. Treat underlying
	   cause
		1. Reduce fluid
		   retention by salt and
		   fluid restriction
		2. Diuretics to increase
		   fluid excretion
		3. Treat underlying
		   cause

GI = Gastrointestinal; CHF = congestive heart failure; CVP = central venous pressure; SOB = shortness of breath; BUN = blood urea nitrogen.
Source: Data from *Critical Care Nursing: Clinical Management Through the Nursing Process* (pp. 436, 442) by J. Dolan, 1991, Philadelphia: F.A. Davis Company. Copyright 1991 by F.A. Davis Company. Reprinted by permission.

PHYSICAL ASSESSMENT

The nurse must use a systems approach to assess for fluid and electrolyte imbalances related to intravenous (I.V.) therapy. A head-to-toe system assessment should include vital signs, infusion rate, intake, and output and an awareness of agency policy and procedure to prevent complications associated with I.V. therapy (refer to Chapter 8 for complications). The following body systems should be assessed at the beginning of each shift and as needed to monitor the patient's reactions to infusions: neurologic, cardiovascular, respiratory, and integumentary. The special senses and body weight also should be assessed.

Neurologic

There is a progressive loss of central nervous system cells with advancing age, along with decreases in olfactory and tactile sense. The thirst mechanism in the aged may be diminished and is thus a poor guide for fluid needs in such patients. An ill patient may not be able to verbalize thirst or to reach for a glass of water. Sensation of thirst depends on excitation of the cortical centers of consciousness. The use of antianxiety agents, sedatives, or hypnotics can lead to confusion and disorientation, causing the patient to forget to drink fluid. Changes in orientation can also be an indicator of fluid volume deficit.

45

Cardiovascular

The quality and rate of the pulse is an indicator of how the patient is tolerating ECF volume. The peripheral veins in the extremities provide a way of evaluating plasma volume. Examination of hand veins can evaluate the plasma volume. Peripheral veins empty in 3 to 5 seconds when the hand is elevated and fill in the same amount of time when the hand is lowered to a dependent position. Peripheral vein filling takes longer than 3 to 5 seconds in patients with sodium depletion and extracellular dehydration (Metheny, 1984, p 41). Slow emptying of the peripheral veins indicates overhydration and excessive blood volume. A 10 mm Hg fall in systolic blood pressure when shifting from the lying to the standing position usually indicates fluid volume deficit. The jugular vein provides a built-in manometer for evaluation of central venous pressure (CVP). Changes in fluid volume are reflected by changes in neck vein filling.

The external jugular veins, with the patient supine, fill to the anterior border of the sternocleidomastoid muscle. Flat neck veins in the supine position indicate a decreased plasma volume. When the patient is in a 45-degree position the external jugular distends no higher than 2 cm above the sternal angle. Elevated venous pressure is indicated by neck veins distending from the top portion of the sternum to the angle of the jaw.

Fluid Volume Excess	Fluid Volume Deficit
Bounding pulse	Decreased pulse rate
Jugular vein distention	Decreased blood pressure
Increase in blood pressure	Narrow pulse pressure
	Cardiac arrhythmia
	Potassium deficit

Respiratory

A key to assessment of circulatory overload is assessing the lung fields. Changes in respiratory rate and depth may be a compensatory mechanism for acid-base imbalance. Moist rales, in the absence of cardiopulmonary disease, indicates fluid volume excess.

Fluid Volume Excess	Fluid Volume Deficit
Moist rales	Clear lungs
Increased respiratory rate	
Dyspnea	
Pulmonary edema	

✎ **Note:** Shallow, slow breathing could indicate metabolic alkalosis or respiratory acidosis. Deep, rapid breathing could indicate respiratory alkalosis or metabolic acidosis. Refer to Chapter 4 for further information on acid-base imbalances.

Integumentary

The temperature and skin surface assessment are key in determining fluid volume changes. Turgor of the skin should be assessed by pinching the areas over the hands, sternum, or forehead. In a normal person the pinched skin will immediately fall back to its normal position when released. This elastic property, referred to as turgor, partially depends on interstitial fluid volume. In an individual with a fluid volume deficit the skin may remain slightly elevated for many seconds. This can be assessed by placing your fingers firmly on the patient's sternum; if imprints of your fingers remain, a condition called *fingerprinting* is present. Fingerprinting is associated with fluid volume excess.

✎ **Note:** The skin turgor in people 55 years and older is reduced primarily because of reduced skin elasticity. Skin turgor in these patients is probably most valid on the skin over the sternum.

ASSESSMENT OF INTEGUMENTARY SYSTEM

	Fluid Volume Excess	Fluid Volume Deficit
Temperature		Decrease in temperature
Skin surfaces	Warm moist skin	
	Sternum fingerprinting	Decreased turgor over sternum and forehead (tenting of the skin)

✎ **Note:** An increase in temperature can indicate a sodium excess, and flushing of the skin surfaces can indicate a magnesium deficit. Refer to Chapter 4 for more detail on electrolyte imbalances.

Special Senses

The eyes, mouth, lips, and tongue are also key indicators of fluid volume imbalances. The absence of tearing and salivation in a child is a sign of fluid volume deficit. In a normal, healthy individual the tongue has one longitudinal furrow. In the person with fluid volume deficit there are additional longitudinal furrows and the tongue is smaller because of fluid loss (Metheny, 1984, p 32).

SPECIAL SENSES ASSESSMENT

	Fluid Volume Excess	Fluid Volume Deficit
Eyes	Periorbital edema	Dry conjunctiva
		Sunken eyes
		Decreased tearing
Mouth		Sticky, dry mucous membranes coating in mouth
Lips		Dry, cracked lips
Tongue		Extra longitudinal furrows

✎ **Note:** Good oral hygiene is imperative with mouth-breathing patients. Also, if you are giving good oral care and the crusted, dry, furrowed tongue is not getting better, fluid volume deficit must be remedied to aid in solving this problem.

Body Weight

It is an important clinical tool to monitor daily the weight of patients with potential fluid imbalances. Accurate body weight measurement is a better indicator of gains or losses than intake and output records.

BODY WEIGHT ASSESSMENT

Fluid Volume Excess	Fluid Volume Deficit
Gains	*Losses*
1–5% TBW or below 5% TBW = Mild overhydration	Below 5% TBW = Mild dehydration
5–10% TBW = Moderate overhydration	5–10% TBW = Moderate dehydration
Above 15% TBW = Severe overhydration	Above 15% TBW = Severe dehydration

✎ **Note:** A loss or gain of 1 kg (2.2 lb) reflects a loss or gain of 1 liter of body fluid. The following assessment tool may be copied and used as a pocket reference for assessing patients for fluid volume disorders.

NURSE'S QUICK ASSESSMENT GUIDE

System Assessed	Fluid Volume	
	Excess	Deficit
Neurologic		
Change in orientation or confusion		X
Special Senses		
Eyes		
Dry conjunctiva		X
Decreased tearing		X
Sunken eyes		X
Mouth		
Sticky, dry mucous membrane		X
Lips		
Dry, cracked		X
Tongue		
Extra longitudinal furrows		X
Cardiovascular		
Decreased pulse rate		X
Decreased blood pressure		X
Narrow pulse pressure		X
Hand vein filling slow, > 3–5 s		X
Bounding pulse	X	
Increase pulse rate	X	

NURSE'S QUICK ASSESSMENT GUIDE (Continued)

System Assessed	Fluid Volume	
	Excess	Deficit
Cardiovascular (Continued)		
Jugular distension	X	
Overdistended hand veins slow to empty, $> 3-5$ s	X	
Pulmonary (Lung Fields)		
Moist rales	X	
Increase respiratory rate > 20	X	
Dyspnea	X	
Pulmonary edema	X	
Integumentary		
Turgor: Decreased over sternum and forehead		X
Skin Surfaces: Warm and moist	X	
Temperature: Decreased temperature		X
Body Weight		
Decrease		*% LOSS* <5% mild FVD 5–10% moderate FVD >15% severe FVD
Increase	*% GAINS* <5% mild FVE 5–10% moderate FVE >15% severe FVE	

FVD = Fluid volume deficit; FVE = fluid volume excess.

NURSING DIAGNOSES RELATED TO FLUID BALANCE

1. Altered oral mucous membrane related to dehydration
2. Altered tissue perfusion: cardiopulmonary, renal, peripheral related to hypovolemia
3. Altered thought process related to confusion, disorientation resulting from chemical imbalance
4. Fluid volume deficit related to failure of regularity mechanism
5. Fluid volume deficit related to loss of body fluid and inadequate fluid intake (Poyss, 1987)
6. Fluid volume excess related to infusion of sodium chloride solution
7. Fluid volume excess related to compromised regulatory function (kidney)
8. Hyperthermia related to dehydration
9. Impaired skin integrity related to altered circulation, edema
10. Risk of injury related to confusion

SUMMARY OF CHAPTER 3

FUNDAMENTALS OF FLUID BALANCE

Fluid is distributed in three compartments as follows:

Intracellular	40 percent
Intravascular	5 percent
Interstitial	15 percent
TBW in water	60 percent

Fluid Balance Intake and Output

Intake — Liquids, food, and oxidation (2500 mL in 24 hours)
Output — Insensible loss: Sweat, respirations (500 to 1000 mL in 24 hours)
Sensible loss: Urine, feces (1500 mL in 24 hours)

Fluid Functions

Maintains blood volume
Regulates body temperature
Transports material to and from cells
Serves as aqueous medium for cellular metabolism
Assists digestion of food through hydrolysis
Acts as solvent in which **solutes** are available for cell function
Serves as medium for excretion of waste

Fluid is transported passively by filtration, diffusion, and osmosis. Electrolytes are actively transported by ATP on cell membrane and the sodium-potassium pump. The definition of osmosis is movement of water from a lower concentration to a higher concentration across a semipermeable membrane.

Tonicity

Isotonic solutions: range, 250 to 375 mOsm/liter
Hypotonic solutions: less than 250 mOsm/liter
Hypertonic solutions: more than 375 mOsm/liter

Homeostatic Organs

Kidneys
Heart
Blood vessels
Lungs
Glands: adrenal, parathyroid, and pituitary

Systems Assessment

Neurologic
Cardiovascular
Respiratory
Integumentary
Special senses
Body weight

Fluid Imbalance

ECF volume deficit
ECF volume excess

Activity Journal

1. Within your work environment, identify the patients at risk for fluid volume deficit or excess. Remember, even outpatient units see patients at risk.

2. Using the six body systems to assess for fluid volume excess or deficit, pick four patients on your unit to assess and check for fluid volume changes.

3. Check the I.V. solutions infusing on your patients and identify whether the solutions are isotonic, hypotonic, or hypertonic.

Quality Assessment Model

Instructions: Use this quality assessment model to conduct retrospective audits of charts, establish quality control standards, or develop outcome criteria for quality assurance. Refer to Chapter 2 for details on quality assessment.

STRUCTURE

(Resources that affect outcome)
Human Resource: Nurse
↓

PROCESS

(Actual giving and receiving of care)
Therapist activities related to the assessment of fluid balance excess and deficit are:

1. Assess integumentary system for temperature, elasticity, and edema every 8 hours.
2. Assess cardiovascular system every 8 hours.
3. Auscultate lungs every 8 hours and document respiratory rate and depth.
4. Assess orientation every 8 hours.
5. Assess eyes, mouth, tongue, and lips for signs and symptoms of fluid volume deficit or excess.
6. Weigh patient daily.
7. Record accurate intake and output (I & O), including sensible and insensible losses.
8. Maintain I.V. solutions at prescribed rate.
9. Monitor blood serum and urine specific gravity.
↓

OUTCOME STANDARDS

(Effects of care)
Documentation will reflect standards of care for monitoring patient for fluid balance disorders:

1. Documentation of adequate intake of fluid and electrolytes as evidenced by I & O and dietary records.
2. Evidence of documented daily weights.
3. Evidence of documented assessment of the five body systems (neurologic, cardiovascular, respiratory, integumentary, and special senses), which are indicators of fluid volume disturbances.
4. Documentation of specific gravity on graphic record.

Post-test, Chapter 3

Match the definition in column 2 to the correct term in column 1.

Term

1. _____ Isotonic
2. _____ Hypertonic
3. _____ Hypotonic
4. _____ Osmolarity
5. _____ Homeostasis
6. _____ ADH
7. _____ Intravascular fluid
8. _____ Intracellular fluid
9. _____ Interstitial fluid
10. _____ Insensible loss

Definition

A. Output that is difficult to measure, such as perspiration

B. Hormone secreted from the pituitary that causes kidneys to conserve water.

C. Having an osmotic pressure equal to blood.

D. Ability to restore equilibrium under stress.

E. Fluid portion of the blood

F. Having an osmotic pressure higher than 375 mOsm/liter.

G. Fluid between the cells.

H. Fluid inside the cells.

I. Having an osmotic pressure less than 250 mOsm/liter.

J. A measure of solute concentration.

Keeping the principle of osmosis in mind, answer the following three questions about fluid shift:

11. A physician orders 5% dextrose in 0.9% sodium chloride (mOsm 559).

    Fluid will move from the _____ space to the _____ space
    A. Intracellular to vascular
    B. Vascular to interstitial
    C. Interstitial to cellular

12. A physician orders 0.45% sodium chloride (mOsm 154).

    Fluid will move from the _____ space to the _____ space.
    A. Intracellular to vascular
    B. Vascular to intracellular
    C. Interstitial to cellular

13. A physician orders lactated Ringer's solution (mOsm 273). Fluid will _____.

    A. Move from the intracellular space to the vascular space
    B. Move from the vascular space to the cellular space
    C. Stay in the vascular space

14. List two functions of body fluids.

    1. _____

    2. _____

15. List three homeostatic organs.

    1. _____

    2. _____

    3. _____

16. Fluid is transported passively by the mechanism(s) of:
    A. Diffusion
    B. Osmosis
    C. Filtration
    D. All of the above

17. Identify one nursing diagnosis for fluid volume deficit.

    _____

18. A nurse has just completed a physical assessment on Mr. Marx, age 68.
    The results include the following:

    He knows who he is but is unsure of where he is (previous orientation was
        normal).
    His eyes are sunken.
    His mouth is coated and has an extra longitudinal furrow, and his lips are
        cracked.
    His hand vein filling time is more than 5 seconds.
    Tenting is present over his sternum.
    Vital signs: BP 128/60, P 78 R 16 (prior vital signs were BP 150/78, P 76
        R 16)

Your assessment would lead you to suspect _____.

Answers to Post-test, Chapter 3

1. C
2. F
3. I
4. J
5. D
6. B
7. E
8. H
9. G
10. A
11. A
12. B
13. C
14. Maintains blood volume, regulates body temperature, transports material to and from cells, acts as aqueous medium for cellular metabolism, assists in digestion of food, serves as a solvent in which solutes are available for cell function and as a medium for excretion of waste.
15. Kidneys, heart, blood vessels; lungs; adrenal, parathyroid, and pituitary glands
16. D
17. Fluid volume deficit related to failure of regulatory mechanism.
Fluid volume deficit related to loss of body fluid and inadequate fluid intake.
18. Fluid volume deficit

References

Carson, R. (1961). *The sea around us.* New York: New American Library.

Chenevey, B. (1987). Overview of fluids and electrolytes. *Nursing Clinics of North America, 22*(4), 749–759.

Dolan, J.T. (1991). *Critical care nursing: Clinical management through the nursing process.* Philadelphia: F.A. Davis.

Goldberger, E. (1986). *A primer of water, electrolytes and acid-base syndromes* (7th ed.). Philadelphia: Lea & Febiger.

Mathewson-Kuhn, M. (1991). *Pharmacotherapeutics: A nursing process approach* (2nd ed.). Philadelphia: F.A. Davis.

Metheny, N.M. (1984). *Quick reference to fluid balance.* Philadelphia: J.B. Lippincott.

Metheny, N.M. (1987). *Fluids and electrolyte balance: Nursing considerations.* Philadelphia: J.B. Lippincott.

Metheny, N.M. (1990). Why worry about IV fluids? *American Journal of Nursing, 90*(6), 50–55.

Poyss, A.S. (1987). Assessment and nursing diagnosis in fluid and electrolyte disorders. *Nursing Clinics of North America, 22*(4), 773–783.

Bibliography

Berger, E. (1984). Nutrition in hypodermoclysis. *Journal of American Geriatric Society, 32,* 199.

Burgess, R.E. (1965). Fluids and electrolytes. *American Journal of Nursing, 65*(10), 1310–1316.

Gahart, B.L. (1991). *Intravenous medications: A handbook for nurses and other allied health personnel* (7th ed.). St. Louis: C.V. Mosby.

Maxwell, M., & Kleeman, C. (1980). *Clinical disorders of fluid and electrolyte metabolism* (3rd ed.). New York: McGraw-Hill.

Merck, Sharp, & Dohme (1989). *Critical care quick reference*. California: Merck.

Rolls, B.J. & Phillips, P.A. (1990). Aging and disturbances of thirst and fluid balance. *Nutrition Reviews, 48*(3), 137–143.

Rutherford, C. (1989). Fluid and electrolyte therapy: Considerations for patient care. *Journal of Intravenous Therapy, 12*(3), 173–184.

Vanatta, J., & Fogelman, M. (1982). *Moyers fluid balance* (3rd ed.). Chicago: Year Book Medical.

CHAPTER 4

Fundamentals of Electrolyte Balance

CHAPTER CONTENTS

Glossary

Acidosis: Increase in hydrogen ion concentration; blood pH below normal (less than 7.35)

Alkalosis: Decrease in hydrogen ion concentration; blood pH above normal (greater than 7.45)

Anion: Negatively charged electrolyte

Antidiuretic hormone (ADH): A hormone secreted from the pituitary mechanism that causes the kidney to conserve water, sometimes referred to as the "water-conserving hormone"

Cation: Positively charged electrolyte

Chvostek's sign: A sign elicited by tapping the facial nerve 2 cm anterior to the earlobe, just below the zygomatic process; the response is a spasm of the muscles supplied by the facial nerve, which is seen in tetany

ECF: Extracellular fluid

Hypercalcemia: An excess of calcium in the blood

Hyperchloremia: An excess of chloride in the blood

Hyperkalemia: An excess of potassium in the blood

Hypermagnesemia: An excess of magnesium in the blood

Hypernatremia: An excess of sodium in the blood

Hyperphosphatemia: An excess of phosphate in the blood

Hypocalcemia: A low calcium concentration in the blood

Hypochloremia: A low chloride concentration in the blood

Hypokalemia: A low potassium concentration in the blood

Hypomagnesemia: A low magnesium concentration in the blood

Hyponatremia: A low sodium concentration in the blood

Hypophosphatemia: A low phosphate concentration in the blood

ICF: Intracellular fluid

pH: Hydrogen ion (H^+) concentration

SIADH: Syndrome of inappropriate antidiuretic hormone, a condition in which excessive antidiuretic hormone is secreted, resulting in hyponatremia

Tetany: Continuous tonic spasm of a muscle

Trousseau's sign: A spasm of the hand elicited when the blood supply to the hand is decreased or the nerves of the hand are stimulated by pressure; it is elicited within several minutes by applying a blood pressure cuff inflated above systolic pressure

LEARNING OBJECTIVES

Upon completion of this chapter, the reader will be able to:

☐ Define terminology related to electrolytes.
☐ State the seven major electrolytes within the body fluids.
☐ Differentiate between cations and anions.
☐ Contrast each of the seven electrolytes and their major roles in body fluids.
☐ Identify signs and symptoms of deficits of sodium, potassium, calcium, magnesium, chloride, and phosphorus.
☐ Identify signs and symptoms of excesses of sodium, potassium, calcium, magnesium, chloride, and phosphate.
☐ Identify patients at risk for electrolyte imbalance.
☐ State the normal pH range of body fluids.
☐ Compare clinical manifestations of metabolic acidosis and alkalosis.
☐ Identify regulatory organs of acid-base balance.
☐ Determine nursing diagnoses appropriate for patients experiencing an electrolyte imbalance.

Pre-test, Chapter 4

Instructions: The pre-test is to review prior knowledge of the theory of electrolyte balance. Each question in the pre-test is based on the learning objectives of the chapter. Match the definition in column 2 to the correct term in column 1.

Column 1

1. _____ Acidosis
2. _____ Hyperkalemia
3. _____ pH
4. _____ Cation
5. _____ ECF
6. _____ Alkalosis
7. _____ Ion
8. _____ ICF
9. _____ Tetany
10. _____ Anion

Column 2

A. Electrolyte
B. Hydrogen ion concentration
C. An excess of potassium in the blood
D. Continuous tonic spasm of a muscle
E. Positively charged electrolyte
F. H^+ ion concentration increases
G. Extracellular fluid
H. H^+ ion concentration decreases
I. Intracellular fluid
J. Negatively charged electrolyte

True-False

11. **T F** The normal pH range for arterial blood is 7.35 to 7.45.

12. **T F** The major function of sodium is to maintain extracellular fluid volume.

13. **T F** Calcium and phosphate have a reciprocal relationship.

14. **T F** Magnesium is a major intracellular electrolyte.

15. **T F** The kidneys and liver are the organs that regulate acid-base balance.

16. Which of the following are positively charged electrolytes?
    A. Potassium, sodium, bicarbonate
    B. Potassium, sodium, calcium
    C. Bicarbonate, phosphate, chloride
    D. Chloride, magnesium, bicarbonate

Match the signs and symptoms of the deficit with the electrolyte imbalance.

Electrolyte Imbalance	Signs and Symptoms
17. _____ Hypokalemia	A. Anorexia, exhaustion, muscle cramps, ataxia
18. _____ Hypocalcemia	B. Irritability, diminished reflexes, anorexia, nausea, vomiting
19. _____ Hypomagnesemia	C. Numbness of fingers, cramps, mental changes, Chvosteks's sign
20. _____ Hyponatremia	D. Neuromuscular and nervous system irritability, paresthesia, cardiac arrhythmias, disorientation

21. Which of the following signs and symptoms would indicate alkalosis (bicarbonate excess)?
    A. Kussmaul's breathing, confusion, increased respiratory rate
    B. Tetany, soft tissue calcification, Kussmaul's breathing
    C. Dizziness, tingling of fingers and toes, carpopedal spasm

---

ANSWERS TO PRE-TEST, Chapter 4

1. F   2. C   3. B   4. E   5. G   6. H   7. A   8. I   9. D

10. J   11. T   12. T   13. T   14. T   15. F   16. B   17. B

18. C   19. D   20. A   21. C

Chemical compounds in solution behave in one of two ways — they either separate and combine with other compounds or remain intact. One group of compounds remain intact; these are called nonelectrolytes (e.g., urea, dextrose, and creatinine). These compounds do not separate from their complex form when added to a solution. The second group of compounds, electrolytes, dissociate or separate in solution. These compounds break up into individual particles known as ions, in a process called ionization. (Refer to Table 4–1 for a list of the major electrolytes in body fluid).

Ions, which are the dissociated particles of an electrolyte, each carry an electrical charge, either positive or negative. Negative ions are called **anions** and positive ions, **cations** (Table 4–2).

Table 4–1 □ **MAJOR ELECTROLYTES IN BODY FLUID**

Sodium
Potassium
Calcium
Magnesium
Chloride
Phosphorus
Bicarbonate

Electrolytes are active chemicals that unite. The ions are expressed in terms of milliequivalents (mEq) per liter rather than milligrams (mg). A milliequivalent measures chemical activity rather than weight. The total cations and anions in a given compartment are equal. There are 154 mEq of anions and 154 mEq of cations in the plasma. Each water compartment of the body contains electrolytes. The concentration and composition of electrolytes vary from compartment to compartment. Refer to Table 4–3 for a diagrammatic comparison of electrolyte composition in the fluid compartments.

ELECTROLYTE FUNCTION, DEFICIT, EXCESS, AND TREATMENT

Sodium

Normal laboratory value: 135 to 145 mEq/liter

Function

The major function of sodium is to maintain extracellular fluid (**ECF**) volume. Extracellular sodium level affects the cellular fluid volume, based on the principle of osmosis. A low serum sodium level results in dilute ECF, which allows water to be drawn into the cells (lower to higher concentration). The normal daily requirement for sodium in adults is approximately 100 mEq.

✎ **Note:** Sodium does not easily cross the cell-wall membrane; therefore, sodium is the most abundant cation of ECF.

Deficit: Hyponatremia

Hyponatremia refers to a condition in which the sodium level is below normal (less than 135 mEq/liter). Low sodium can be the result of an excessive loss of

Table 4–2 □ **POSITIVE AND NEGATIVE IONS IN BODY FLUIDS**

Cations	Anions
Sodium (Na^+)	Chloride (Cl^-)
Potassium (K^+)	Phosphate (HPO_4^{2-})
Calcium (Ca^{2+})	Bicarbonate (HCO_3^-) (also SO_4^{2-}, proteinates, and organic acids)
Magnesium (Mg^{2+})	

Table 4-3 □ COMPARISON OF ELECTROLYTE COMPOSITION IN FLUID COMPARTMENTS

Intracellular Water (approx. mEq/L)		Extracellular Water (approx. mEq/L)			
		PLASMA		INTERSTITIAL FLUID	
Cations	Anions	Cations	Anions	Cations	Anions
205 mEq	205 mEq	154 mEq	154 mEq	154 mEq	154 mEq

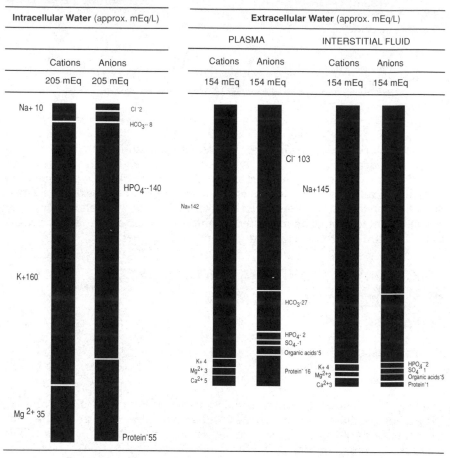

Intracellular Water:
- Na+ 10
- K+ 160
- Mg $^{2+}$ 35
- Cl $^-$ 2
- HCO$_3$-- 8
- HPO$_4$--140
- Protein 55

Plasma:
- Na+142
- K+ 4
- Mg^{2+} 3
- Ca^{2+} 5
- Cl$^-$ 103
- HCO$_3$-27
- HPO$_4$- 2
- SO$_4$-1
- Organic acids 5
- Protein 16

Interstitial Fluid:
- Na+145
- K+ 4
- Mg^{2+}2
- Ca^{2+}3
- HPO$_4$--2
- SO$_4$-1
- Organic acids 5
- Protein 1

sodium or an excessive gain of water; in either event, hyponatremia is due to a relatively greater concentration of water than of sodium.

Etiology

LOSS OF SODIUM
✓ Gastrointestinal fluid loss
✓ Excessive sweating, coupled with excessive water consumption
✓ Use of diuretics (especially dangerous with low-salt diets)
✓ Adrenal insufficiency (aldosterone deficiency causes sodium loss)

GAINS OF WATER
✓ Excessive use of dextrose and water solutions
✓ Compulsive water drinking (psychogenic polydipsia)
✓ Labor induction with oxytocin (oxytocin has been shown to have an in-

trinsic **antidiuretic hormone (ADH)** effect, acting to increase water reabsorption from the glomerular filtrate)

✓ Syndrome of inappropriate antidiuretic hormone (**SIADH**) secretion (Metheny, 1987, p 53).

✎ **Note:** "The syndrome of inappropriate antidiuretic hormone has progressed from a rare occurrence to the most common cause of hyponatremia seen in a general hospital" (Anderson, Chung, & Kluge, 1985). SIADH occurs in patients with inflammatory disorders such as pneumonia; tuberculosis; abscess; oat cell cancer of the lung; and central nervous system disorders such as meningitis, trauma, stroke, or degenerative disease (Lamb, 1986).

Pharmacologic Agents

Chemical agents may impair renal water excretion and thereby lead to sodium deficit. Drugs that contribute to sodium deficit are:

✓ Nicotine
✓ Diabinase
✓ Cytoxan
✓ Morphine
✓ Barbiturates
✓ Acetaminophen

Signs and Symptoms

CHRONIC HYPONATREMIA
- Impaired sensation of taste: anorexia
- Muscle cramps
- Feeling of exhaustion
- Apprehension: feeling of impending doom (Na^+ less than 115)
- Focal weaknesses: hemiparesis, ataxia

✎ **Note:** Dehydration and chronic hyponatremia can lead to confusional states that interfere with fluid intake in the elderly. The elderly are very susceptible to dehydration (Rolls & Phillips, 1990).

ACUTE HYPONATREMIA (DUE TO WATER OVERLOAD)
- Same as for chronic hyponatremia
- Fingerprint edema (sign of intracellular water excess)
- Specific gravity: 1.002 to 1.004

✎ **Note:** Fingerprint edema is demonstrated by pressing a finger firmly over the sternum or other body surface for 15 to 30 seconds. A positive sign is a visible fingerprint remaining after the finger is removed, similar to that seen when a fingerprint is made on paper with ink (Vanatta & Fogelman, 1982, pp 33–34).

Treatment

The treatment of hyponatremia is to provide sodium through diet or parenterally. Patients able to eat and drink can easily replace sodium by consuming a normal diet. Those unable to take sodium orally must be given the electrolyte parenterally. An isotonic sodium chloride solution or lactated Ringer's solution may be ordered to replace sodium.

✎ **Note:** When the primary problem is water retention, it is safer to restrict water than to administer sodium. An example of an intravenous (I.V.) solution that can contribute to hyponatremia is excessive administration of 5% dextrose and water.

Excess: Hypernatremia

The serum level of sodium is above 145 mEq in **hypernatremia**. This elevation can be caused by a gain of sodium without water, or a loss of water without loss of sodium.

Etiology

✓ Deprivation of water, occurring when a patient cannot respond to thirst
✓ Hypertonic tube feeding with inadequate water supplements
✓ Watery diarrhea (higher risk in infants)
✓ Increased insensible loss
✓ Ingestion of sodium in unusual amounts
✓ Excessive parenteral administration of sodium-containing solutions
✓ Profuse sweating
✓ Heatstroke
✓ Drowning in sea water

Signs and Symptoms

- Thirst
- Elevated body temperature
- Swollen red tongue with dry, sticky mucous membranes
- Severe hypernatremia: disorientation, irritability and hyperactivity when stimulated

Treatment

Goal is *gradually* to lower the serum sodium level, infusing a hypotonic electrolyte solution such as 0.45% normal saline or 5% dextrose and water. Gradual reduction is necessary to decrease the risk of cerebral edema. It is recommended that the sodium level should not be lowered more than 15 mEq/liter in an 8-hour period for adults (Rose, 1984, p 536)

✎ **Note:** Patients who are debilitated need to be offered fluids at regular intervals. The literature states hypodermoclysis via infusion is a short-term method to aid the elderly in reducing sodium levels (Berger, 1984).

Potassium

Normal laboratory value: 3.5 to 5.5 mEq/liter

Function

Potassium is considered an intracellular electrolyte (98 percent is found in intracellular fluid [ICF], 2 percent in the ECF). Potassium is a dynamic electrolyte. ICF potassium will replace ECF potassium if it becomes depleted. Potassium is acquired through diet and must be ingested daily, as the body has no effective method of storage. The daily requirement is 40 mEq. Potassium influences both skeletal and cardiac muscle activity. Alteration in the concentration of plasma potassium changes myocardial irritability and rhythm. Potassium moves easily into the intracellular space when glucose is being metabolized by the body. It moves into the plasma space during strenuous exercise, when cellular metabolism is impaired, or when the cell dies. Potassium, along with sodium, is responsible for transmission of nerve impulses. During nerve cell innervation these ions exchange places, creating an electrical current (Metheny, 1987, p 65)

There is a relationship between acid-base imbalance and potassium balance. **Hypokalemia** can cause alkalosis, which in turn can further decrease serum potassium. **Hyperkalemia** can cause **acidosis**, and acidosis can cause hyperkalemia.

Deficit: Hypokalemia

Hypokalemia refers to a below-normal serum potassium level. It usually reflects a real deficit in total potassium stores; however, it may occur in patients with normal potassium stores when alkalosis is present. Hypokalemia is a common disturbance: many factors are associated with this deficit, and many clinical conditions contribute to it.

Etiology

Many conditions can lead to potassium deficit: gastrointestinal loss, increased use of diuretics, increased perspiration, and poor dietary intake.

GASTROINTESTINAL LOSS
✓ Diarrhea or laxative overuse
✓ Prolonged gastric suction
✓ Protracted vomiting

RENAL LOSS
✓ Diuretic therapy
✓ Excessive use of glucocorticoids
✓ Drugs such as sodium penicillin, carbenicillin, or amphotericin B
✓ European licorice abuse

SWEAT LOSS
✓ Heavy perspiration in clients acclimated to heat

ELECTROLYTE SHIFT
✓ Hyperalimentation therapy without adequate potassium supplement
✓ **Alkalosis**
✓ Excessive administration of insulin

POOR INTAKE
✓ Anorexia nervosa, bulimia
✓ Alcoholism

Signs and Symptoms

- Fatigue
- Anorexia, nausea, vomiting
- Muscle weakness
- Irritability (early)
- Diminished deep tendon reflexes
- Increased sensitivity to digitalis
- Electrocardiographic (ECG) changes: ST-segment depression; broad, inverted, progressively flattening T waves
- Flaccid paralysis (late)
- Death, in severe hypokalemia (resulting from cardiac arrest)

✎ **Note:** Clinical signs and symptoms rarely occur before the serum potassium level has fallen below 3 mEq/liter.

Treatment

Replacement of potassium is the key concept in potassium deficit.

1. Mild hypokalemia is usually treated with dietary increases of potassium or oral supplements.
2. Salt substitutes contain potassium and can be used to supplement potassium intake (Morton's salt substitute, Co-salt, Adolph's salt substitute).
3. If the serum potassium is below 2 mEq/liter, monitor the patient's ECG and administer 10 to 20 mEq of potassium chloride (KCl) via a secondary piggyback set in a volume of 100 mL (Metheny, 1990). Caution should be used in this replacement method and the patient should receive continuous ECG monitoring. *Never give potassium in an I.V. push.*

KCl should be added to a nondextrose solution such as isotonic saline to treat severe hypokalemia because administration of KCl in a dextrose solution may cause a small reduction in the serum potassium level.

✎ **Note:** Potassium replacement must occur slowly to prevent hyperkalemia. Extreme caution should be used when the replacement of KCl exceeds 120 mEq in 24 hours. The patient must be monitored for dysrhythmias.

Excess: Hyperkalemia

Although hyperkalemia is rarer than hypokalemia, this condition can be more dangerous for the patient. It seldom occurs in patients with normal renal function. Hyperkalemia is defined as a serum plasma level of potassium above 5.5 mEq/liter.

Etiology

✓ Excessive administration of potassium parenterally or orally
✓ Severe renal failure
✓ Release of potassium from damaged cells, as occurs in burns and crushing injuries
✓ Pseudohyperkalemia (occurs with prolonged tourniquet application during blood withdrawal)
✓ Acidosis

Signs and Symptoms

• Cardiac: widened QRS complex, prolonged PR interval, and ventricular arrhythmias
• Neuromuscular: vague muscle weakness, flaccid paralysis
• Gastrointestinal: nausea

Treatment

1. Restrict dietary potassium in mild cases.
2. Discontinue potassium supplements.
3. Administer calcium gluconate intravenously (I.V.) if necessary for cardiac symptoms.
4. Administer sodium bicarbonate I.V., which alkalinizes the plasma and causes a temporary shift of potassium into the cells.
5. Administer regular insulin (10 to 25 U) and hypertonic dextrose (10%), which causes a shift of potassium into the cells. This form of treatment begins to act in 15 to 60 minutes and lasts 2 to 4 hours.
6. Peritoneal dialysis or hemodialysis may be ordered.

Calcium

Normal laboratory value: 8.5 to 10.5 mg/dL

Function

The calcium ion is most abundant in the skeletal system, with 99 percent residing in the bones and teeth. Only 1 percent is available for rapid exchange in the circulating blood, bound to protein. The parathyroid hormone (PTH) is responsible for transfer of calcium from the bone to plasma. PTH also augments the intestinal absorption of calcium and enhances net renal calcium reabsorption. Calcium is acquired through dietary intake. Adults require approximately 1 g of calcium daily, along with vitamin D and protein, which are required for absorption and use of this electrolyte.

Calcium is instrumental in activating enzymes and stimulating essential chemical reactions. It plays an important role in maintaining normal transmission of nerve impulses and has a sedative effect on nerve cells. Calcium is most important in the conversion of prothrombin to thrombin, a necessary sequence in the formation of a clot.

Calcium and phosphorus have a reciprocal relationship; that is, a rise in the serum calcium level causes a drop in the serum phosphorus concentration, and a drop in calcium causes a rise in phosphorus.

Deficit: Hypocalcemia

Etiology

✓ Loss in diarrhea or wound exudate
✓ Inadequate secretion of PTH (most common cause) (McFadden & Zaloga, 1983)
✓ Surgical hypoparathyroidism
✓ Acute pancreatitis
✓ Hyperphosphatemia, usually associated with renal failure
✓ Inadequate vitamin D or minimal exposure to the sun
✓ Metabolic alkalosis: nasogastric (NG) tube, prolonged suctioning

Signs and Symptoms

- Numbness of the fingers
- Muscle cramps (especially in extremities)
- Hyperactive deep tendon reflexes
- Mental changes
- **Trousseau's sign**
- **Chvostek's sign**
- Convulsions (late sign)

✎ **Note:** The most dangerous symptom is the development of laryngospasm and tetanylike contractions.

✎ **Note:** The presence of a low magnesium level and a high potassium level potentiates the cardiac and neuromuscular irritability produced by a low calcium level. However, a low potassium level can protect the patient from hypocalcemic **tetany** (McFadden, Zaloga, & Chernow, 1983).

Treatment

1. Oral calcium supplements
2. I.V. calcium gluconate (10 to 20 mL of a 10% solution in 5% dextrose and water over 20 minutes) (McFadden & Zaloga, 1983)

Excess: Hypercalcemia

Hypercalcemia can be very dangerous, with 50% mortality, if untreated.

Etiology

✓ Hyperparathyroidism
✓ Neoplastic disorders: solid tumors with metastasis (breast, prostate, and malignant melanomas); hematologic tumors (lymphomas, acute leukemia, and myeloma); certain chemotherapeutic regimens (use of androgens and estrogens)
✓ Paget's disease
✓ Multiple fractures
✓ Thiazide diuretics
✓ Overuse of calcium-containing antacids

Signs and Symptoms

- Neuromuscular changes: muscle weakness, incoordination, lethargy
- Constipation
- Deep bony pain, flank pain
- Anorexia, nausea, and vomiting
- Polyuria-polydipsia, leading to uremia if not treated
- Renal colic, stones
- Pathologic fractures (due to bone weakening)
- Cardiac manifestations

Treatment

1. Treat underlying disease.
2. Fluids should be forced to help eliminate the source of the hypercalcemia; 0.45% NaCl or 0.9% NaCl I.V. dilutes the serum calcium level. Rehydration is important to dilute the calcium and promote renal excretion.
3. Inorganic phosphate salts can be given orally (Neutra-Phos) or rectally (Fleet enema).
4. Hemodialysis or peritoneal dialysis should be performed to reduce serum calcium levels in life-threatening situations.
5. Lasix (e.g., 20 to 40 mg every 2 hours) may be used to prevent volume overloading during saline administration.
6. Calcitonin will temporarily lower the serum calcium level by 1 to 3 mg/100 mL.
7. In severe hypercalcemia ethylene diaminetetra-acetic acid (EDTA) 15 to 50 mg/kg I.V. over 4 hours is recommended; EDTA chelates calcium and lowers Ca^+ levels in 30 minutes (Calloway, 1987).

Magnesium

Normal laboratory value: 1.5 to 2.5 mEq/liter

Function

The same factors that regulate calcium balance also have an influence on magnesium balance. Magnesium balance is also affected by many of the same agents that decrease or influence potassium balance. The normal diet supplies approximately 25 mEq of magnesium. Magnesium is a major intracellular electrolyte. Approximately one third of serum magnesium is bound to protein; the remaining two thirds exist as free cations.

Magnesium acts directly on the myoneural junction and affects neuromuscular irritability and contractility; therefore, it may have a sedative effect. Magnesium activates many enzymes and plays a role in carbohydrate and protein metabolism. Magnesium affects the cardiovascular system, acting peripherally to produce vasodilation. Magnesium can lower blood pressure and cause cardiac arrest in diastole (Goldberger, 1986, p 341). Imbalances in magnesium predispose the heart to ventricular arrhythmias (Shrier, 1986, p 334).

Deficit: Hypomagnesemia

Hypomagnesemia is an often-overlooked problem in critically ill patients (Zaloga & Chernow, 1983).

Etiology

✓ Chronic alcoholism
✓ Malabsorption syndromes, especially in small bowel
✓ Prolonged malnutrition or starvation
✓ Prolonged diarrhea
✓ Administration of magnesium-free solutions for more than 1 week
✓ Certain drug administration: gentamicin, diuretics, and cisplatin et al., (McFadden, et al., 1983)
✓ Acute pancreatitis
✓ Prolonged gastric suction

Signs and Symptoms

- Neuromuscular and nervous system irritability

  Hyperactive reflexes
  Coarse tremors
  Muscle cramps
  Positive Chvostek's and Trousseau's signs
  Convulsions

- Paresthesias of feet and legs
- Painfully cold hands and feet
- Cardiac signs

  Arrhythmias
  Tachycardia
  Increased potential for digitalis toxicity

- Disorientation

Treatment

1. Administer oral magnesium salts.
2. Administer 40 mEq (5 g) magnesium sulfate I.V. added to 1 liter of 5% dextrose and water or 5% dextrose and saline.

3. Administer 1 to 2 g of 10% solution of magnesium sulfate, direct I.V. push at a rate of 1.5 mL/minute (Gahart, 1991).

✎ **Note:** Be aware that other central nervous system depressants could cause further depressed sensorium when magnesium sulfate is being administered. Therefore, be prepared to deal with respiratory arrest should hypermagnesemia inadvertently occur during administration of magnesium sulfate.

Excess: Hypermagnesemia

The most common cause of **hypermagnesemia** is renal failure.

Etiology

✓ Renal failure
✓ Addison's disease
✓ Excessive magnesium administration during treatment of eclampsia
✓ Hemodialysis with excessively hard water or with a dialysate inadvertently high in magnesium content
✓ Hyperparathyroidism or hypothyroidism

Signs and Symptoms

EARLY
• Flushing and sense of skin warmth
• Lethargy and sedation
• Hypotension
• Nausea and vomiting

LATE
• Hypoactive reflexes
• Depressed respirations
• Coma (12–15 mEq/L) at serum levels
• Cardiac abnormalities: sinus bradycardia, heart block, and cardiac arrest in diastole (at serum levels of 7.1–10 mEq/L).
• Weak or absent cry in newborn

Treatment

1. Decrease oral magnesium intake.
2. Administer calcium gluconate to antagonize the action of magnesium.
3. Support respiratory function.
4. Peritoneal dialysis or hemodialysis may be ordered in severe cases of hypermagnesemia.

Phosphorus

Normal laboratory value: 3.0 to 4.5 mg/dL

Function

Approximately 80 percent of the phosphorus is found in the bones and teeth, and 20 percent is abundant in the ICF. PTH plays a major role in homeostasis of phosphate owing to PTH's ability to vary phosphate reabsorption in the proximal tubule of the kidney. PTH also allows for shift of phosphate from bone to plasma.

Phosphate plays an important role in delivery of oxygen to tissues by regulating the level of 2,3-diphosphoglycerate (2,3-DPG), a substance in red cells that decreases the affinity of hemoglobin for oxygen.

Because phosphate and calcium have a reciprocal relationship, an increase in phosphorus level frequently causes hypocalcemia.

Deficit: Hypophosphatemia

Etiology

✓ Hyperalimentation if inadequate amounts of phosphorus are supplied (tissue synthesis requires phosphate)
✓ Malabsorption syndromes
✓ Alcohol withdrawal
✓ Treatment of diabetic ketoacidosis
✓ Overuse of phosphate-binding antacids (e.g., Amphojel, Basalgel, or Dialume)
✓ Prolonged respiratory alkalosis
✓ Hyperparathyroidism

Signs and Symptoms

- Paresthesia (early symptoms)
- Profound muscle weakness
- Tremor
- Ataxia and incoordination
- Dysarthria
- Dysphagia
- Disorientation and confusion
- Convulsions

Treatment

1. For mild to moderate deficiency, oral phosphate supplements such as Neutra-Phos or Phospho-Soda can be administered.
2. For severe deficiency I.V. phosphate solutions should be given.

✑ Note: In treating **hypophosphatemia**, be aware that calcium levels should be monitored closely (Calloway, 1987).

Excess: Hyperphosphatemia

Etiology

✓ Renal insufficiency
✓ Hypoparathyroidism

✓ Increased catabolism
✓ Myelogenous leukemia
✓ Lymphoma

Signs and Symptoms

- Short-term: tetany
- Long-term: soft tissue calcification

Treatment

1. Identify the underlying cause of **hyperphosphatemia**.
2. Restrict dietary intake of phosphorus.
3. Administer phosphate-binding gels (e.g., Amphojel, Basalgel, or Dialume).

Chloride

Normal laboratory value: 95 to 108 mEq/liter

Functions

Chloride is the major anion in the ECF. Changes in serum Cl concentration are usually secondary to changes in one or more of the other electrolytes. Cl^- has a reciprocal relationship with bicarbonate (HCO_3^-). If there is a drop in bicarbonate concentrations, there is a reciprocal rise in Cl^-; when Cl^- decreases, bicarbonate will increase in compensation. Chloride exists primarily combined as NaCl or hydrochloric acid (HCl). Serum Cl^- is most frequently measured for its inferential value.

Reabsorption of chloride by the renal tubules is one of the major regulatory functions of the kidneys. As NaCl is reabsorbed, water follows through osmosis. It is through this function that vascular blood volume is maintained.

Chloride plays its most important role in acid-base balance. Its role in the pH balance of the ECF is referred to as the "chloride shift." The chloride shift is an ionic exchange that occurs within red blood cells. This shift preserves the electrical neutrality of the red blood cells and maintains a 1:20 ratio of carbonic acid and bicarbonate that is essential for pH balance of the plasma.

Deficit: Hypochloremia

Etiology

✓ Severe vomiting
✓ Severe diarrhea
✓ Pyloric obstruction
✓ Acute infection
✓ Chlorothiazide diuretics

Signs and Symptoms

- Tetany
- Hypertonic reflexes
- Depressed respiration
- Excessive loss of chloride results in alkalosis because of increase in bicarbonate ion
- Signs and symptoms of alkalosis

✎ **Note: Hypochloremia** reflects a deficiency in potassium. When replacing potassium, use a potassium chloride solution.

Treatment

1. Treat underlying cause (patient in alkalosis).
2. Administer saline solutions.

Excess: Hyperchloremia

Etiology

✓ Any condition that causes a decrease in bicarbonate ions: acidosis
✓ Some kidney disorders

Signs and Symptoms

- Deep, rapid breathing
- Stupor
- Weakness
- Signs and symptoms of acidosis

Treatment

1. Treat underlying cause of acidosis.
2. Administer solutions free of NaCl.

SUMMARY OF ELECTROLYTE IMBALANCE

Patients at Risk for Electrolyte Imbalance		
Patient Care Units	Conditions That Can Lead to Imbalance	Potential Electrolyte Imbalances
Geriatric	Prolonged diarrhea Prolonged malnutrition Diuretic therapy	FVD Hypernatremia Hypokalemia
Medical	Anorexia nervosa Profuse sweating Overuse of antacids Gastroenteritis Hyperparathyroidism Diabetic ketoacidosis Alcoholism Renal failure SIADH	FVD Hyponatremia Hypomagnesemia Hypocalcemia Hyperkalemia Hypermagnesemia Hypokalemia
Surgical	Infections Surgical hypoparathyroidism Nasogastric tube to suction causing alkalosis Postoperative complications Pharmacologic agents: morphine, penicillin, and carbenicillin Ileus	FVD or FVE Hypokalemia Hypomagnesemia Hypocalcemia Hypochloremia
Oncology	Myelogenous leukemia Lymphoma Pharmacologic agents: cytoxan Hypertonic tube feeding Neoplastic disease Solid tumors: breast, prostate Malignant melanoma	Hyponatremia Hypercalcemia Hypernatremia Hypermagnesemia
Critical Care	Crushing injuries TPN administration Hypertonic tube feeding Burns Drowning in sea water Head injuries	Hypomagnesemia Hypercalcemia Hypernatremia Hyponatremia Hypophosphatemia Hyperkalemia

FVD = Fluid volume deficit; FVE = fluid volume excess; TPN = total parenteral nutrition.

Summary Worksheet No. 1: Electrolytes

CATIONS

SODIUM (Na$^+$)   **Normal lab:**
Key points:

Deficit:

    Etiology   *Signs and Symptoms*

Excess:

    Etiology   *Signs and Symptoms*

POTASSIUM (K$^+$)   **Normal lab:**
Key points:

Deficit:

    Etiology   *Signs and Symptoms*

Excess:

    Etiology   *Signs and Symptoms*

CALCIUM (Ca²⁺)

Normal lab:

Key points:

Deficit:

    Etiology   *Signs and Symptoms*

Excess:

    Etiology   *Signs and Symptoms*

MAGNESIUM (Mg²⁺)

Normal lab:

Key points:

Deficit:

    Etiology   *Signs and Symptoms*

Excess:

    Etiology   *Signs and Symptoms*

ANIONS

CHLORIDE (Cl⁻)

Normal lab:

Key points:

ANIONS

CHLORIDE (Cl⁻) (*Continued*)   **Normal lab:**
Deficit:

  Etiology   *Signs and Symptoms*

Excess:

  Etiology   *Signs and Symptoms*

PHOSPHATE (HPO₄⁻)   **Normal lab:**
Key points:

Deficit:

  Etiology   *Signs and Symptoms*

Excess:

  Etiology   *Signs and Symptoms*

ACID-BASE BALANCE

The regulation of the hydrogen ion concentration of body fluids actually is the key component of acid-base balance. The **pH** of a fluid reflects the hydrogen ion concentration of that fluid. The normal pH of arterial blood ranges from 7.35 to 7.45.

The inverse proportion of the pH to the concentration of hydrogen ions is reflected in the concept that the higher the pH value, the lower the hydrogen

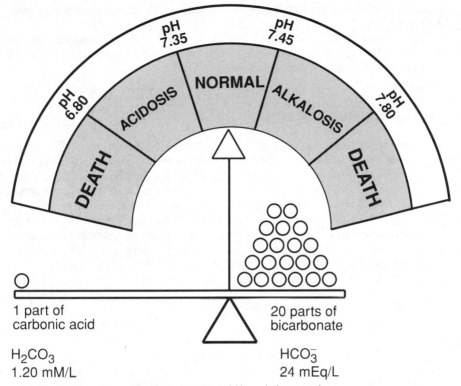

Figure 4–1 □ Acid-base balance scale.

ion concentration. Conversely, the lower the pH value, the higher the hydrogen ion concentration. Therefore, a pH of below 7.35 reflects an acidotic state. A pH greater than 7.45 indicates alkalosis and a lower hydrogen ion concentration. A variation of 0.4 above or below the range of 7.35 to 7.45 can be fatal. Figure 4–1 shows the pH scale.

Three mechanisms operate to maintain the appropriate pH of the blood:

1. Chemical buffer systems in the ECF and ICF
2. Respiratory regulation: removal of carbon dioxide by the lungs
3. Renal regulation of the hydrogen ion concentration

Chemical Buffer Systems

These systems act like a sponge, combining with any acid or alkali to prevent excessive change in the hydrogen ion concentration. The bicarbonate buffer system is just one.

The pH of the plasma is determined by the ratio of sodium bicarbonate ($NaHCO_3$) to carbonic acid (H_2CO_3), which is the main buffer pair. Because the body has a strong tendency toward acidity, it requires a buffering system that is more basic than acidic. The ratio of bicarbonate, a base, to carbonic acid is normally 20 : 1. The sodium bicarbonate – carbonic acid buffer system is responsible for approximately 45 percent of all hydrogen ion buffering.

Two other buffer systems present in the body are the phosphate buffer system and the protein buffer system. Both act in a manner identical to that of the bicarbonate buffer system (Chenevey, 1987).

Respiratory Regulation

When carbon dioxide combines with water, carbonic acid is formed. Therefore, an increase in the acid carbon dioxide lowers the pH of blood, creating an acidotic state; a decrease in the carbon dioxide increases the pH, causing the blood to become more alkaline. After carbonic acid is formed, it dissociates into carbon dioxide and water. The carbon dioxide is transferred to the lungs, where it diffuses into the alveoli and is eliminated via exhalation. Therefore, the rate of respiration affects the hydrogen ion concentration. An increase in respiratory rate will cause carbon dioxide to be blown off by the lungs, resulting in an increase in the pH. Conversely, a decrease in respiratory rate will cause retention of carbon dioxide and thus a decrease in the pH.

Renal Regulation

The kidneys regulate the hydrogen ion concentration by increasing or decreasing the bicarbonate ion concentration in the body fluid through a series of complex chemical reactions that occur in the renal tubules. The regulation of acid-base balance by the kidney occurs chiefly by increasing or decreasing the bicarbonate ion concentration in body fluids. Hydrogen is secreted into the tubules of the kidney, where it is eliminated in the urine. At the same time sodium is reabsorbed from the tubular fluid into the ECF in exchange for hydrogen, and combines with bicarbonate ions to form the buffer sodium bicarbonate.

The kidneys help to regulate the extracellular concentration of bicarbonate. There are two buffer systems that aid the kidney in eliminating excess hydrogen in the urine: the phosphate buffer system and the ammonia buffer system. With each of these, an excess of hydrogen is secreted and bicarbonate ions are formed; sodium is reabsorbed, thus forming sodium bicarbonate.

The time it takes for a change to occur in the acid-base balance can range from a fraction of a second to more than 24 hours. Although the kidneys are the most powerful of all regulating mechanisms, they are slow to make major changes in the acid-base balance (Chenevey, 1987).

MAJOR ELECTROLYTE IMBALANCES

1. Metabolic (base bicarbonate deficit and excess) acidosis and alkalosis
2. Respiratory (carbonic acid deficit and excess) acidosis and alkalosis

Metabolic Acid-Base Imbalance

Normal laboratory value: bicarbonate 22 to 26 mEq/liter

Base Bicarbonate Deficit: Metabolic Acidosis

Metabolic acidosis (HCO_3^- deficit) is a clinical disturbance characterized by a low pH and a low plasma bicarbonate level. This condition can occur by a gain of H^+ ion or a loss of HCO_3^-.

✎ **Note:** Compensation mechanisms are not discussed in this chapter.

Etiology

✓ Diarrhea
✓ Fistulas
✓ Hyperalimentation administration increases risk
✓ Diabetic ketoacidosis
✓ Starvation ketoacidosis
✓ Lactic acidosis
✓ Renal failure
✓ Ingestion of acids (acetylsalicylic acid [ASA], ethylene alcohol)

✎ **Note:** Hyperkalemia is usually present in clinical cases of acidosis (Metheny, 1987, pp 112–114).

Signs and Symptoms

- Headache
- Confusion
- Drowsiness
- Increased respiratory rate
- Nausea and vomiting
- Decreased cardiac output
- pH below 7, causing bradycardia
- Kussmaul's breathing
- Arterial blood gases (ABGs)
  pH less than 7.35
  HCO_3^- less than 22
  $Paco_2$ less than 38

Treatment

1. Reverse underlying cause.
2. If cause of metabolic acidosis is excessive administration of sodium chloride, eliminate source.
3. Administer sodium bicarbonate (7.5% 44.4 mEq/50 mL or 8.4% 50 mEq/50 mL I.V.) per physician's order adjusted according to pH, clinical response, and fluid limitations of the patient (Gahart, 1991, p 457).

Base Bicarbonate Excess: Metabolic Alkalosis

Metabolic alkalosis (HCO_3^- excess) is a clinical disturbance characterized by a high pH and a high plasma bicarbonate concentration. It can result from a gain of bicarbonate or a loss of hydrogen ion.

Etiology

✓ Gastric suctioning
✓ Vomiting
✓ Hypokalemia
✓ Potassium-losing diuretics
✓ Excessive alkali ingestion (antacids, Alka-Seltzer)
✓ Parenteral $NaHCO_3$ administration for cardiopulmonary resuscitation (CPR)

Signs and Symptoms

CALCIUM IONIZATION
- Dizziness
- Tingling of fingers and toes
- Circumoral paresthesia
- Carpopedal spasm
- Hypertonic reflexes
- Depressed respirations
- ABGs
  pH greater than 7.45
  HCO_3^- greater than 26 mEq
  $Paco_2$ greater than 42 mm Hg

✎ **Note:** In alkalosis hypokalemia is often present, along with serum Cl^- level proportionately lower than serum Na^+ level.

Treatment

1. Reverse underlying cause.
2. Administer sufficient chloride for the kidney to excrete the excess bicarbonate.
3. Restore normal fluid volume by administration of saline fluids.

Respiratory Acid-Base Imbalance

Normal laboratory value: partial pressure carbonic acid $Paco_2$ 38 to 42 mm Hg

Carbonic Acid Excess: Respiratory Acidosis

Respiratory acidosis is due to inadequate excretion of carbon dioxide and inadequate ventilation resulting in increase of plasma carbon dioxide levels and carbonic acid levels. Acute respiratory acidosis is usually associated with emergency situations.

Etiology

ACUTE
✓ Pulmonary edema
✓ Aspiration of foreign body
✓ Pneumothorax
✓ Overdose of sedatives
✓ Cardiac arrest
✓ Severe pneumonia

CHRONIC
✓ Emphysema
✓ Bronchial asthma
✓ Bronchiectasis

OTHER
✓ Postoperative pain
✓ Obesity
✓ Tight abdominal binders or dressing

Characteristics

ACUTE
- Mental cloudiness
- Dizziness
- Palpitations
- Convulsions
- Warm, flushed skin
- Ventricular fibrillation
- ABGs
  pH less than 7.35
  $Paco_2$ greater than 42 mm Hg
  HCO_3 normal/slight increase

CHRONIC
- Weakness
- Dull headache
- ABGs
  pH less than 7.35
  $Paco_2$ greater than 42 mm Hg
  HCO_3 greater than 26 mEq/liter

Treatment

1. Improve ventilation.
2. Administer bronchodilators or antibiotics for respiratory infections as ordered.
3. Administer oxygen as needed.
4. Administer adequate fluid 2 to 3 liters/day) to keep mucous membranes moist and help to remove secretions.

Carbonic Acid Deficit: Respiratory Alkalosis

Respiratory alkalosis is usually due to hyperventilation, which causes "blowing off" of carbon dioxide and a decrease in H_2CO_3 content. Acute or chronic alkalosis can occur.

Etiology

✓ Anxiety (most common cause)
✓ Hypoxemia
✓ High fever
✓ Early salicylate overdose
✓ Gram-negative bacteremia
✓ Pulmonary emboli
✓ Excessive ventilation by mechanical ventilators
✓ Central nervous system lesions involving respiratory center

Characteristics

- Lightheadedness
- Inability to concentrate
- Numbness and tingling of extremities, circumoral paresthesia
- Hyperventilation syndrome, which includes:
  Tinnitus
  Palpitations
  Epigastic pain
  Blurred vision
  Precordial pain (tightness)
  ABGs: pH greater than 7.45
  $\quad\quad$ Paco$_2$ less than 38 mm Hg
  $\quad\quad$ HCO$_3$ less than 22 mEg/liter
  Sweating
  Dry mouth
  Tremulousness
  Convulsions and loss of consciousness

Treatment

1. Treat source of anxiety; instruct patient to breathe slowly into a paper bag.
2. Administer sedative as ordered.
3. Treat other underlying cause (Metheny, 1987, pp 108–119).

Summary Worksheet No. 2: Acid-Base Balance

METABOLIC ACID-BASE IMBALANCE: BASE BICARBONATE DEFICIT AND EXCESS

Bicarbonate   **Normal lab:**

Key points:

Deficit: base bicarbonate deficit, acidosis

Etiology   *Signs and Symptoms*

Excess: Base bicarbonate excess, alkalosis

Etiology   *Signs and Symptoms*

RESPIRATORY ACID-BASE IMBALANCE: CARBONIC ACID EXCESS AND DEFICIT

Carbonic Acid   **Normal lab:**

Key points:

Summary Worksheet No. 2: (*Continued*)

RESPIRATORY ACID-BASE IMBALANCE: CARBONIC ACID EXCESS AND DEFICIT

Carbonic Acid (*Continued*)   **Normal lab:**

Deficit: carbonic acid deficit, respiratory alkalosis

    Etiology   *Signs and Symptoms*

Excess: carbonic acid excess, respiratory acidosis

    Etiology   *Signs and Symptoms*

Physical Assessment Related to Electrolyte Balance

The nurse must use a systems approach to assess for fluid and electrolyte imbalances related to I.V. therapy. A head-to-toe system assessment should include vital signs, infusion rate, intake and output, and an awareness of agency policy and procedures to prevent complications associated with I.V. therapy (refer to Chapter 8 for complications). The following body systems should be assessed at the beginning of each shift and as needed to monitor the patient's reactions to infusions. All laboratory findings should be monitored. Symptoms listed with each system may indicate an electrolyte imbalance.

NEUROMUSCULAR
Disorientation
Confusion
Irritability
Hyperactivity
Apprehension: feelings of doom
Headache
Fatigue
Lethargy
Sedation
Convulsions
Lack of coordination
Hyperactivity or hypoactivity of the reflexes
Tremors
Tetany
Dysarthria
Dysphagia
Paresthesia of the extremities
Paralysis of the extremities
Muscle weakness—general or focal
Ataxia
Numbness of extremities
Chvostek's sign
Trousseau's sign

CARDIOVASCULAR
Irregular pulse
Decreased blood pressure
Increased sensitivity to digitalis
ECG changes

RESPIRATORY
Change in respiratory rate
Tachypnea
Kussmaul's respirations

GASTROINTESTINAL
Anorexia
Nausea
Vomiting
Constipation

RENAL
Polyuria
Oliguria
Stones
Complaints of flank pain
Specific gravity 1.002 to 1.004

INTEGUMENTARY
Edema
Fingerprint edema
Flushing and feeling warm
Increased body temperature

SPECIAL SENSES
Thirst
Impaired taste sensation
Red swollen tongue
Dry sticky mucous membrane

SUMMARY OF CHAPTER 4

FUNDAMENTALS OF ELECTROLYTE BALANCE

Electrolyte Function, Deficit, Excess, and Treatment

The seven major electrolytes and their symbols are:

CATIONS
Sodium (Na^+)
Potassium (K^+)
Calcium (Ca^{2+})
Magnesium (Mg^{2+})

ANIONS
Chloride (Cl^-)
Phosphate (HPO_4^{2-})
Bicarbonate (HCO_3^-)

The prefix "hypo" means deficit in an electrolyte; "hyper" means excess in an electrolyte.

Acid-base Balance

Three mechanisms that control the pH of body fluids are:

1. Chemical buffer systems
2. Lungs
3. Kidneys

The H^+ ion concentration is reflected in the pH. The normal pH of body fluids is 7.35 to 7.45; a variation in 0.4 in either direction can be fatal. Deficit in base bicarbonate results in acidosis; excess results in alkalosis. Laboratory values of importance in screening for acid-base problems are pH, HCO_3^-, and $Paco_2$.

Activity Journal

1. In your work environment, list the types of patients who are at risk for potassium deficit.

2. If you have a patient who is receiving total parenteral nutrition, read the I.V. solution container and write down the contents. Is this patient receiving phosphorus and magnesium?

3. Review the chemistry laboratory report on one patient. Write the patient's chemistry values down and compare the slip to the normal laboratory values. Did you pick up any deficits or excesses?

4. Conduct a conference on your unit on the relationship between NG tubes and the effects on electrolyte imbalances. What was the response of the nurses? How many nurses knew there was such a risk in patients with NG tubes?

5. Why are patients who have NG tubes at risk for alkalosis?

Quality Assessment Model

Instructions: Use this quality assessment model to conduct retrospective audits of charts, establish quality control standards, or develop outcome criteria for quality assurance. Refer to Chapter 2 for details on quality assessment.

STRUCTURE

(Resource that affects outcome)
Human Resource: Primary Nurse

↓

PROCESS

(Actual giving and receiving of care based on standards of practice)
Therapist activities related to assessment of electrolyte balance are:

1. Assessment of musculoskeletal system for signs of hyperactive reflexes.
2. Daily review of serum laboratory data to detect electrolyte imbalances.
3. Monitoring of high-risk patient for ECG changes.
4. Assessment of patients every 4 hours for objective or subjective changes.
5. Accurate intake and output every 8 hours.

↓

OUTCOME STANDARDS

(Effects of care)
Documentation reflects standards of care for evaluation of the patient for electrolyte imbalance:

1. Evidence of documented assessments of body systems.
2. Evidence of documented accurate intake and output on patients with NG tubes to suction.
3. Evidence of documented reference to laboratory data that are not within the normal range.
4. Evidence of documented ECG tracings on monitored patients.

Post-test, Chapter 4

Match the definition in column 2 to the correct term in column 1.

Term

1. _____ Acidosis
2. _____ SIADH
3. _____ Ion
4. _____ Anion
5. _____ Alkalosis
6. _____ Cation
7. _____ Trousseau's sign
8. _____ pH
9. _____ Chvostek's sign
10. _____ Intravascular fluid

Definition

A. Electrolyte

B. H^+ ion concentration decreases, pH greater than 7.45

C. Positively charged ion

D. Syndrome of inappropriate antidiuretic hormone

E. H^+ ion concentration increases, pH less than 7.35

F. Negatively charged ion

G. Hydrogen ion concentration

H. Fluid in the plasma

I. Spasm of muscle supplying facial nerve

J. Spasm of hand, elicited when blood supply is decreased

11. List the four cations in body fluids.
    1. _____
    2. _____
    3. _____
    4. _____

12. A nurse completes an assessment that includes the following signs and symptoms: Fatigued muscles, diminished deep tendon reflexes, and the patients' complaints of nausea and anorexia. The patient is irritable. Upon review of the serum electrolytes, the nurse finds a chloride level of 92, potassium 3.1 mEq/L, and sodium 135 mEq/L. The nurse would anticipate that the patient has the following electrolyte imbalance:
    A. Hyponatremia
    B. Hyperchloremia
    C. Hypokalemia
    D. Hypernatremia

13. A patient has an NG tube for continuous suction. What electrolytes could potentially be in deficit with an NG tube for continuous suction?
    A. Sodium
    B. Potassium
    C. Chloride
    D. All of the above

True-False

14. **T F** The normal pH of body fluid is 7.35 to 7.45.

15. **T F** The major electrolytes in the *intracellular* compartment are sodium and chloride.

16. **T F** Potassium influences skeletal and cardiac muscle activity.

17. **T F** Normal potassium level is 3.5 to 5.0 mEq/L.

18. List one nursing diagnosis for electrolyte balance.

19. Which of the following organs are the regulatory organs in acid-base balance?
    A. Lungs and liver
    B. Lungs and kidneys
    C. Pituitary and adrenal glands

20. In the medical-surgical setting, what is one patient diagnosis that could lead to an electrolyte imbalance, and explain why

21. On the oncology unit, what is one patient diagnosis that could lead to an electrolyte imbalance? Explain why.

22. A patient presents with the following signs and symptoms: Respirations 30, blood pressure 100/70, confusion, prior admission for renal failure. Upon review of the ABGs, the nurse finds the pH at 7.32, HCO_3^- 20 mEq/L, $Paco_2$ 34 mm Hg. What is the anticipated diagnosis?
    A. Metabolic acidosis
    B. Metabolic alkalosis
    C. Respiratory acidosis

23. What is the most common cause of hypermagnesemia?
    A. NG tubes to suction
    B. Renal failure
    C. Overzealous administration of I.V. potassium chloride
    D. Respirators

24. In critical care units, patients are at risk for which of the following electrolyte imbalances:
    A. Hypomagnesemia, hypercalcemia, and hypophosphatemia
    B. Hyperkalemia, hypernatremia, and hyperchloremia
    C. Hyponatremia, hypernatremia, and hyperkalemia

Answers to Post-test, Chapter 4

1. E
2. D
3. A
4. F
5. B
6. C
7. J
8. G
9. I
10. H

11. Magnesium (Mg^+)
    Sodium (Na^+)
    Potassium (K^+)
    Calcium (Ca^{2+})
12. C
13. D
14. T
15. F
16. T
17. F

18. Alteration in health maintenance related to poor dietary habits.
Alteration in nutrition, related to lack of adequate food intake.
Potential impaired verbal communication, related to confusion, lethargy, and electrolyte balance.
Potential for injury related to tetany.

19. B
20. Patient with NG tube to suction
21. Patient with myelogenous leukemia, lymphoma
22. A
23. B
24. A

References

Anderson, R.J., Chung, H., & Kluge, R. (1985). Hyponatremia: A prospective analysis of its epidemiology and the pathogenetic role of vasopressin. *Annals of Internal Medicine, 102,* 164–168.

Berger, E. (1984). Nutrition in hypodermoclysis. *Journal of American Geriatric Society, 32,* 199.

Calloway, C. (1987). When the problem involves magnesium, calcium or phosphate. *RN, 5,* 30–35.

Chenevey, B. (1987). Overview of fluids and electrolytes. *Nursing Clinics of North America, 22*(4), 749–759.

Gahart, B.L. (1991). *Intravenous medications: A handbook for nurses and other allied health personnel* (6th ed.). St. Louis: C.V. Mosby.

Goldberger, E. (1986). *A primer of water, electrolytes and acid-base syndromes* (7th ed.). Philadelphia: Lea & Febiger.

Lamb, C. (1986). SIADH: Why is the serum sodium low? Interviews with Culpepper, M., Porter, G.A., & Roddam, R. *Patient Care,* 94–110.

McFadden, E., & Zaloga, G.P. (1983). Calcium regulation. *Critical Care Quarterly, 12,* 12–21.

McFadden, E., Zaloga, G., & Chernow, B. (1983). Hypocalcemia: A medical emergency. *American Journal of Nursing, 80,* 226–230.

Metheny, N.M. (1987). *Fluids and electrolyte balance: Nursing considerations.* Philadelphia: J.B. Lippincott.

Metheny, N.M. (1990). Why worry about IV fluids? *American Journal of Nursing,* (6), 50–55.

Rolls, B.J., & Phillips, P.A. (1990). Aging and disturbances of thirst and fluid balance. *Nutrition Reviews, 48*(3), 137–143.

Rose, B. (1984). *Clinical physiology of acid-base and electrolyte disorders* (2nd ed.). New York: McGraw-Hill.

Shrier, R. (1986). *Renal and electrolyte disorders* (3rd ed.). Boston: Little, Brown.

Vanatta, J., & Fogelman, M. (1982). *Moyers fluid balance* (3rd ed.). Chicago: Year Book Medical.

Zaloga, G., & Chernow, B. (1983). Magnesium metabolism in critical illness. *Critical Care Quarterly 4,* 22–27.

Bibliography

Chernow, B., Smith, J., Rainey, T., & Finton, C. (1982). Hypomagnesemia: Implications for the critical care specialist. *Critical Care Medicine, 10,* 193.

Fuller, E. (1984). Endocrine emergencies: Crises of calcium imbalance. Roundtable Discussion: Davidson, M.D., Mecklenburg, R.S., Pont, A.B., & Schneider.

Huerta, B., & Lemberg, L. (1985). Potassium imbalances in the coronary unit. *Heart and Lung, 14*(2), 193–195

Maxwell, M., & Kleeman, C. (1980). *Clinical disorders of fluid and electrolyte metabolism* (3rd ed.). New York: McGraw-Hill.

Merck, Sharp, & Dohme (1989). *Critical care quick reference.* California: Merck & Company.

Rutherford, C. (1989). Fluid and electrolyte therapy: Considerations for patient care. *Journal of Intravenous Therapy, 12*(3), 173–184.

Toto, K.H. (1987). When the patient has hyperkalemia. *RN, 4*, 34–37.

Toto, K.H. (1987). When the patient has hypokalemia. *RN, 3*, 38–41.

Parenteral Fluids

CHAPTER 5

Parenteral Fluids

Glossary

Balanced fluid: Parenteral fluid containing portions of electrolytes similar to those of plasma (these solutions also contain bicarbonate or acetate ion)

Catabolism: The breakdown of chemical compounds by the body; an energy-producing metabolic process

Colloid: A substance that does not dissolve into a true solution and is not capable of passing through a semipermeable membrane (e.g., blood, plasma, albumin, and dextran)

Crystalloid: A substance that forms a true solution and is capable of passing through a semipermeable membrane. (e.g., lactated Ringer's, isotonic saline)

Dehydration: A deficit of body water; can involve one fluid compartment or all three

Hydrating fluids: Solution of water, carbohydrate, Na^+, and Cl^- used to determine adequacy of renal function

Maintenance therapy: Providing all nutrients necessary to meet daily patient requirements

Normal saline: Solution of salt

Plasma substitute: A solution of a synthetic product such as dextran used as a substitute for plasma

Replacement therapy: Replenishment of losses when maintenance cannot be met, when patient is in a deficit state

Restoration therapy: Reconstruction of fluid and electrolyte needs on a continuing basis until homeostasis returns

LEARNING OBJECTIVES

Upon completion of this chapter, the reader will be able to:

☐ Define terminology related to parenteral fluids.
☐ Identify the three objectives of parenteral therapy.
☐ List the key elements in intravenous fluids.
☐ List the uses of maintenance fluids.
☐ List the four functions of glucose as a necessary nutrient when administered parenterally.
☐ Explain the roles of vitamins C and B complex in maintenance therapy.
☐ Describe the uses of hypotonic, isotonic, and hypertonic fluids.
☐ Identify the major groupings of intravenous fluids.
☐ Compare the advantages and the disadvantages of dextrose, sodium chloride, hydrating, and multiple electrolyte fluids.
☐ Identify the main role of hydrating fluids.
☐ List one hydrating fluid.
☐ State two uses of lactate fluids.
☐ State the most commonly used multiple electrolyte fluid.
☐ Determine nursing diagnosis appropriate for patients receiving parenteral solutions.

Pre-test, Chapter 5

Instructions: The pre-test is to review prior knowledge of the theory of parenteral fluids. Each of the questions in the pre-test is based on the learning objectives of the chapter.

Match the definition in column 2 to the correct term in column 1.

Column 1

1. _____ Maintenance therapy

2. _____ Replacement therapy

3. _____ Restoration therapy

Column 2

A. Objective required to meet daily needs; usually includes water, carbohydrates, and electrolytes

B. Objective for continuing (ongoing) losses; reassess every 4 hours

C. Objective for meeting previous losses

4. List four of the seven key elements in intravenous fluids.

1. _____

2. _____

3. _____

4. _____

Match the definition in column 2 to the correct glossary term in column 1.

Column 1

5. _____ Normal saline

6. _____ Oliguria

7. _____ Hydrating solution

8. _____ Colloid

9. _____ Crystalloid

Column 2

A. A substance that does not dissolve into a true solution

B. Solution of salt

C. Diminished amount of urine

D. A substance that forms a true solution

E. Solution of water, carbohydrate, Na^+, and Cl^- used to determine adequacy of renal function

10. Hypotonic fluids are used to:
    A. Hydrate cells
    B. Increase vascular space
    C. Supply sodium and chloride in deficit states

11. Hypertonic fluids are used to:
    A. Shift extracellular fluid from interstitial fluid to plasma
    B. Hydrate cells
    C. Supply free water to vascular space

12. What is/are the function(s) of parenteral glucose?
    A. Improve hepatic function
    B. Supply necessary calories for energy
    C. Spare body protein
    D. Minimize ketosis
    E. All of the above

13. What is the role of vitamin C in parenteral therapy?
    A. To increase tensile strength of collagen
    B. To protect cells against oxidation
    C. To promote wound healing
    D. To help with metabolism of carbohydrate

14. The *main* role of a hydrating fluid is to:
    A. Check kidney function
    B. Expand the extracellular fluid compartment
    C. Hydrate the cells
    D. Supply sodium and potassium in deficit states

15. What is the most commonly used multiple electrolyte fluid?
    A. 5% dextrose in water
    B. 0.9% sodium chloride
    C. Lactated Ringer's solution
    D. 5% dextrose in sodium chloride

ANSWERS TO PRE-TEST, Chapter 5

1. A   2. C   3. B   4. Free water, carbohydrates, electrolytes, protein, vitamins, trace elements, and pH   5. B   6. C   7. E   8. A   9. D
10. A   11. A   12. E   13. C   14. A   15. C

This chapter introduces the reader to parenteral fluids and their content and application in today's practice.

In the mid-1950s less than 20 percent of hospital patients received intravenous (I.V.) therapy. The primary use of I.V. fluids during the 1950s was in surgery and to treat **dehydration**. Fluids for the surgical patients were infused over 3- to 4-hour periods and discontinued at night. The only solutions available then were 5% dextrose in water and 5% dextrose in sodium chloride saline. Today more than 80 percent of hospitalized patients receive I.V. therapy, and more than 200 different types of parenteral fluids are available.

Intravenous fluids are mistakenly referred to as "intravenous solutions." In this chapter, all parenteral fluids will be referred to as "fluids" or "injections." The term solution is defined in the *United States Pharmacopeia* (*USP*) as "liquid preparations that contain one or more soluble chemical substances usually dissolved in water. They are distinguished from injection, for example, because they are not intended for administration by infusion or injection." The *USP* refers to parenteral fluids as injections, and methods of preparation must follow standards for injection. IV fluids must meet tests for pyrogens and sterility, as well as for pH standards (*USP*, 1980, p 803).

RATIONALES AND OBJECTIVES OF PARENTERAL THERAPY

To understand the use of parenteral fluids the nurse must know: (1) the rationale for the physician's order of I.V. therapy and (2) the type of solution ordered, as well as the composition and clinical use of that solution.

Objectives or rationales for administration of I.V. therapy fall into three broad categories:

1. **Maintenance therapy** for daily body fluid requirements
2. **Replacement therapy** for present losses
3. **Restoration therapy** for concurrent or continuing losses (Table 5–1)

These three objectives differ in the time necessary to complete the therapy, the purpose of the I.V. fluid and the type of patient who may receive it. Factors affecting choice of objective in prescribing parenteral fluids and rate of administration by the physician are:

Patient's renal function
Patient's daily maintenance requirements
Patient's existing fluid and electrolyte imbalance
Patient's clinical status
Disturbances in homeostasis as a result of parenteral therapy (Metheny, 1984, p 57)

Table 5–1 ☐ **THREE MAIN OBJECTIVES OF I.V. THERAPY**

1. Maintain daily requirements.
2. Replace previous losses (deficits).
3. Restore daily concurrent losses.

Maintenance Therapy

In maintenance therapy water has priority. The body needs water to replace insensible loss, which can occur as perspiration from the skin and as moisture from respirations. The average adult loses 500 to 1000 mL of water over 24 hours through insensible loss. Water is also important in diluting waste products excreted by the kidney. Approximately 30 mL of fluid is needed per kilogram of body weight (15 mL/lb) for maintenance needs (Metheny, 1984, p 58). Also, an individual's fluid requirements are based on age, height, weight, and amount of body fat.

Maintenance therapy provides nutrients that meet the daily needs of a patient for water, electrolytes, and dextrose. As previously mentioned, water has priority. The typical patient profile for maintenance therapy is one who is allowed nothing by mouth (NPO) or has restricted oral intake for any reason. Remember, insensible loss is approximately 500 to 1000 mL per 24 hours. Maintenance therapy according to Metheny (1984) should be 1500 mL per square meter (m^2) of body surface over 24 hours.

Calculation of Adult Maintenance Therapy

Example

A male weighing 85 kg (187 lb) has a body surface area of 2 (m^2).

1500 mL $\times$ 2 = 3000 mL for maintenance therapy.

(Refer to Appendix A for nomogram of body surface areas.)

A **balanced fluid** for maintenance therapy contains water; daily needs of sodium, magnesium, and potassium; and glucose. Glucose, a necessary component in maintenance therapy, is converted to glycogen by the liver and has four main uses in parenteral therapy:

1. Improves hepatic function
2. Supplies necessary calories for energy
3. Spares body protein
4. Minimizes ketosis

✎ **Note:** The basic caloric requirement for an adult is 1600 calories/day for a 70-kg adult at rest. Approximately 100 to 150 g of carbohydrates are needed daily to minimize protein catabolism and prevent starvation. In 1 liter of 5% dextrose and water, there are 50 g of dextrose. (Metheny, 1984, p 59).

Hospitalized patients receiving additional saline or glucose infusions are prone to potassium deficiency. Hospitalized patients are usually under stress.

Solutions	Na	K	Ca	Mg	Cl	HCO₃ Precursor
Plasma Lyte M (Baxter)	40	16	5	3	40	Lactate 12
Normosol M (Abbott)	40	16	5	3	40	Lactate 12
Isolyte R (McGraw)	41	16	5	3	40	Acetate 24

*5% dextrose is usually added to balanced multiple electrolyte solutions.

Excretion of potassium in urine can rise to 60 to 120 mEq/day even with limited intake. Tissue injury significantly increases the loss of potassium. Normal dietary intake of potassium is 80 to 200 mEq.

Vitamins are necessary for use of other nutrients. Vitamins C and B complex are used frequently in parenteral therapy, especially in postoperative patients. Vitamin C promotes wound healing, and vitamin B complex has a role in metabolism of carbohydrates and maintenance of gastrointestinal function (Plumer, 1987, p 85).

Refer to Table 5-2 for a list of the balanced maintenance fluids.

Replacement Therapy

Replacement therapy is necessary to meet the fluid, electrolyte, or blood product deficits of patients in acute distress and is supplied within 48 hours. Examples of conditions of patients needing replacement infusion therapy are:

Hemorrhage (replace cells and plasma)
Low platelets (replace clotting factors)
Vomiting and diarrhea (replace losses of electrolytes and water)
Starvation (replace loss of water and electrolytes)

When maintenance of body requirements cannot be met, the physician institutes replacement therapy. The physician must figure the losses and calculate replacement over a 48-hour period. *The very first thing to check before replacement therapy can begin is kidney function.* Patients requiring replacement therapy, except those in shock, need potassium. Patients under stress from tissue injury, wound infection, or gastric or bowel surgery also require potassium. Potassium, 20 mEq/liter, achieves adequate replacement (Metheny, 1987, p 68).

✎ **Note:** Never give more than 120 mEq of potassium chloride per infusion in 24 hours, unless cardiac status is monitored continuously. More than this amount can be life threatening.

Carefully monitor balanced solutions with potassium given to the following individuals:

1. Patients with dysfunction of:

Renal system
Cardiovascular system
Adrenal glands

106

Pituitary gland
Parathyroid gland

2. Patients with deficits of:

Sodium
Calcium
Base bicarbonate
Blood volume (hypovolemic)

3. Patients with excess of:

Base bicarbonate
Extracellular potassium
Extracellular calcium

✎ **Note:** *Key nursing assessment:* Check kidney function before administration of potassium in replacement therapy.

Restoration Therapy (Concurrent Losses)

Restoration therapy is achieved on an ongoing *daily* basis. Critical evaluation of concurrent losses of fluids and electrolytes is done at least every 24 hours. Of extreme importance in this type of management of fluid and electrolyte therapy is accurate documentation of intake and output. Restoring homeostasis depends on the nursing assessment of intake of I.V. fluids, as well as on the documentation of all bodily fluid losses. The types of clinical patients who require 24-hour evaluation are those with:

Draining fistulas
Abscesses
Nasogastric (NG) tubes
Burns
Abdominal wounds

As you can see, the fluid and electrolyte management of these patients cannot be completed in 48 hours; therefore, maintenance therapy and replacement therapy do not meet these patients' needs. A day-by-day restoration of vital fluids and electrolytes is necessary. With these types of patients you will see frequent changes in the types of fluid ordered, the amount of electrolytes ordered based on laboratory values, and the rate of infusion.

The type of restoration fluid ordered depends on the type of fluid being lost. For example, excessive loss of gastric fluid must be replaced by solutions resembling that fluid; with NG suctioning, chloride, potassium, and sodium are lost continually. Restoration of electrolyte balance is imperative for proper homeostatic management therapy. Rather than waiting to make daily rounds to evaluate the 24-hour totals and change infusion orders, physicians are ordering multiple electrolyte solutions to be used as a replacement solution via the main infusion system on an ongoing basis. This replacement need is reevaluated every 1 to 8 hours.

Example

The physician orders 1000 mL of 5% dextrose/0.45% sodium chloride every 8 hours as a primary fluid. A multiple electrolyte fluid, such as lactated Ringer's, is

Table 5-3 □ **EXAMPLE OF NG MILLILITER-FOR-MILLILITER RESTORATION THERAPY**

0800 (400 mL gastric)	0900	1000	1100	1200 (300 mL gastric)	1300	1400
125 mL primary	125	125	125	125	125	125
100 mL lactated	100	100	100	75	75	75
225 mL	225	225	225	200	200	200

ordered in addition to the primary fluid to replace NG output mL for mL over 4 hours. The primary I.V. fluid continuously infuses at 125 mL/hour. If the NG suction container is emptied and there is 400 mL of gastric secretions, the nurse will need to infuse 400 mL of lactated Ringer's over the next 4 hours, or 100 mL/hour. The primary fluid (5% dextrose/0.5% NS) will infuse at 125 mL, and the lactated Ringer's will infuse at 100 mL/hour, for a total of 225 mL/hour. The nurse will then empty the NG suction container 4 hours later and recalculate the replacement fluid (Table 5-3).

This type of restoration of fluids and electrolytes is challenging for nurses. One must be on time and accurate so as not to overload the patient or get behind in fluid therapy.

Summary Worksheet No. 1: Objectives of I.V. Therapy

1. MAINTENANCE THERAPY FOR DAILY BODY FLUID REQUIREMENTS

Time   Purpose   Patient Profile

2. REPLACEMENT THERAPY FOR PREVIOUS LOSSES

Time   Purpose   Patient Profile

Key nursing assessment: _____

3. RESTORATION THERAPY FOR CONCURRENT OR CONTINUING LOSSES

Time   Purpose   Patient Profile

KEY ELEMENTS IN PARENTERAL FLUIDS

This section examines the following key elements in parenteral fluids:

Water
Carbohydrates (glucose)
Protein
Vitamins
Trace elements
Electrolytes
pH

Water

Normal adult maintenance requirements for water are roughly 1000 mL/day. These water needs are increased in patients with excessive insensible water loss, such as those with respirations above 20, fever, and diaphoresis, and in low humidity; in patients with decreased renal concentration ability; and in the elderly. The average adult loses 500 to 1000 mL in the form of insensible water loss per 24 hours. Sufficient water must be provided for adequate kidney function.

✎ **Note:** High humidity, such as that in an incubator, minimizes insensible water loss (Metheny, 1987, p 145).

Carbohydrates (Glucose)

Glucose, a nutrient included in maintenance, restoration, and replacement therapies, is converted into glycogen by the liver, improving hepatic function. By supplying calories for energy, it spares body protein. Sources of carbohydrate (CHO) include dextrose (glucose) and fructose. When glucose is supplied via infusion, all the parenteral glucose is bioavailable.

✎ **Note:** The addition of 100 g of glucose a day minimizes starvation. Every 2 liters of 5% dextrose and water contains 100 g of glucose (Plumer, 1987, p 84).

Protein

The body-building nutrient protein contributes to tissue growth and repair, replacement of body cells, healing of wounds, and synthesis of vitamins and enzymes. Amino acids are the basic units of protein. Current parenteral proteins are elemental, provided as synthetic crystalline amino acids. They are available in concentrations of 3 to 11.4 percent and are used in total parenteral nutrition centrally or peripherally. When administered per infusion, protein bypasses the gastrointestinal and portal circulation (Metheny, 1987, p 151).

✎ **Note:** The usual daily requirement is 1 g protein per kilogram of body weight. For example, 54-kg female needs 54 g protein.

Vitamins

Vitamins are added to restorative and replacement therapies. Certain vitamins are necessary for growth and as catalysts for metabolic processes. These are fat-soluble vitamins A, D, E, and K and water-soluble vitamins B and C. Some disease conditions alter vitamin requirements (Metheny, 1984, p 153). Vitamins B and C are the most frequently used in parenteral therapy. Vitamin B complex is important in metabolism of carbohydrates and maintaining gastrointestinal function, which is especially important in postoperative patients. Vitamin C promotes wound healing.

Trace Elements

Many trace elements have become "essential" nutrients. Trace elements have various functions and their actions often work together. The trace elements important in restorative therapy are:

1. Zinc, which contributes to wound healing by increasing tensile strength of collagen
2. Copper, which assists iron's incorporation of hemoglobin
3. Selenium, which protects cells against oxidation

Other important trace elements include

Iron
Chromium
Manganese

Electrolytes

The major additives to replacement and restorative therapies are electrolytes. The correction of electrolyte imbalances is important in prevention of serious complications associated with excess or deficit of electrolytes. Because seven major electrolytes exist in normal body fluids, seven major elements are supplied by manufactured I.V. solutions (refer to Chapter 4 for a review of electrolyte functions). The electrolytes of major importance in parenteral therapy are:

Potassium
Sodium
Chloride
Magnesium
Phosphate
Calcium
Bicarbonate or acetate ion (important for acid-base balance)

pH

The pH reflects the degree of acidity or alkalinity of a solution. For routine parenteral therapy blood pH is not a significant problem. Normal kidneys can achieve an acid-base balance as long as enough water is supplied. The *USP* standards require that fluids must be slightly acidic, between a pH of 3.5 and a pH of 6.2. Many solutions have a pH of 5. The acidity of solutions allows them to have a longer shelf life (Plumer, 1987, p 104).

✎ **Note:** As the acidity of a solution increases, irritation to the vein wall increases.

HYPOTONIC, ISOTONIC, AND HYPERTONIC FLUIDS

The choice of I.V. fluid depends on the amount of solutes in the solution and the osmolarity of the infusant. The effect of I.V. fluids on the body fluid compartments depends on how its osmolarity compares with the patient's serum osmolarity. I.V. fluids can change the fluid compartments in one of three ways; they can expand the intravascular compartment; they can expand the intravascular compartment and deplete the intracellular and interstitial compartments; or they can expand the intracellular compartment and deplete the intravascular compartment. I.V. fluids are hypotonic, isotonic, or hypertonic, depending on the amount of solutes in the solution (Gasparis, Murray & Ursomanno, 1989)

Hypotonic Fluids

Hypotonic fluids have an osmolarity less than 250 mOsm/liter. Hypotonic fluids lower the serum osmolarity and cause the body fluid to shift out of blood vessels and into cells and interstitial spaces, where osmolarity is higher. Hypotonic fluids hydrate cells while depleting the circulatory system.

Examples: 0.45% sodium chloride, mOsm/liter = 154.
Uses: To hydrate cells and lower serum sodium levels.
Caution: Hypotonic solutions cause depletion of circulatory system.

✎ **Note:** Do not give hypotonic solutions to patients with low blood pressure, as this will exacerbate a hypotensive state.

Isotonic Fluids

Isotonic fluids have an osmolarity of 250 to 375 mOsm/liter and are used to expand the extracellular fluid (ECF) compartment. Isotonic fluids do not affect the intracellular and interstitial compartments, because the fluid does not alter serum osmolarity. Isotonic fluids can be used for hypotension caused by hypovolemia. Many isotonic fluids are available.

Examples: lactated Ringer's 275 mOsm/liter, 0.9% sodium chloride 308 mOsm/liter.
Use: Expand the intravascular compartment.
Cautions: The danger with the use of isotonic fluids is circulatory overload. These fluids do not cause fluid shifts into other compartments. The problem with overexpanding the vascular compartment is that

the fluid dilutes the concentration of hemoglobin and lowers hematocrit.

Hypertonic Fluids

Hypertonic fluids have an osmolarity of 375 mOsm/liter or higher. These fluids are used to replace electrolytes. When hypertonic dextrose fluids are used alone they also are used to shift ECF from interstitial space to plasma.

> Examples: 5% dextrose in 0.45% sodium chloride 406 mOsm, 5% dextrose in 0.9% sodium chloride 560 mOsm, 5% dextrose in lactated Ringer's 575 mOsm.
> Uses: To replace electrolytes and to shift fluid from interstitial and cellular spaces to plasma to expand the intravascular compartment
> Cautions: These I.V. fluids are irritating to vein walls and may cause hypertonic circulatory overload.

✎ **Note:** Give hypertonic fluids slowly to prevent circulatory overload.

TYPES OF PARENTERAL FLUIDS

Crystalloid Solutions

Crystalloid solutions consist of electrolyte solutions that are hypotonic, isotonic, or hypertonic. Because crystalloid solutions are "true" solutions, they are capable of passing through a semipermeable membrane. All the fluids included in this chapter are crystalloid.

Colloid Solutions

Colloid solutions are solutions that do not dissolve and thus are not true solutions. These solutions do not flow freely between fluid compartments. When you infuse a colloid solution you increase intravascular colloid osmotic pressure (pressure of plasma proteins). Colloid solutions are further discussed in the chapter on blood and blood products.

Dextrose and Water Fluids

Carbohydrates can be administered by parenteral route as dextrose, fructose, or invert sugar. Approximately 1600 calories are needed daily for an adult at bedrest; however, this is a basal figure and does not allow for fever or other causes of increased metabolism (Metheny, 1984, p 67). When CHO needs are inadequate, the body will use its own fat to supply calories.

Carbohydrates perform the following functions:

✓ Provide calories for energy
✓ Reduce catabolism of protein
✓ Reduce protein breakdown of glucose
✓ Help prevent a negative nitrogen balance (Plumer, 1987, p 91)

113

TYPES OF DEXTROSE AND WATER FLUIDS AVAILABLE

2.5% dextrose	Hypotonic
5% dextrose	Isotonic
10% dextrose	
20% dextrose	Hypertonic
50% dextrose	

It is difficult to administer enough calories via I.V. infusion, especially with 5% dextrose and water, which provides only 170 calories per liter. One would have to give 9 liters to meet calorie requirements and most patients cannot tolerate the administration of 9000 mL of fluid in 24 hours. Concentrated CHO solutions in 20% or 50% dextrose are useful for supplying calories. The solutions containing high percentages of dextrose must be administered slowly for adequate absorption and use by the cells (Metheny, 1984, p 67).

Glucose via infusion is usually supplied as dextrose. Dextrose is thought to be the closest to the ideal CHO available because it is well metabolized by all tissue. The tonicity of the dextrose solutions depends on the particles of sugar in the solution. Dextrose 5% is rapidly metabolized and has no osmotically active particle once in the plasma. Dextrose is a nonelectrolyte, and the total number of particles in a solution does not depend on ionization. The osmolarity of a dextrose solution is determined differently from that of an electrolyte solution. Dextrose is distributed inside and outside the cells, with 8 percent remaining in the circulation to increase blood volume. The *USP* pH requirement for dextrose is 3.5 to 6.5 (Plumer, 1987, p 107).

✎ **Note:** Hypotonic fluids hydrate the interstitium more than they do the intravascular space.

The other two types of carbohydrates used for infusions, fructose and invert sugar, have their own specific uses. Fructose is similar to glucose but is less irritating to veins. The important point about fructose is that it can be metabolized by adipose tissue independent of insulin. However, fructose cannot be used if the patient is in acidosis. Invert sugar contains the same equimolar quantities of glucose and fructose, but less invert sugar is lost in the urine (Metheny, 1984, p 68).

ADVANTAGES

✓ Acts as vehicle for administration of medications
✓ Provides nutrition
✓ Can be used as treatment for hyperkalemia (using high concentrations of dextrose)
✓ Can be used in treatment of dehydration

DISADVANTAGE

✓ I.V. fluids of 20% to 50% dextrose, if infused rapidly, act as an osmotic diuretic and pull interstitial fluid into plasma, causing severe cellular dehydration. Any solution of dextrose infused rapidly can place the patient at risk for dehydration. To prevent this adverse reaction to dextrose, infuse the solution at the prescribed rate.

114

STOP Do not play "catch up" if the solution infusion is behind schedule. Make sure I.V. fluids do not "run away" and infuse rapidly into patient.

If 20% to 50% dextrose solution is infused too rapidly it can irritate the vein wall. Rapid infusion of 20% to 50% dextrose solutions can also lead to transient hyperinsulin reaction. The pancreas secretes extra insulin to metabolize the infused dextrose. Sudden discontinuation of any hypertonic dextrose solution may result in a temporary excess of insulin. To prevent hyperinsulinism, an isotonic (5% to 10%) dextrose solution should be infused to wean the patient from the hypertonic dextrose. The infusion rate should be gradually decreased over 48 hours.

✓ Dextrose and water does not provide any electrolytes. These CHO solutions cannot replace or correct electrolyte deficits. Continuous infusion of 5% dextrose and water places the patient at risk for deficits in sodium, potassium, and chloride.
✓ Dextrose cannot be mixed with blood infusions because this causes hemolysis.

Sodium Chloride Fluids

Sodium chloride injection (0.9%), *USP* (**normal saline**), is an isotonic fluid. It is isotonic owing to the higher than normal amount of sodium and chloride ions. Normal saline has 154 mEq of both sodium and chloride or about 9% higher than normal plasma levels of Na^+ and Cl^-, without other plasma electrolytes.

TYPES OF AVAILABLE SALINE SOLUTIONS
0.2% NaCl (quarter strength)	Hypotonic
0.45% NaCl (half strength)	Hypotonic
0.9% NaCl (full strength)	Isotonic
3% NaCl (hypertonic saline)	

ADVANTAGES

✓ Provides ECF replacement when chloride loss is greater than or equal to sodium losses (e.g., patients on NG suctioning)
✓ Treats metabolic alkalosis in the presence of fluid loss (the 154 mEq of chloride will help compensate for the increase in bicarbonate ions)
✓ Treats sodium depletion
✓ Initiates or terminates a blood transfusion (the saline solutions are the *only* solutions to be used with any blood product)

DISADVANTAGES

✓ Provides more sodium and chloride than a patient needs, causing hypernatremia (excess sodium). The adult dietary sodium requirement is 90 to 250 mEq daily. Three liters of 0.9% NS provides the patient with 462 mEq of sodium, a level that exceeds normal tolerance. To prevent this overload of electrolytes, assess for signs and symptoms of sodium retention.

✎ **Note:** During stress the body retains sodium, adding to hypernatremia.

✓ Can cause acidosis in patients receiving continuous infusions of sodium chloride because sodium chloride fluids contain a third more chloride than is present in ECF. The excess chloride leads to loss of bicarbonate ions, leading to an imbalance of acid.

✓ May cause low potassium levels (hypokalemia) owing to lack of the other important electrolytes over time.

✓ Can lead to circulatory overload. Isotonic fluids expand the ECF compartment, which could lead to overload of the cardiovascular compartments.

✎ **Note:** Hypotonic (0.45%) sodium chloride can be used to supply normal daily salt and water requirements safely. Hypertonic (3%) saline is used only to correct severe sodium depletions and water overload (Keithley & Fraulini, 1982).

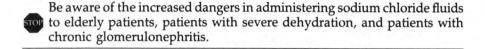 Be aware of the increased dangers in administering sodium chloride fluids to elderly patients, patients with severe dehydration, and patients with chronic glomerulonephritis.

Dextrose and Sodium Chloride Fluids

When sodium chloride is infused, the addition of 100 g of dextrose prevents formation of ketone bodies and aids in the increased demand for water the ketone bodies impose for renal excretion. Dextrose prevents **catabolism** and consequently the loss of potassium and intracellular water (Plumer, 1987, p 111).

TYPES OF AVAILABLE DEXTROSE AND SODIUM CHLORIDE COMBINATIONS

0.2% dextrose + 0.9% NaCl	Isotonic
5% dextrose + 0.45% NaCl	Hypertonic
5% dextrose + 0.9% NaCl	Hypertonic

ADVANTAGES

✓ Temporarily treats circulatory insufficiency and shock due to hypovolemia, in the immediate absence of a plasma expander
✓ Provides early treatment of burns, along with plasma or albumin
✓ Replaces nutrient and electrolytes
✓ Acts as hydrating solution to check kidney function before replacement of potassium

DISADVANTAGES

✓ Same as for sodium chloride fluids (see earlier section): hypernatremia, acidosis, and circulatory overload

116

Hydrating Fluids

Fluids that contain dextrose and hypotonic sodium chloride provide more water than is required for excretion of salt and are useful as hydrating fluids. **Hydrating fluids** are used to assess the status of the kidneys. The administration of a hydrating fluid at a rate of 8 mL/m² of body surface per minute for 45 minutes is called a fluid challenge. When urinary flow is established, it indicates that the kidneys have begun to function; the hydrating fluid may then be replaced with a specific electrolyte solution. If after 45 minutes the urinary flow is not restored, the rate of infusion should then be reduced and monitoring of the patient should continue without electrolyte additives (especially potassium) (Plumer, 1987, p 113). Carbohydrates in hydrating solutions reduce depletion of nitrogen and liver glycogen and are also useful in rehydrating cells.

TYPES OF AVAILABLE HYDRATING SOLUTIONS

2.5% dextrose/0.45% NaCl	Hypotonic
5% dextrose/0.45% NaCl	Hypertonic
5% dextrose/0.9% NaCl	Hypertonic

ADVANTAGES

✓ Assesses the status of the kidneys *before* replacement therapy is started
✓ Hydrates medical and surgical patients
✓ Promotes diuresis in dehydrated patients (Plumer, 1987, p 112)

DISADVANTAGES

✓ Must be used cautiously in edematous patients (e.g., those with cardiac, renal, or liver disease)

✎ **Note:** Do not give potassium to any patient unless kidney function has been established.

Multiple Electrolyte Fluids

Multiple electrolyte fluids are available as balanced hypotonic or isotonic maintenance and replacement solutions (Tables 5–4 and 5–5). The Ringer's injection fluids are also considered multiple electrolyte fluids. The maintenance fluids approximate normal body electrolyte needs; replacement fluids contain one or more electrolytes in amounts over those found in maintenance fluids. Multiple electrolyte fluids contain potassium because this electrolyte is often the main one in imbalance. Lactate or acetate (yielding bicarbonate) is often lost by the body when combating acidosis; therefore, this element is included in multiple electrolyte fluids.

Balanced Hypotonic Maintenance Fluids

Hypotonic balanced multiple electrolyte fluids contain 5% dextrose for its protein-sparing effect. Dextrose does increase tonicity of solutions. The balancing

117

Table 5-4 □ **TYPES OF PARENTERAL FLUIDS**

Dextrose + water
Sodium chloride
Hydrating
Multiple electrolyte
    Maintenance: Hypotonic and isotonic
    Replacement: Hypertonic
Specialty fluids
    Alkalizing
    Acidifying
    Plasma expanders
    Potassium

of hypotonic electrolyte (lower than within normal body levels) is ideal to maintain body homeostasis. Balanced I.V. fluids contain sodium, potassium, calcium, magnesium, chloride, and lactate. Potassium is usually not added to maintenance multiple electrolyte fluids.

Balanced Isotonic Maintenance Fluids

Isotonic multiple electrolyte solutions do not contain dextrose. Caution must be used when infusing isotonic maintenance fluids because of fluid overload (Plumer, 1987, p 114).

Replacement Fluids (Hypertonic)

Hypertonic multiple electrolyte fluids are used as replacement fluids and usually have the addition of 5% dextrose, which raises the osmolarity of the solution. There are many types of replacement fluids available. The hazard in using hypertonic multiple electrolyte fluids is fluid overload. Replacement multiple electrolyte fluids are recommended for the following conditions:

Trauma
Alimentary tract fluid losses

Table 5-5 □ **ISOTONIC AND HYPERTONIC REPLACEMENT MULTIPLE ELECTROLYTE FLUID (mEq/L)**

Solution	Na	K	Cl	Ca	Mg	HCO$_3$ Precursor
Plasma Lyte (Baxter)	140	10	103	5	3	55
Isolyte E (McGraw)	140	10	103	5	3	55
Lactated Ringer's	130	4	109	3	0	28
Normosol R (Abbott)	140	5	98	0	3	27

Dehydration
Sodium depletion
Acidosis
Burns (Keithley & Fraulini, 1982)

Hypotonic balanced multiple electrolyte solutions contain 5% dextrose for its protein-sparing effect. Dextrose *does* increase tonicity of solutions. The balancing of hypotonic electrolytes (lower than within normal body levels) is ideal to maintain body homeostasis. Balanced solutions contain sodium, potassium, calcium, magnesium, chloride, and lactate. Potassium is usually not an additive found in maintenance multiple electrolyte solutions.

Isotonic multiple electrolyte solutions do not contain dextrose. Hypertonic multiple electrolyte solutions usually have the addition of 5% dextrose, which raises the osmolarity of the solution. Many types of replacement fluids are available. The hazard in using isotonic or hypertonic multiple electrolyte solutions is fluid overload (Plumer, 1987, p 114).

Ringer's Fluids

The Ringer's fluids (Ringer's injection and lactated Ringer's) used today are classified as balanced or isotonic fluids because their fluid and electrolyte content is similar to that of plasma. They are basically to replace electrolytes at physiologic levels in the ECF compartment. They can, for a short time, be used as replacement for blood.

Ringer's Injection

Ringer's injection is similar to 0.9% sodium chloride in electrolyte levels with the substitute of potassium and calcium for some of the sodium ions in concentrations equal to those of plasma. Ringer's injection, however, is superior to 0.9% sodium chloride as a fluid and electrolyte replenisher, and it is preferred over 0.9% sodium chloride for treatment of dehydration after drastically reduced water intake or water loss.

Ringer's Injection (Total: 309 mOsm/liter)		Normal Saline (Total: 310 mOsm/liter)	
Na	147.5	Na	154
K	4.0	Cl	154
Cl	156.0		
Ca	4.5		

USES
✓ Dehydration
✓ Vomiting
✓ Diarrhea
✓ Fistula drainage

ADVANTAGES

Ringer's injection is similar to NS with the substitution of potassium and calcium for some of the sodium ions in concentrations equal to those of plasma. Ringer's injection, however, is superior to NS as a fluid and electrolyte replenisher, and it is preferred over NS for treatment of dehydration after drastically reduced water intake or water loss, as occurs with vomiting, diarrhea, or fistula drainage.

DISADVANTAGES

Ringer's injection does not contain enough potassium and calcium to be used in maintenance of these ions or to correct a deficit of these electrolytes (Remington, 1980, pp 761–762).

Lactated Ringer's

Lactated Ringer's is probably the most commonly prescribed solution on the market. Although it contains less sodium, calcium, and chloride than Ringer's injection, it *does* contain the bicarbonate precursor (lactate) to assist in acidotic states (Table 5–6).

USES
✓ Treatment of any type of dehydration
✓ Restoration of fluid balance before and after surgery
✓ Replacement of fluids lost in burns
✓ Peritoneal irrigation
✓ Treatment of metabolic acidosis that occurs with mild renal insufficiency
✓ Treatment of infant diarrhea
✓ Treatment of diabetic ketoacidosis
✓ Treatment of salicylate overdose

DISADVANTAGES

✓ Lactated Ringer's should not be used in patients with impaired lactate metabolism, such as those with:

Liver disease
Addison's disease
Severe metabolic acidosis and alkalosis
Profound hypovolemia
Profound shock or cardiac failure

In these patients blood lactate levels may already be elevated (Griffith, 1986).

120

Table 5–6 □ **COMPARISON CHART: ACIDIFYING, ALKALYZING FLUIDS, AND RINGER'S INJECTION TO PLASMA (mEq/L)**

Solution	mOsm/liter	Tonicity	Na	K	Ca	Cl	HCO₃ Precursor	Use
Lactated Ringer's	273	Iso	130	4	3	109	Lactate 28	Dehydration, any type; restore fluid balance before and after surgery
Ringer's injection	309	Iso	147.5	4	4.5	156	None	Dehydration associated with vomiting, diarrhea, fistula drainage
5% dextrose/lactated Ringer's	527	Hyper	130	4	3	109	Lactate 28	Same as lactated Ringer's injection, dextrose added, spares body protein
1/6 molar sodium lactate injection	335	Iso	167				Lactate 167	Acidosis resulting from sodium deficit
Plasma	290	Iso	142	5	5	103	HCO₃ 26	

Summary Worksheet No. 2: Parenteral Fluids

DEXTROSE FLUIDS

ADVANTAGES	DISADVANTAGES
1.	1.
2.	2.
3.	3.
4.	4.

SALINE SOLUTIONS

ADVANTAGES, USES	DISADVANTAGES
1.	1.
2.	2.
3.	3.
4.	4.

DEXTROSE AND SALINE SOLUTIONS

ADVANTAGES, USES	DISADVANTAGES
1.	1.
2.	2.
3.	3.
4.	

MULTIPLE ELECTROLYTE SOLUTIONS

ADVANTAGES, USES
Ringer's injection, lactated Ringer's injection
1.
2.
3.
4.
5.
6.
7.
8.

DISADVANTAGES
Ringer's injection
1.

Lactated Ringer's injection
1.

SPECIALTY FLUIDS

Plasma expanders
Alkalizing and acidifying fluids
Potassium fluids

Plasma Expanders

Plasma substitutes are used to increase blood volume. Dextran is a synthetic plasma volume expander used to treat hypovolemic shock. This fluid is a macromolecular polymer of glucose, which increases the blood's osmotic pressure, thereby drawing interstitial fluid into the vessels and increasing blood volume. Dextran has two advantages, no storage problems and no danger of hepatitis.

Dextran should be used with caution in patients with heart or renal disease because a rapid rate could cause congestive heart failure and pulmonary edema. Allergic reactions can occur for Dextran administration. Dextran is available as dextran 6% in normal saline solution or dextran 5% in water for patients requiring low sodium intake. The usual dose is 500 mL at a rate of 20 mL/kg per 24 hours.

✎ **Note:** Dextran may interfere with typing and cross-matching by causing red cell aggregation (Keithley & Fraulini, 1982).

Alkalizing and Acidifying Fluids

Alkalizing

Metabolic acidosis can occur in clinical situations in which dehydration, shock, liver disease, starvation, or diabetes causes retention of chlorides, ketone bodies, or organic salts or when excessive bicarbonate is lost. Treatment consists of infusion of an alkalizing fluid. Two I.V. fluids may be used when excessive bicarbonate is lost and metabolic acidosis occurs: one sixth molar isotonic sodium lactate and one sixth bicarbonate injection. The lactate ion must be oxidized in the body to carbon dioxide before it can affect acid-base balance. Sodium lactate to bicarbonate requires 1 to 2 hours. Oxygen is needed to increase bicarbonate concentrations.

Advantages

The one-sixth sodium lactate solution is useful whenever acidosis has resulted from sodium deficiency, as in:

✓ Vomiting
✓ Starvation
✓ Uncontrolled diabetes mellitus
✓ Acute infections
✓ Renal failure

The isotonic solution sodium bicarbonate injection provides bicarbonate ions in clinical situations in which excessive bicarbonate is lost:

123

✓ Severe acidosis with severe hyperpnea

The reason this solution is useful to relieve dyspnea and hyperpnea is that the bicarbonate ion is released in the form of carbon dioxide through the lungs, leaving an excess of sodium ion behind.

Disadvantages

The one-sixth molar sodium lactate solution is contraindicated in patients suffering from lack of oxygen or in patients with liver disease. Patients receiving this solution should be watched for signs of hypocalcemic tetany (Plumer, 1987, p 116).

✎ **Note:** Administer sodium bicarbonate injection slowly, as rapid administration may induce cellular acidity and result in death.

Acidifying

Metabolic alkalosis is a condition associated with excess bicarbonate and loss of chloride. Isotonic sodium chloride (0.9% sodium chloride) provides conservative treatment of metabolic alkalosis.

Ammonium chloride is used as an acidifying solution in severe metabolic alkalosis due to loss of gastric secretions or pyloric stenosis. The ammonium ion is converted by the liver to hydrogen ion and to ammonia, which is excreted as urea. Ammonium chloride must be infused at a slow rate to enable the liver to metabolize the ammonium ion. Rapid infusion can result in toxic effects, causing irregular breathing and bradycardia. This solution must be used with caution in patients with severe hepatic disease or renal failure.

✎ **Note:** This I.V. fluid is contraindicated in any condition with a high ammonium level.

Potassium Chloride Fluids

Several premixed potassium chloride (KCl) I.V. fluids are available. Potassium 20 mEq or 40 mEq is added to 5% dextrose or 5% dextrose in 0.45% sodium chloride. Follow special nursing considerations in administration of intravenous potassium chloride.

Nursing Considerations in Administration of Intravenous Potassium Chloride

1. Potassium should *never* be directly administered in concentrated form by I.V. push because of the danger of cardiac arrest.
2. Prevent "layering" of KCl additive by thoroughly mixing KCl to the I.V. fluid. Do not add the KCl to a container that is in the hanging position.
3. Limit the concentration of KCl to 30 to 40 mEq/liter to prevent acci-

dental rapid infusion of large amounts of potassium. (No more than 80 mEq of potassium should ever be added to 1 liter of fluid.)

4. Establish that the patient has adequate kidney function before administration of potassium.
5. I.V. potassium replacement guidelines are as follows:
   5 to 10 mEq/hour (diluted) per continuous infusion.
   10 to 20 mEq/hour (diluted) in extreme hypokalemia while continuously monitoring the ECG.
6. Potassium replacement should be slow; a rapid rise in serum potassium causes hyperkalemia.
7. I.V. fluids containing 20 to 40 mEq/liter of potassium chloride are associated with pain along the vein and phlebitis.
8. Tissue damage can occur if the solution of KCl infiltrates, particularly if the solution exceeds 10 mEq of KCl (Metheny, 1984, p 66).

NURSING DIAGNOSES RELATED TO PARENTERAL FLUID ADMINISTRATION

1. Anxiety (mild, moderate, severe) related to threat to or change in health status; misconceptions regarding therapy
2. Altered nutrition (less than body requirements) related to inability to ingest or digest food or absorb nutrients; inadequate nutrient replacement
3. Decreased cardiac output related to reaction to parenteral solution; contamination
4. Fluid volume excess related to infusion of I.V. fluid
5. Knowledge deficit related to new procedure and maintaining I.V. therapy
6. Fluid volume deficit related to deviations affecting intake or absorption of fluids; factors influencing fluid needs (e.g., hypermetabolic state)
7. Impaired tissue integrity related to irritating fluids
8. Risk for infection related to broken skin or traumatized tissue
9. Sleep pattern disturbance related to external sensory stimuli (e.g., I.V. fluid and tubing)

SUMMARY OF CHAPTER 5

PARENTERAL FLUIDS

I.V. therapy has three objectives:

Maintain daily requirements
Replace previous losses
Restore concurrent losses

The key elements in parenteral therapy are water, carbohydrates, protein, vitamins, trace elements, and electrolytes. The pH is important with respect to the acidity of the fluid and its stability.

QUICK GLANCE CHART OF COMMON I.V. FLUIDS

Product	Osmolarity		pH	Nonelectrolyte		Cations/Liter				Anions/Liter			Uses
				Dext.	Cal./100 mL	Na	K	Ca	Mg	Cl	Acetate	Lactate	
Dextrose Solutions													
5% dextrose and water	Iso	252	4.8	5	17								Supplies calories as carbohydrates; prevents dehydration; maintains water balance; promotes sodium diuresis
10% dextrose and water	Hyper	505	4.7	10	34								
20% dextrose and water	Hyper	1010	4.8	20	68								
50% dextrose and water	Hyper	2525	4.6	50	170								
Saline Solutions													
0.45% NaCl	Hypo	154	5.9			77				77			Treats alkalosis; corrects fluid loss; treats sodium depletion
0.9% NaCl	Iso	308	6.0			154				154			
3% NaCl	Hyper	1026	6.0			513				513			

Dextrose and Saline Solutions

Solution	Tonicity	Osmolality	pH	Dextrose (g)	Cal	Na⁺	K⁺	Ca²⁺	Mg²⁺	Cl⁻	Acetate	Lactate	Action
5% dextrose/0.2% NaCl	Iso	320	4.6	5	17	34				34			Promotes diuresis; corrects moderate fluid loss; prevents alkalosis; provides calories and sodium chloride
5% dextrose/0.45% NaCl	Hyper	406	4.6	5	17	77				77			
5% dextrose/0.9% NaCl	Hyper	559	4.4	5	17	154				154			
10% dextrose/0.9% NaCl	Hyper	812	4.8	10	34	154				154			

Multiple Electrolyte Solutions

Solution	Tonicity	Osmolality	pH	Dextrose (g)	Cal	Na⁺	K⁺	Ca²⁺	Mg²⁺	Cl⁻	Acetate	Lactate	Action
Ringer's solution	Iso	304	6.0			147	4	4	0	155	0	0	Replaces fluid lost through vomiting or gastrointestinal suctioning; treats dehydration; restores normal fluid balance
Lactated Ringer's	Iso	273	6.5			130	4	3	0	109	0	28	
Normosol R (Abbott)	Iso	295	6.4		18	140	5	5	3	98	27	0	
Plasma Lyte M with dextrose* (Baxter)	Hyper	383	5.2		18	40	16	5	3	40	12	12	

*The additon of dextrose to any multiple electrolyte solution renders the solution hypertonic.

PARENTERAL FLUIDS ARE:
Hypotonic: 250 mOsm/liter or below
Isotonic range 250 to 375 mOsm/liter
Hypertonic above 375 mOsm/liter

TYPES OF PARENTERAL FLUIDS
Dextrose and water
Sodium chloride
Dextrose and sodium chloride
Multiple electrolyte
    Ringer's injection
    Lactated Ringer's
    Hypotonic maintenance
    Isotonic maintenance
    Replacement
Specialty Fluids
    Plasma substitutes
    Alkalizing fluids
    Acidifying fluids
    Potassium chloride solutions

The most commonly administered fluid is lactated Ringer's. The nursing concentrations for potassium chloride administration include

- Potassium chloride should never be directly administered in concentrated form by I.V. push.
- Prevent layering of potassium chloride additive by thoroughly mixing KCl to the fluid. Do not add the KCl to a container that is in the hanging position.
- Limit the concentration of KCl to 30 to 40 mEq/liter to prevent administration of large amounts of potassium.
- Establish that the patient has adequate kidney function.

    I.V. potassium replacement guidelines.

- 5 to 10 mEq/hour diluted per continuous infusion.
- 10 to 20 mEq/hour diluted in extreme hypokalemia while continuously monitoring the ECG.
- Potassium replacement should be slow; a rapid rise in serum potassium causes hyperkalemia.
- I.V. Fluids containing 20 to 40 mEq/liter of potassium chloride are associated with pain along the vein and phlebitis.
- Tissue damage can occur if the solution of KCl infiltrates, particularly if the solutions exceed 10 mEq of KCl.

Activity Journal

1. Describe a situation in which you observed I.V. fluid administered too rapidly.

2. Become familiar with the I.V. fluids available in your work environment. Are they primarily fluids without additives? If they are multiple electrolyte solutions, are they arranged on the shelf so as not to be mistaken for each other?

3. The solutions with red lettering on the top are usually fluids with additives such as lidocaine or aminophylline. How are these solutions dispensed at your facility? Are they in such a place that they could be grabbed by mistake and hung in an emergency?

4. You discover that a fluid has rapidly been infused into a patient. Is this a situation that could potentially harm the patient? What would you do to remedy this situation?

129

Quality Assessment Model

Instructions: Use this quality assessment model to conduct retrospective audits of charts, establish quality control standards, or develop outcome criteria for quality assurance. Refer to Chapter 2 for details on quality assessment.

STRUCTURE

(Resources that affect outcome)
Human Resource: I.V. Therapist

↓

PROCESS

(Actual giving and receiving of care)
Therapist activities related to administration of parenteral solution are:

1. Knowledge of the contents of each I.V. fluid hung.
2. Identification of patients at risk for fluid overload.
3. Maintenance of I.V. fluid at 10 percent of prescribed rate.

↓

OUTCOME STANDARDS

(Effects of care)
Evaluation of nursing interventions
   Documentation reflects standards of care for the practice of safe delivery of parenteral solutions:

1. The I.V. fluid infusing must match the physician's order.
2. The I.V. fluid is within 10 percent of the prescribed rate.

Post-test, Chapter 5

Match the definition in column 2 to the correct term in column 1.

Column 1

1. _____ Crystalloid
2. _____ Hydrating solution
3. _____ Homeostasis
4. _____ Colloid
5. _____ Catabolism

Column 2

A. A substance that does not dissolve

B. Ability to restore equilibrium

C. Solution of water, carbohydrate, and sodium chloride used to check kidney function

D. An energy-producing metabolic process

E. A substance that forms a true solution

6. What are the three objectives of I.V. therapy?
   A. Maintenance therapy, replacement therapy, and restoration therapy
   B. Peristaltic therapy, restoration therapy, and maintenance therapy
   C. Replacement therapy, restoration therapy, and transfusion therapy

7. What is the function of glucose in parenteral therapy?
   A. To provide calories for energy
   B. To provide extracellular electrolyte replacement
   C. To provide a vehicle for blood administration
   D. To provide a source for catabolism of potassium

8. Maintenance fluid are used for the patient who is:
   A. NPO for a short period of time
   B. Hemorrhaging from a trauma
   C. Dehydrated from gastrointestinal losses
   D. Dehydrated from diarrhea

Match the definition in column 2 to the correct term in column 1.

Column 1

9. _____ Hypotonic
10. _____ Isotonic
11. _____ Hypertonic

Column 2

A. Osmolarity greater than 375 mEq/liter; replaces electrolytes

B. Equal to blood plasma

C. Used for cellular dehydration; osmolarity less than 250 mEq/liter

12. The average adult insensible loss is between _____ and _____ mL/day.

13. The main role of a hydrating solution is to _____.

14. Identify two uses of lactated Ringer's.
    1. _____
    2. _____

15. The most commonly used multiple electrolyte solution is _____.

16. List one advantage and one disadvantage of the following three groups of solutions:

Dextrose Fluids

Advantage   **Disadvantage**

Sodium Chloride Fluids

Advantage   **Disadvantage**

Multiple Electrolyte Fluids

Advantage   **Disadvantage**

17. A physician orders 1000 mL of 5% dextrose in 0.45% sodium chloride to infuse every 8 hours for Mrs. Black. Mrs. Black has an NG tube to suction. The physician additionally orders lactated Ringer's as a replacement of gastric losses milliliter for milliliter every 4 hours. How many total milliliters per hour will the nurse be infusing if the NG tube container is emptied of 500 mL of output at 8 AM?

_____ mL/hour primary
_____ mL/hour NG replacement
_____ total mL/hour

Answers to Post-test, Chapter 5

1. E
2. C
3. B
4. A
5. D
6. A
7. A
8. A
9. C
10. B
11. A

12. 500 to 1000
13. Check kidney function before administration of potassium.
14. Treat dehydration.
    Restore fluid balance before and after surgery.
    Treat infant diarrhea.
    Treat diabetic ketoacidosis.
    Use as short-term replacement for blood.
15. Lactated Ringer's injection

16. **Dextrose Solutions**

ADVANTAGES
Use as vehicle for administration of medication
Provide nutrition
Treat hyperkalemia
Treat dehydration

DISADVANTAGE
Acts as osmotic diuretic if infused too rapidly

Sodium Chloride Solutions

ADVANTAGES
Extracellular replacement
Treat metabolic alkalosis
Treat sodium depletion
Initiate blood transfusion

DISADVANTAGES
Hypernatremia
Overload of sodium and chloride
Circulatory overload

Multiple Electrolyte Solutions

ADVANTAGES
Treat acidosis
Replace fluids and electrolytes

DISADVANTAGES
Circulatory overload

17. 125 mL/hour of primary solution
    125 mL/hour of replacement solution
    250 mL/hour total

References

Gasparis, L., Murray, E.B., & Ursomanno, P. (1989). I.V. solutions—Which one's right for your patient? *Nursing 89, 4,* 62–64.

Griffith, C.A. (1986). The family of Ringer's solutions. *Journal of Intravenous Therapy Association, 9,* 480–483.

Keithley, J.K., & Fraulini, K.E. (1982). What's behind that I.V. line? *Nursing 82, 3,* 34–42.

Metheny, N.M. (1984). *Quick reference to fluid balance.* Philadelphia: J.B. Lippincott.

Metheny, N.M. (1987). *Fluid and electrolyte balance: Nursing considerations.* Philadelphia: J.B. Lippincott.

133

Plumer, A.L. (1987). *Principles and practices of I.V. therapy* (4th ed.). Boston: Little, Brown.

Remington, J.P. (1980). *Remington's pharmaceutical sciences* (16th ed.). Easton: Mack Publishing.

Sommers, M. (1990). Rapid fluid resuscitation. *Nursing 90, 1,* 52–59.

United States Pharmacopeia (20th ed.). (1980). Easton, PA: Mack Publishing.

Equipment

CHAPTER 6

Equipment

CHAPTER CONTENTS

136

Glossary

Cannula: A tube or sheath used for infusing fluids

Coring: Visible, as well as microscopic, particles of rubber bung displaced by the spike during piercing of the glass container

Drip chamber: Area of the intravenous tubing usually found under the spike where the solution drips and collects before running through the intravenous tubing

Filter: A special porous device used to prevent the passage of undesired substances

Gauges: Sizes of cannula opening

Groshong catheter: Surgically implanted, long-term, indwelling catheter; unique in that it has a two-way valve adjacent to the closed tip that prevents backflow of blood

Heparin lock: Intermittent intravenous device used to maintain patent venous access

Hickman catheter: Long-term indwelling catheter inserted surgically via an incision in the deltopectoral groove through the superior vena cava, terminating near the right atrium

Hub: Female connection point of an intravenous cannula where the tubing or other equipment will attach

Infusate: Intravenous solution

Lumen: The space within an artery, vein, or catheter

Macrodrip: Drop factor of 10 to 20 drops/mL based on manufacturer

Microaggregates: Microscopic collection of particles, such as platelets, leukocytes, and fibrin that can occur in stored blood

Microdrip: Drop factor of 60 drops/mL

137

Multilumen: Venous access device that has more than one lumen

PCA: Patient-controlled analgesia

Ports: Points of entry

Primary port: First port of entry along intravenous tubing

Radiopaque: Material used in intravenous catheter, which can be identified on x-ray examination

Rubber bung: Stopper of glass container composed of numerous substances including rubber, chemical particles, and cellulose fibers

LEARNING OBJECTIVES

Upon completion of this chapter, the reader will be able to:

☐ Identify the terminology related to intravenous equipment.

☐ Identify types and characteristics of three infusate containers.

☐ Describe gravity flow systems.

☐ Compare vented and nonvented administration sets.

☐ Identify types and characteristics of peripheral and central infusion devices.

☐ State the major complications associated with over-the-needle catheters and scalp vein needles.

☐ Identify the characteristics and uses of controllers and pumps to regulate infusions.

☐ Describe the use of filters in the infusion of solutions and blood products.

☐ Describe the use of miscellaneous adjuncts to aid in administration of safe infusions.

☐ Identify Intravenous Nurses Society and Centers for Disease Control recommendations for standards of practice related to equipment safety and use.

Pre-test, Chapter 6

Instructions: The pre-test is to review prior knowledge of equipment for safe delivery of infusions. Each question in the pre-test is based on the learning objectives of the chapter.

1. When using a closed glass system, the administration set should be:
   A. Vented
   B. Nonvented

2. What are the three types of systems manufactured for the delivery of intravenous solutions?
   A. Plastic, open glass, and closed glass
   B. Open glass, vented, and nonvented plastic
   C. Closed glass, open glass, and filtered plastic

3. What are inline filters useful for?
   A. Filtering nonviable contaminants such as particles of metal, lint, and glass
   B. Filtering viable contaminants such as bacteria and fungi
   C. Filtering air from the administration set
   D. All of the above

4. A major hazard of using Teflon over-the-needle catheters for peripheral infusion is:
   A. The risk of phlebitis
   B. The risk of infiltration
   C. That they can be used only for 24 hours
   D. The risk of septicemia

5. The infusate solution containers should be inspected for:
   A. Clarity, expiration date, and air vents
   B. Clarity, expiration date, and punctures or cracks
   C. Punctures or cracks, presence of ports, and clarity

6. Volumetric pumps require:
   A. A 170-micron filter
   B. A 0.22-micron filter
   C. Special cassette (cartridge) tubing
   D. Microdrip tubing

True-False

7. **T F** Scalp vein needles have a higher rate of infiltration than do over-the-needle catheters.

8. **T F** According to the Intravenous Nursing Standards of Practice, primary tubing changes should coordinate with catheter changes at 48 hours.

9. **T F** Controllers eliminate the need for frequent monitoring of the patient by the nurse.

10. **T F** Controllers are gravity dependent.

Match the definition in column 2 to the correct term in column 1.

Column 1	Column 2
11. ____ Port	A. Porous device used to prevent passage of undesirable substances
12. ____ Lumen	
13. ____ Radiopaque	B. Size of cannula opening
14. ____ Gauge	C. Space within an artery, vein, or catheter
15. ____ Filter	D. Material used in catheters that can be identified on x-ray examination
	E. Point of entry

ANSWERS TO PRE-TEST, Chapter 6

1. A	2. A	3. D	4. A	5. B	6. C	7. T	8. T	9. F
10. T	11. E	12. C	13. D	14. B	15. A			

INFUSATE SYSTEMS

Three systems are available for the delivery of intravenous (I.V.) fluids: the open glass system, closed glass system, and plastic system. Sterile evacuated glass containers became available in 1929. The rigid glass containers contain a standard mix of materials, glass, metal, and rubber. The combination of materials can be a disadvantage because of incompatibilities with other fluids or additives and breakdown of the materials during heat sterilization. In 1950, plastic containers became accessible for the storage and delivery of blood products. Today, the plastic system is used 90 to 95 percent of the time for administration of solutions and blood products (Ausman, 1984).

Glass System

The glass system, open and closed, has a partial vacuum and requires air vents. In the open glass system air enters through a plastic tube in the container and collects in the air space in the bottle, allowing for displacement of the solution. In the closed glass system air is filtered into the container via vented tubing. The closed glass system must use vented tubing in order to allow air into the container.

✎ **Note:** In the open glass system the straw must extend above the fluid level to prevent bubbling of the air through the **infusate**. Bubbling increases the risk of contamination.

The glass system has a stopper, also called the **rubber bung**. During insertion of the administration set **coring** can occur, which causes fragments of the rubber core to be introduced into the solution. Visible and microscopic particles of the rubber bung can be displaced by twisting the spike through the rubber bung (Delaney & Lauer, 1988, pp 75–79).

Because of the combination of materials in the glass system there have been some disadvantages to this system during heat sterilization procedures (Table 6–1). Openings between the external environment and the internal container occur at peak heating and early cooling phases of sterilization. Recalls of endogenously contaminated fluids in the United States were caused by the expansion of metal, rubber, and glass during the sterilization procedure (Ausman, 1984).

Checking the Glass System for Clarity

In order to ensure safety in the administration of solutions the nurse must check the solution's clarity and expiration date before connection to the administration set. To check the glass system, hold the glass bottle up to the light and

Table 6–1 ☐ **ADVANTAGES AND DISADVANTAGES OF GLASS SYSTEM**

Advantages	Disadvantages
Crystal clear: allows for good visualization of contents	Breakage and shattering of glass
Fluid level easily read	Storage space
Inert, has no plasticizers	Coring (due to rubber bung)
	Cumbersome disposal
	Rigidity
	Container constructed of mixed materials

check for flashes of light, floating particles, or discoloration. The glass system should be crystal clear; if it is not, mark the container contaminated and return to central supply. Check the expiration date on the label.

Plastic System

Flexible and Rigid Plastic (Fig. 6–1)

The majority of I.V. fluids are packaged in plastic containers (Fig. 6–2). The flexible plastic container has several unique features. The entire structure that comes in contact with the fluid, including the closure, is made of the same material; it is all polyvinyl chloride or other suitable material. There is no combination of metal, rubber, or glass as in the rigid glass system. The stability and compatibility with additives is relatively safe. This is a truly closed system. The plastic system does not contain a vacuum; therefore, the containers must be flexible and collapsible. The plastic system does not need air to replace fluid flowing from the container. Either a vented or a nonvented administration set is acceptable for delivery of the infusate. A membrane seals both the medication and administration ports of the container, and there is no entry of air into this system. Because there is no rubber bung on the plastic system, spiking the system is simplified. A twisting motion can be used with this system (Fig. 6–3).

The semirigid, hard plastic unit is also a closed system. The advantage of the rigid container is that it contains no plasticizers, and the container has marks that make it easier to read fluid levels. This system is also impermeable to moisture. However, a disadvantage to the rigid system is that it does not completely collapse; therefore, the last 50 mL of the solution may have difficulty infusing.

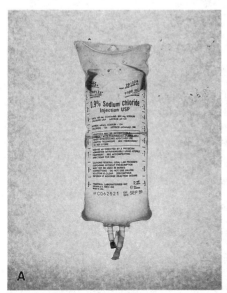
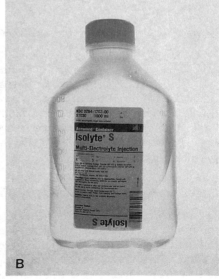

Figure 6–1 ☐ Plastic infusion system. (Courtesy of D. Andersen, Chico, California.)

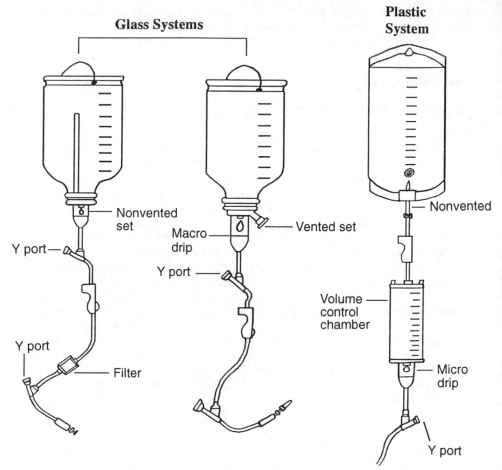

Figure 6 – 2 ☐ Comparison of infusate containers and administration sets. (Drawing by Timothy D. Mitas.)

A study by Moorhatch & Chiou in 1974 found that leaching of the plasticizers into the infusate can possibly contribute to increased phlebitis rates. Both the flexible and semirigid plastic systems, when used in a series with other similar containers, may promote movement of residual air into the I.V. line (Delaney & Lauer, 1988). Table 6 – 2 list the advantages and disadvantages to the plastic system.

Checking the Plastic System for Clarity

The plastic container should be held up to the light and checked for clarity. If the plastic system is not crystal clear, any discoloration or floating particles in the solution should be identified and labeled as contaminated. The plastic system must be squeezed to check for pinholes. Check expiration date on the label to ensure patient safety. The outer wrap of the plastic system should be free of pooled solution.

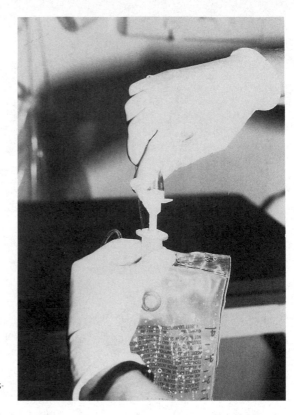

Figure 6-3 ☐ Spiking the plastic system.

ADMINISTRATION SETS

Administration sets vary among manufacturers. The sets vary in drop factor but all have the basic component parts (Fig. 6-4). Administration sets that are most frequently used are:

> Primary (standard) set
> Secondary set
> > Piggyback
> > Volume-controlled sets
> Blood administration sets

Table 6-2 ☐ **ADVANTAGES AND DISADVANTGES OF PLASTIC SYSTEM**

Advantages	Disadvantages
Closed system	Punctures easily
Flexible	Fluid level difficult to determine
Lightweight	Composed of plasticizers
Container composed of one substance	Not completely inert (leaching)
Better storage	

143

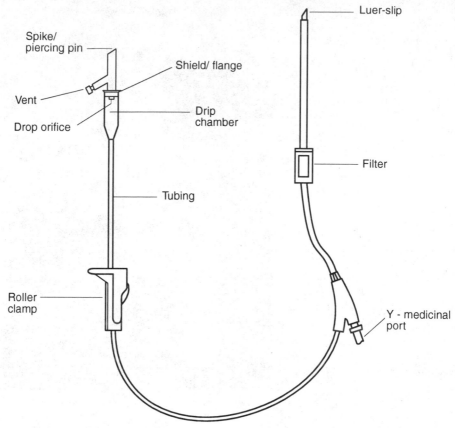

Figure 6–4 ☐ Basic administration set. (Drawing by Timothy D. Mitas.)

BASIC COMPONENT PARTS TO ADMINISTRATIONS SETS

1. **Spike/piercing pin:** The spike/piercing pin is a sharply tipped plastic tube designed to be inserted into the infusate container. It is connected to the flange, drop orifice, and drip chamber.
2. **Flange:** The flange is a plastic guard that helps prevent touch contamination during insertion of the spike.
3. **Drop orifice:** The drop orifice is an opening that determines the size and shape of the fluid drop. The size of this drop orifice determines the drop factor.
4. **Drip chamber:** The **drip chamber** is a pliable, enlarged clear plastic tube that contains the drop orifice. It is connected to the tubing.
5. **Tubing:** The plastic tubing connects to the drip chamber. Depending on the manufacturer, the tubing may have a variety of clamps, ports, connectors, or filters built into the system. The average length of primary tubing is usually 66 to 100 in. The length of secondary administration sets averages from 32 to 42 in.
6. **Clamp:** The flow clamp control device operates on the principle of compression of the tubing wall. Each manufacturer supplies a clamp

(roller, screw, or slide) and all operate on the principle of compression. The roller and screw clamps are equally reliable. The slide clamp is viewed as less reliable in controlling flow.

7. **Injection ports:** Injection **ports** serve as an access into the tubing and are located at various points along the administration set. Usually the ports are used for administration of medication. Small needles should be used to access these ports (21- to 25-gauge) to ensure resealing. The **primary port** is the first injection port along the intravenous tubing.

8. **Final filter:** The final **filter** removes foreign particles from the infusate. It can be purchased as a part of the administration set tubing, or filters can be added on.

The primary sets are supplied as vented or nonvented. In vented sets an air filter is attached to the spike pin, which allows for air to enter the container. Vented sets must be used on the closed glass system. Nonvented sets have a straight spike pin without an air vent device. Nonvented sets can be used on any open glass or plastic system.

Primary

Primary sets are referred to as standard sets. Primary sets are available in **macrodrip** form (10 to 20 drops/mL) or in **microdrip** form (60 drops/mL). The calibration is clearly specified on the box of each administration set, as well as on the accompanying literature. The microdrip set, also called a minidrip or pediatric set, is used when small amounts of fluid are required, as in keep vein open (KVO) rates (Fig. 6–5).

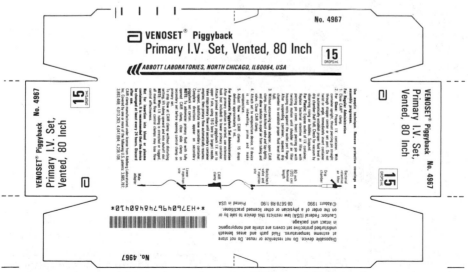

Figure 6–5 □ Primary administration set package. (Courtesy of Abbott Laboratories, Hospital Products Division, Abbott Park, Illinois.)

145

Intermittent

There are two ways to deliver intermittent fluids: piggyback or volume-controlled administration sets. The piggyback or secondary set is used for delivery of 50 to 100 mL of infusate and has short tubing with a standard drop factor of 10 to 20 drops/mL. In setting up the piggyback line the primary infusate is positioned lower than the secondary container, using the extension hook provided in the secondary line box. The secondary tubing connects to the primary line at the Y port.

The volume-controlled set is designed for intermittent administration of measured volumes of fluid with a calibrated chamber. This set is most frequently used for pediatric patients and critically ill patients when small amounts and/or well-controlled delivery of medication or fluid are needed (Fig. 6–6).

Large-Bore Tubing Sets

Large-bore tubing sets are available for trauma care. These sets provide up to 514 mL/minute for rapid flow rates, along with a 55 percent faster packed cell flow rate than standard blood administration sets (Plumer & Cosentino, 1987, p 146).

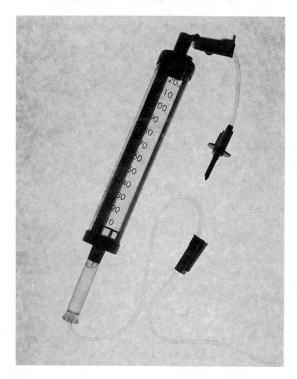

Figure 6–6 □ Volume chamber control set for intermittent infusion. (Courtesy of D. Anderson, Chico, California.)

Blood

Blood components are administered through a straight or Y blood set to allow for filtering of debris. A Y set allows for normal saline to be used as a primer for the administration set before the blood is administered. Most blood administration sets contain inline filters with a pore size of 170 microns. Blood sets have a drop factor of 10 to allow for the safe infusion of blood cells (Delaney & Lauer, 1988, pp 85–86).

STANDARDS OF PRACTICE FOR ADMINISTRATION SETS

INTRAVENOUS NURSING STANDARDS OF PRACTICE 1990 (S54)

1. Peripheral and central primary sets shall be changed every 48 hours and immediately upon suspected contamination or when the integrity of the product has been compromised.
2. Peripheral and central secondary sets shall be changed every 48 hours and immediately upon suspected contamination or when the integrity of the product has been compromised.
3. Primary intermittent administration sets shall be changed every 24 hours and immediately upon suspected contamination or when the integrity of the product has been compromised.

CENTERS FOR DISEASE CONTROL STANDARDS OF PRACTICE RECOMMENDATIONS 1981 (pp 4–5)

1. I.V. administration tubing, including piggyback tubing, should be routinely changed every 48 to 72 hours (Category I).
2. Tubing used for hyperalimentation should be routinely changed every 24 to 48 hours (Category II).
3. Tubing should also be changed after the administration of blood, blood products, or lipid emulsions (Category III).
4. Between changes of components, the I.V. system should be maintained as a closed system as much as possible (Category I).

INFUSION DEVICES (TABLE 6–3)

Scalp Vein Needles

The winged-tip or butterfly needle are types of scalp vein needles. Scalp vein needles are made of stainless steel with odd-numbered **gauges** (17, 19, 21, 23, 25) and lengths of 1/2 in to 1-1/4 in. The wings attached to the shaft are made of rubber or plastic, and the flexible tubing extending behind the wings varies from 3 in to 12 in long (Fig. 6–7). Most commonly these needles are used in clinical situations when short-term therapy is needed, such as to provide single-dose therapy, to administer I.V. push medication, or to obtain blood samples. These needles are also used for pediatric patients. Because of their rigidity, the use of steel needles limits the patient's mobility and may cause more discomfort than other infusion devices (Delaney & Lauer, 1988, p 92).

147

Table 6–3 □ **COMPARISON OF PERIPHERAL INFUSION DEVICES**

Cannula	Advantages	Disadvantages	Uses
Scalp Vein Needle	Excellent for one-time I.V. medication, blood withdrawal, in patients allergic to nylon or Teflon Wings allow for ease of insertion and secure taping Attached extension permits easy tubing change	Needle increases risk of infiltration Not recommended for use in flexor areas Needle not flexible Repuncture by contaminated needle possible	Infants and children Elderly and other adults with small veins Adults receiving short-term therapy
Over-the-Needle Catheter	Easy to insert Patent longer Catheter tip tapered to prevent peelback Radiopaque feature makes x-ray detection easy Infiltration rare If using winged cannula, easy to tape Stable: allows for greater patient mobility	Depending on hub, sometimes difficult to secure with tape Long inflexible stylet increases risk of accidental puncture; pressure marks from hub Some catheters drag through the skin on insertion Increased risk of phlebitis	Long-term therapy Delivery of viscous liquids—blood and hyperalimentation Arterial monitoring
Inside-the-Needle Catheter	Permits insertion into superior vena cava Less likely to damage vein Stable Plastic sleeve reduces risk of touch contamination	Needle remains secured outside skin; risk of catheter embolus Plastic catheter may support infection or trigger phlebitis	Long-term therapy Delivery of viscous liquid Delivery of drugs to central veins Central venous pressure monitoring Rarely used

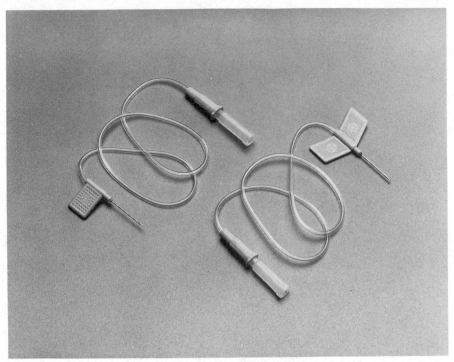

Figure 6–7 □ E-Z scalp vein needle. (Courtesy of Becton Dickinson, Deseret Division, Sandy, Utah.)

Over-the-Needle Catheters

The over-the-needle catheter (ONC) consists of a needle with a catheter sheath (Fig. 6–8). The **cannula** consists of a catheter from 3/4 in to 2 in long with gauges of even numbers ranging from 12 to 24. The point of the needle extends beyond the tip of the catheter. After venipuncture the needle is withdrawn and discarded, leaving a flexible catheter within the vein.

Materials used in ONCs include Teflon (DuPont), Aquavene (Menlo Care, Inc.) (which softens and expands), and vialon (which softens with the body temperature). Teflon, a polyurethane material, provides low cost, low rates of infiltration, and comparatively low rates of phlebitis (Hershey, Tomford, & McLaren, 1984; Larson, Lunche, & Tran, 1984).

Aquavene is different from other venous access materials in that it changes physical properties after insertion. It softens in the vessel, expands two gauge sizes, and reduces thrombogenicity because of its biocompatibility.

Vialon, an elastomer of polyurethane, is a high-strength material that provides a smooth-surfaced catheter for easy insertion. Once inside the vein, vialon becomes soft and pliable, permitting the catheter to float in the vein rather than lying against the intima of the vein wall. Vialon is designed also to minimize local reactions under conditions of extended use (McKee, Shell, Warren, & Campbell, 1989).

149

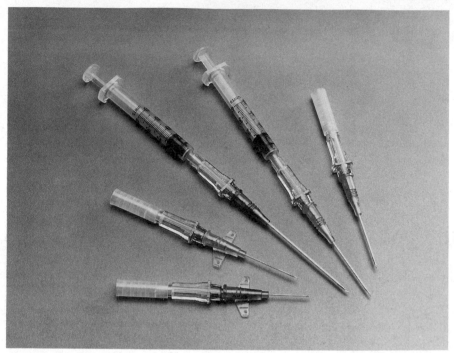

Figure 6–8 □ Minicath, Insyte over-the-needle catheter. (Courtesy of Becton Dickinson, Deseret Division, Sandy, Utah.)

✎ **Note:** Teflon ONCs tend to increase the risk of phlebitis (Millam, 1990; Larson et al., 1984).

Uses for ONCs, as determined by gauge numbers, are listed in Table 6–4.

The Intravenous Nursing Standards of Practice recommends that over-the-needle catheters be replaced every 48 hours and their removal shall coincide with the administration set change (S46). Peripheral arterial catheters should be removed every 96 hours (S46).

Table 6–4 □ **GUIDE TO ONC USE**

Gauge	Use
14–16	Multiple trauma, heart surgery, and transplants
18	Major trauma or surgery, blood administration
20	Minor trauma or surgery, blood administration
22	Pediatric, small veins, platelets, plasma (avoid with packed red blood cells and whole blood, and antibiotic therapy in selected patients)

Inside-the-Needle Catheters

Inside-the-needle catheters (INCs) consist of a catheter between 14 and 19 gauge lying inside a needle. The needle may be from 1-1/2 in to 2 in long, and the catheter 8 in to 36 in long. The clear plastic sleeve over the catheter protects it from touch contamination during insertion. After the catheter is placed, the needle is withdrawn and secured outside the skin. Because the catheter is **radiopaque**, confirmation by x-ray examination can be done before administration of viscous solutions. These catheters are rarely used because of the advances in central line catheters and because shearing of the catheter with the needle is a major risk (Burrows, 1984).

✎ **Note:** With any catheter, use the shortest length and the smallest gauge to deliver the ordered therapy. Also use a vein large enough to sustain sufficient blood flow, as this will decrease irritation to the vein wall.

Midarm Catheters

The midarm catheter is designed for intermediate-term therapies of 2 weeks or more. Landmark, Menlo Care, in Palo Alto, CA, has developed a new technology in vascular access devices. This midarm catheter is made with a new biomaterial called Aquavene. This catheter is 6 in long and is an alternative to central and peripheral venous access. This catheter is useful for intermediate therapies and is placed midline in the antecubital region in the basilic, cephalic, or median antecubital sites and is then advanced into the larger vessels of the upper arm for greater hemodilution. The arm should be measured from the proposed insertion site to the desired placement of the catheter tip. In most adults this will be about 5 to 6 in (Hadaway, 1990). Verification of tip location by x-ray examination is not necessary (Menlo Care, 1989).

CENTRAL INFUSION DEVICES

This is a basic introduction to the various types of central line catheters used today. Central venous access devices (CVADs) are discussed in detail in Chapter 12.

Long-term I.V. therapy may include the need for venous access over weeks, months, or even years. Special central venous catheters have been designed for long-term access, for patient comfort, and to decrease complications associated with multiple therapies. There are three general types of placement of central venous lines: centrally placed percutaneous catheters and tunneled catheters, both inserted by physicians, and the peripherally inserted central catheters, inserted by nurses.

1. Percutaneous catheters

    Subclavian
    Jugular
    Femoral

151

2. Tunneled catheters
   Broviac
   Hickman
   Groshong
   Implanted ports
3. Peripherally inserted central catheters

Percutaneous

In 1961 the first I.V. catheter for accessing the central circulation was introduced (Stewart & Sainslow, 1961). The percutaneous catheter is placed by an infraclavicular approach to the subclavian vein. The percutaneous short-term catheter is secured by suturing and no tunneling is involved. This catheter may remain in place for a few days to several weeks. This catheter provides an access to larger venous circulation for delivery of hypertonic solutions. The percutaneous and central venous tunneled catheters are available as **multilumen** and as single lumen.

Central Venous Tunneled

Broviac

The Broviac (Bard Access Systems) device is a 90-cm long, 1-mm diameter, silicone Silastic, long-term indwelling catheter equipped with cuffs. It allows for infusion of I.V. fluids including parenteral nutrition. Because of the Broviac's diameter, this catheter is used primarily in pediatric patients.

Hickman

The **Hickman (Bard Access Systems) catheter** is 90 cm long, 1.6 mm in diameter, silicone Silastic, long-term indwelling, and is equipped with one or two Dacron cuffs; it is a modified Broviac catheter with a larger diameter. This central catheter allows for central drawing of blood samples.

The Hickman is inserted surgically through an incision in the deltopectoral groove into the superior vena cava and terminates just before the right atrium. The catheter is tunneled subcutaneously and exits in an area that allows the patient to care for the site and port. The surgeon sutures the catheter in place via a Dacron polyester cuff that adheres to the tissues; this further secures the catheter and helps to prevent entrance of bacteria.

Once the cutdown and exit sites heal, only the external catheter is visible. The patient or nurse can infuse medications, chemotherapeutic drugs, or blood through the Hickman. Blood specimens can be obtained via this catheter (Fig. 6–9).

Groshong

The **Groshong (Bard Access Systems) catheter** is a thin-walled translucent silicone rubber catheter with an encapsulated barium sulfate radiopaque stripe and a patented two-way slit valve adjacent to a rounded, closed tip. A small

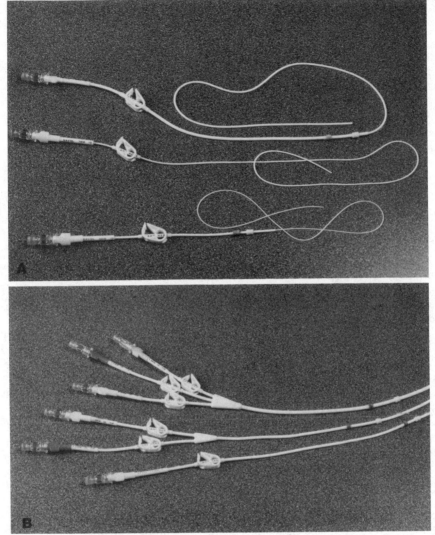

Figure 6–9 ☐ Hickman and Broviac catheters. (Courtesy of Daval Inc., a subsidiary of C. R. Bard, Inc., Specialty Access Products, Salt Lake City, Utah.)

Dacron cuff attached to the catheter promotes ingrowth of fibrous tissue, which helps secure the catheter and reduces the potential for infection. Although similar to the Hickman catheter, its design allows for both fluid administration and blood sampling through the same **lumen**. The Groshong is available in single-or triple-lumen style (Fig. 6–10).

Implantable Venous Access Ports

This is a completely closed system composed of an implanted device consisting of a drug reservoir, or port, with a self-sealing system connected to an outlet

153

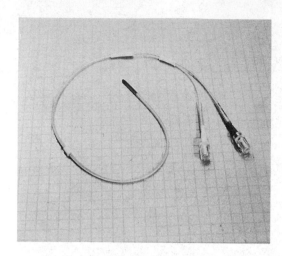

Figure 6-10 ☐ Groshong catheter. (Courtesy of Daval, Inc., a subsidiary of C. R. Bard, Inc., Specialty Access Products, Salt Lake City, Utah.)

catheter that is surgically implanted into a convenient body site in a subcutaneous pocket. The self-sealing septum can withstand 1000 to 2000 needle punctures. This totally implantable port provides venous access for blood withdrawal, I.V. solution infusion, blood transfusion, and chemotherapy.

The implanted port must be accessed with a Huber needle (noncoring). These special needles allow for safe and proper penetration of the septum of the port. Because they are noncoring needles, they contribute to the long lifetime of the port. The needles are sized from 19 to 24 gauge and are 1/2 in to 2-1/2 in long. They are available in 90-degree angle or straight-needle designs (Fig. 6-11).

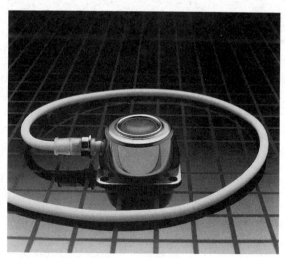

Figure 6-11 ☐ Implanted port. (Port-A-Cath Courtesy of Pharmacia Deltec Inc., St. Paul, Minnesota.)

154

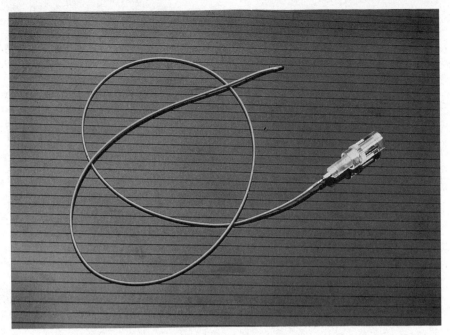

Figure 6–12 ☐ Peripherally inserted central catheter. (Courtesy of Daval, Inc., a subsidiary of C. R. Bard, Inc., Specialty Access Products, Salt Lake City, Utah.)

Peripherally Inserted Central Venous Catheters

The peripherally inserted central venous catheter (PIC, PICC) is also referred to as a long-arm catheter, long-term peripheral catheter, and midclavicular catheter. It usually ranges from 16 to 25 gauge and 20 in to 24 in long. The peripheral catheter is inserted into a peripheral site and advanced into the superior vena cava. To reach the superior vena cava in the average adult, a catheter length of at least 20 in is required. The catheter is made of silicone, polyurethane, polyvinylchloride, or some other polymer material. Silicone has proved its reliability and biocompatibility over the years in central venous catheter application as well as in a variety of implant uses. Silicone elastomer is soft, flexible, nonthrombogenic, and biocompatible (Fig. 6–12).

FILTERS

Final filters are used in delivery of I.V. therapy to filter microorganisms, which, if alive, will multiply in the bloodstream or, if dead, will enter the tissue and cause a sterile abscess. There are two groups of particulate matter: nonviable contaminants such as particles of metal, lint, asbestos, rubber, cotton, dust, or glass; and viable contaminants consisting of bacteria and fungi. Inline filters remove undissolved drug powders or crystals and precipitates from incompatible admixtures as well (Gurevich, 1984; Chrystal, 1985).

Final filters are available in a variety of forms, sizes, and materials. Two

155

commonly used inline filters are the depth filter and the membrane filter. The depth filter is composed of fibers or fragmented materials that have been pressed or bonded to form a maze. Fluid flows through a random path, which absorbs and traps the particles. Depth filters remove particles but do not block the passage of air.

Membrane filters are screen filters with uniformly sized pores. A 5-micron screen will retain on the flat portion of the membrane all particles greater than 5 microns. Filters of 0.2 micron are bacteria-, fungus-, and air-retention fibers. The 0.22- micron air-venting filters automatically vent air through a nonwettable (hydrophobic) membrane and permit uniform high-gravity flow through large wettable (hydrophilic) membrane (Plumer & Cosentino, 1987, p 15) (Fig. 6–13 shows a membrane filter.)

Use a filter whenever:

1. An additive has been combined with the solution.
2. The injection port on the tubing will be used.
3. The patient is susceptible to infusion phlebitis or infection.
4. The infusion is given centrally.

Filter sizes range from 5 microns (largest) to 0.22 micron (smallest). They allow liquids but not particles to pass through them. The finer the membrane, the more fully it will filter the liquid. Refer to Table 6–5 for function of filters.

Standards of Practice for Inline Filters

Intravenous Nursing Standards of Practice (1990) Recommendations

A 0.22-micron filter should be routinely used for the delivery of I.V. therapy. The filter change shall coincide with the administration set change (S57). Refer to Table 6–6 for optimal filter characteristics.

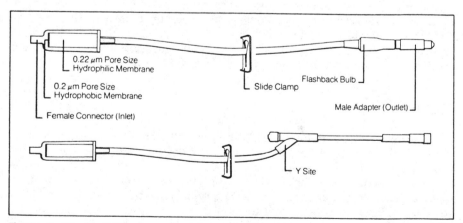

Figure 6–13 □ 0.22 micron filter. (Courtesy of Abbott Laboratories, Hospital Products Division, Abbott Park, Illinois.)

Table 6–5 ☐ **FUNCTION OF FILTERS**

Size	Function
5-micron to 1-micron	Removes most particulate matter; does not remove fungi or bacteria
0.45-micron	Removes fungi and most bacteria
0.22-micron	Removes all fungi and bacteria but reduces flow rate

Centers for Disease Control (1981) Recommendations

The use of I.V. inline filters as a routine infection control measure is not recommended. In the 1970s the *United States Pharmacopeia (USP)*, with input from the National Coordinating Committee on Large Volume Parenterals (NCCLVP), set standard control measures for I.V. fluids. Plain I.V. fluids now have strict guidelines for regulating the amount of particulate matter within the solution. This is the rationale behind the Centers for Disease Control (CDC) recommendations regarding final inline filtration.

✎ **Note:** The drugs creating the greatest problem from incomplete dissolution of reconstituted medications, recrystallization of drugs, and precipitates from incompatible mixtures (Gurevich, 1984) are:

Penicillin G
Potassium
Cephalothin sodium
Ampicillin sodium
Mannitol
Drugs manufactured by the "dry-fill" process

Intravenous Set Saver

This inline set extends the set life and protection from inadvertent microbial, endotoxin, air, and particulate contamination up to 96 hours. Manufactured by Pall Biomedical Products Corporation, Glenn Cove, NY, this filter can also be added to central lines owing to its high flow rate and capacity. This set also has the capability of retaining endotoxin molecules up to 96 hours (Pall Biomedical Corporation, 1990).

Table 6–6 ☐ **OPTIMAL FILTER CHARACTERISTICS**

- Automatically vents air
- Retains bacteria, fungi, and endotoxins
- Prevents binding of drugs
- Allows high-gravity flow rates
- Withstands psi pressure of an infusion pump

157

Blood Filters

Standard Clot

Blood administration sets have a standard clot filter of 170 microns and are intended to remove gross clots found in stored blood. These filters do allow the passage of smaller particles called **microaggregates** that are composed of nonviable leukocytes—primarily granulocytes, platelets, and fibrin strands. The microaggregates can cause pulmonary dysfunction when large quantities of stored bank blood are infused.

Microaggregate

A supplementary filter (transfusion filter) can be added to an in-use administration set, permitting infusion of blood; easy replacement of the filter, should clogging occur; and multiple infusion of blood units. The microaggregate blood filters are 20 to 40 microns. Microaggregate filters are added to blood administration sets for delivery of whole blood and packed red cells stored more than 4 days to eliminate microaggregates.

Leukocyte Removal

Leukocyte-removal blood filters are used to remove leukocytes from the red blood cells and the platelets. Leukocyte-removal filters are classified according to the number of cells left in the bag after filtration. The filters contain several microporous fiber layers that remove microaggregates, clots, and debris in addition to the adsorption of the leukocytes to the surface of the filter (Pall, 1990). Depletion of white blood cells is significant to the reduction of febrile reactions to transfusions of red blood cells (Falchuk, Peterson, & McNeil, 1985) (Fig. 6–14).

INFUSION REGULATION DEVICES

Infusion regulation devices have come a long way since their introduction in 1958. The very early models had serious accuracy and safety problems: air embolisms, fluid containers running dry, and clogged catheters were common. The pumps, which were large and hard to troubleshoot, were limited in their reliability and usability.

IVAC Corporation introduced the concept of the rate controller in 1972. Today many models and types are available. There are various gravity-control devices, volumetric pumps, peristaltic pumps, syringe pumps, and recently small portable units for home care.

Controllers

Nonvolumetric

Nonvolumetric controllers (Fig. 6–15) operate strictly on gravity flow. The gravity flow of fluid is regulated by a drop sensor and electric feedback mecha-

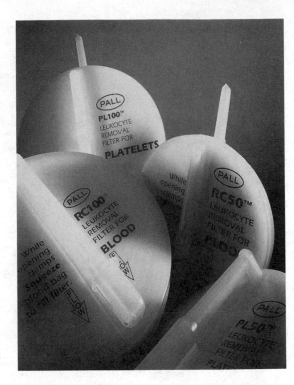

Figure 6–14 □ Microaggregate, platelet, and leukocyte removal filters. (Courtesy of Pall Biomedical Products Corporation, East Hills, New York.)

nism. Controllers reduce the potential for rapid infusion of large amounts of solution (runaways) and empty bottles. Controllers assist the nurse in detecting infiltrations and maintaining accurate flow rates. It is estimated that 80 percent of I.V. fluid and drug administration can safely be regulated by the use of a controller.

✎ **Note:** The maximum flow rate is affected by how high the I.V. container is hung above the I.V. site (Millam, 1990).

The I.V. bag is usually hung 36 in above a patient's head for adequate gravity pressure. When there is resistance to the flow, the controller's alarm will sound, signaling that it cannot maintain the preset rate. Resistance will trip alarms, such as when the patient is restless and frequently changing positions, when the catheter tip is at a flexion point, or when the patient lies on the tubing.

Volumetric

Some controllers and pumps have a linear peristaltic mechanism that squeezes the I.V. tubing. Blood and packed cells should not be given through a controller because the squeezing can damage cells. Most controllers use standard administration sets.

159

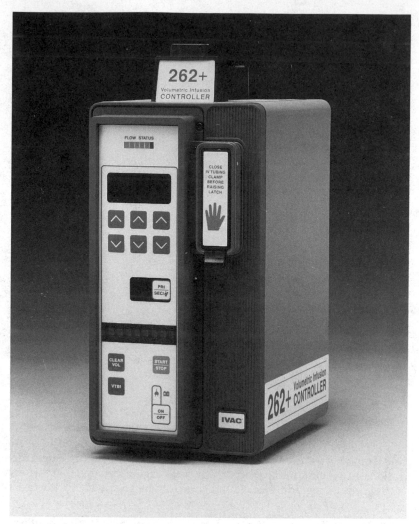

Figure 6-15 ☐ 262+ Controller. (Courtesy of IVAC Corporation, San Diego, California.)

GENERAL INFORMATION ON CONTROLLERS
Rate range: 1 to 99 drops/minute
Increments: Drops
Accuracy: ±2 percent
Maximum occlusion pressure: Gravity
Battery life: 4 to 10 hours
KVO when I.V. complete: Not applicable
Displays: Vary: general alarm indicators, flow alarms, battery alarm, oc-
    clusion, or low-flow alarms

Pumps

Volumetric

An I.V. infusion pump is a device for automatic delivery of fluids at a preselected rate. Pumps are more precise than controllers and have additional features for keeping track of fluid amounts and sounding alarms for various malfunctions. Pumps totally control the flow rate. They usually operate at a pressure of 1.3 pounds per square inch (psi) but can reach an occlusion pressure of 4 to 25 psi. This exceeds normal venous pressure of 0 to 0.4 psi (Engler & Engler, 1986). However, if resistance develops, the pump will exert positive pressure only high enough to overcome the resistance and will not exceed preset limits, which is called the occlusion pressure.

Many nurses prefer the pumps because they are more accurate and have fewer nuisance alarms. Infusion pumps have proved invaluable in neonatal, pediatric, and adult intensive care units, where critical infusions of small volumes of fluid or doses of high-potency drugs are indicated. Volumetric pumps have a cartridge that pumps the solution to be delivered; therefore, blood and red blood cells can be administered without damage to the blood cells.

Many of the pumps use microprocessor technology for a more compact unit and for easier troubleshooting. *Most volumetric pumps require special tubing* (Fig. 6–16).

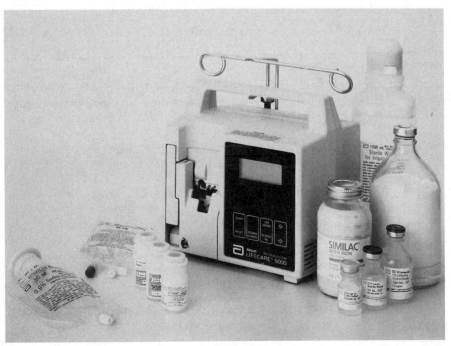

Figure 6–16 ☐ Lifecare 5000 Plum Pump. (Courtesy of Abbott Laboratories, Hospital Products Division, Abbott Park, Illinois.)

Note: Reading the literature, familiarizing oneself with the pump, and observing all precautions are imperative measures to ensure safe, efficient operation.

GENERAL INFORMATION ON VOLUMETRIC PUMPS
Range rate: 1 to 999 mL/hour
Increments: 1 mL
Accuracy: ±2 percent
Maximum occlusion pressure: Varies with manufacturer, 4 to 15 psi
Battery life: Average is 8 hours
KVO when I.V. complete: 1 to 4 mL/hour
Displays: Vary: volume infused, dose delivered, alarm messages (battery low, dose complete), KVO, flow detector, occlusion, malfunction
Alarm indicators: Door open, back pressure, empty bag/air, I.V. complete

Peristaltic

"Peristaltic" refers to the controlling mechanisms: a peristaltic device moves fluid by intermittently squeezing the I.V. tubing. The device may be rotary or linear. In a rotary peristaltic device, a rotating disk or series of rollers compresses the tubing along a curved or semicircular chamber, propelling the fluid when pressure is released. In a linear device, one or more projections intermittently press the I.V. tubing. Hemolysis of cellular blood components can occur when they are infused through a peristaltic pump. However, many newer pumps can deliver cellular blood components, so be sure to check manufacturers' recommendations before using any rate control device.

✎ **Note:** Peristaltic pumps are used primarily for infusion of enteral feedings.

Syringe

Syringe pumps provide precise infusion by controlling the rate by drive speed and syringe size, thus eliminating the variables of the drop rate. Syringe pumps are valuable for critical infusions of small doses of high-potency drugs.

GENERAL INFORMATION ON SYRINGE PUMPS
Rate range: 0.1 to 99.9 mL/hour 5- to 60-mL syringe)
Increments: 0.1 mL
Maximum occlusion pressure: Varies with manufacturer
Battery life: Varies
KVO when I.V. complete: 1 to 4 mL/hour
Displays: Vary

Advanced Systems

The technology related to types of infusion devices is rapidly changing. Patient needs dictate the complicated systems now on the market, a few of which are described here.

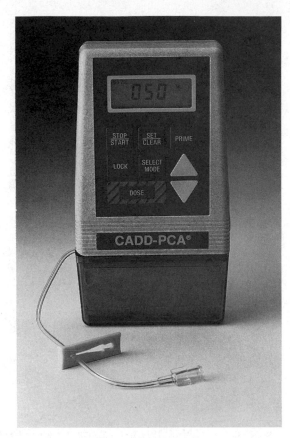

Figure 6–17 □ Portable infusion pump CADD-PCA. (Courtesy of Pharmacia Deltec Inc., St. Paul, Minnesota.)

Disposable Elastomeric Infusion Systems for I.V. Therapy

This system is a portable device designed with an elastomeric reservoir. When the reservoir is filled, it exerts positive pressure to administer the medication with an integrated flow restrictor that controls the flow rate. This system requires no batteries or electronic programming. It is designed for use with chemotherapy, antibiotics, and pain medications.

Implantable Pumps

There has been a sudden surge of implantable infusion pumps because of their convenience and reliability. They are now used to deliver morphine and other pain medications to patients with chronic pain. These pumps can infuse 1 to 6 mL/day.

Portable Pumps

Lightweight, compact infusion pumps have made a significant breakthrough in long-term care. Verifuse by Block Medical is a portable pump that operates

163

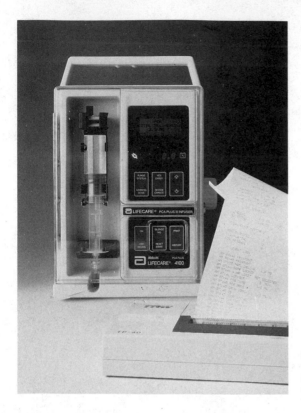

Figure 6–18 ☐ PCA Plus II infuser pump. (Courtesy of Abbott Laboratories, Hospital Products Division, Abbott Park, Illinois.)

by bar codes. This type of pump delivers medication in small doses set manually by the nurse or patient. The patient wears the pump all the time, either on a belt or in a pocket. The pump consists of a syringe or minibag. The battery life depends on the rate of infusion. Figure 6–17 is an example of a portable infusion pump.

Multichannel Fluid and Drug Delivery Systems

Today a major ICU and surgery challenge is multiple fluid and drug administration. Two or three simultaneous infusions may occur. Frequently, cardiac patients and patients who require multiple inotropes, vasodilators, and dysrhythmics receive four or more infusions. Multichannel pumps provide accurate precise delivery while conserving space and simplifying the patient environment. For this reason multichannel devices can be used with a single common infusion tubing from device to patient, decreasing the opportunity for entanglement and mislabeling. Multichannel systems decrease drug compatibility issues and have multifunction capabilities.

Several manufacturers have dual-channel pumps Flo-Gard 6300 (Baxter Healthcare Corporation) and Gemini PC2 Volumetric Pump Controller (IMED Corporation). Three-channel pumps Minimed Ill Infusion system (Siemens Life Support Systems) are also available. Intelliject I.V. Drug Delivery System (Intelligent Medicine, Englewood, CO) is a portable programmable drug infusion system that administers up to four drugs automatically through a single I.V. line.

NURSING CONSIDERATIONS WHEN WORKING WITH PUMPS OR CONTROLLERS

- Peristaltic regulators repeatedly pinch the I.V. tubing and are not appropriate for administration of blood.
- The administration set's drip chamber must be only half full to allow the sensor to monitor the drip accurately; most drip sensors are placed at the top of the chamber.
- Tubing cassettes should be inverted for priming.
- Rate regulation devices do not take the place of nursing assessment but rather verify accurate functioning of the machine at regular intervals. All solutions should be additionally labeled with a flow strip.
- In linear peristaltic devices, polyvinylchloride (PVC) tubing that is in contact with projections may need to be moved slightly every 8 hours.
- Piggyback administration sets increase the risk of introducing air bubbles, so these should be added inline above the air detector.
- Check the package instruction to find out if a filter can be used with a pump or controller.
- Peristaltic throbbing in some infusion lines may cause ECG artifacts. Check this by observing whether there is any change in the ECG when the regulator is stopped.

Patient-Controlled Analgesia

Infusion devices have been developed to assist the patient in control of pain. These patient-controlled analgesia (PCA) pumps can be used at home or in the hospital, usually for delivery of pain medication. They are different from other infusion devices in that they have a remote control bolus mechanism. The patient or nurse can deliver a bolus of medication at set intervals. The PCA pumps in today's market are ambulatory or pole mount models (Fig. 6–18).

GENERAL INFORMATION ON PCA PUMPS
Rate range: 250 mL/hour
Increments: 0.1 mL/hour
KVO rate: 0.1 mL/hour
Programmable concentration: 0.1 mg/mL to 1000 mg/mL
Weight: 400 g (14 oz including batteries)
Alarms: Vary: air-inline, low reservoir, low battery, end of infusion, overuse of prime, occlusion, latch open, cartridge improperly inserted

ACCESSORY EQUIPMENT

Fluid Warmers

These fluid warmers are used primarily for the administration of blood to prevent stress of the cardiac systems, as well as to diminish hypothermia in multiple transfusions. Several companies have devised units consisting of blood-

165

warming coils that are placed in warm-water baths. Warming devices must undergo careful and continuing quality control procedures. Standard blood tubing connected to the coils is usually needed (Plumer & Cosentino, 1987, p 148). The blood tubing must never be placed directly into warm water.

Devices: Latex Resealable Locks

These capped resealable latex diaphragms (Fig. 6–19) may have a Luer lock or Luer slip connection. They convert a continuous I.V. infusion device to an intermittent device by inserting a plug into the cannula **hub**. These devices are used for saline or heparin flush. One disadvantage is that the locking devices can separate at the hub or plug junction, allowing bacteria to enter the system. Another disadvantage is that an occlusion or blood clot can occur within the locking device.

Intravenous Loops

A J- or U-shaped device may be used at the injection site to turn the tubing in a different direction. This is useful in home I.V. therapy. The disadvantages of I.V. loops are that they can increase cost and add a site for bacteria to enter the system.

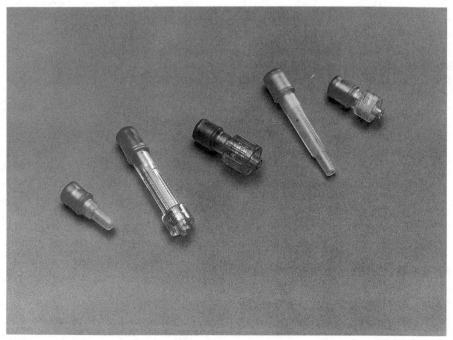

Figure 6–19 ☐ PRN adapters (Courtesy of Becton Dickinson, Deseret Division, Sandy, Utah.)

Microbore Extension Tubing

These add-on sets are available in various lengths to add I.V. line for active patients. The extension sets aid in tubing changes without site manipulation. These are frequently used as primary tubing for syringe pumps and ambulatory pumps. Their disadvantage is that when extension tubing is connected to a primary set, costs increase and another site is added for bacteria to enter the system.

Needle Protector Systems

The Occupational Safety and Health Administration (OSHA) Final Blood-borne Pathogens Standard (1992) has had a large impact on the delivery of I.V. medications. Owing to needle-stick injury risks in the health care delivery system, many companies are developing protection devices. The products available include needle recapping devices, needle sheaths, blunt needle/injection ports, and needleless systems.

The needle protection system covers the needle and protects against accidental needle sticks while sampling blood and administering I.V. push medications and intermittent I.V. medications, as well as during other catheter access procedures.

The needle-free access systems (Fig. 6–20) have also entered the market and provide alternatives to needles to perform medical procedures.

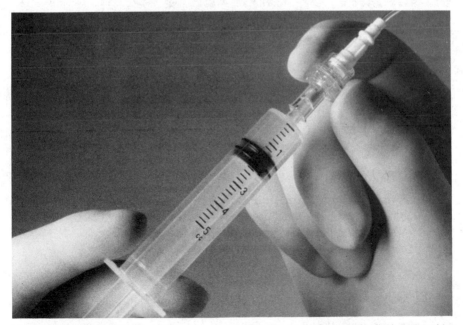

Figure 6–20 ☐ Safsite Needle-Free Access System. (Courtesy of Burron Medical, Inc., Bethlehem, Pennsylvania.)

Disposable syringes: Becton-Dickinson Safety Lock Syringe, Becton-Dickinson and Company, Rutherford, NJ.

I.V. Tubing needle assembly devices: Safsite Needle-free I.V. Access System, Burron Medical, Inc., Bethlehem, PA.

Baxter Protective Needle Lock, Baxter Healthcare Corporation, Deerfield, IL.

InterLink, I.V. Access System, Baxter Healthcare Corporation, Deerfield, IL.

ICU Click-Lock, ICU Medical, Inc., Mission Viejo, CA.

For a complete list of safer medical devices write to: SEIU Health and Safety Department, 1313 L Street, NW, Washington, DC 20005.

The Safsite Needleless System (Burron Medical, Inc) is a two-way valve used in place of a male adaptor cap on a **heparin-locked** I.V. catheter. The valve is opened when accessed by a syringe or tubing. The luer taper on the syringe or tubing opens the valve diaphragm and allows for infusion or aspiration of fluids. The diaphragm closes when the syringe or tubing is removed.

ADVANTAGES TO THE SAFSITE (BURRON MEDICAL, INC.) NEEDLELESS SYSTEM

✓ No needle to recap or remove
✓ Valve facilitates line use
✓ Valve protects patient
✓ Valve protects nurse
✓ No needle disposal necessary

SUMMARY OF CHAPTER 6

EQUIPMENT

Infusate Systems

Open glass
Closed glass
Plastic

Administration Sets

1. **Primary (Standard):** Vented or nonvented (vented used for closed glass)
2. **Secondary (Intermittent):** Piggyback

Key Parts to Administration Sets

Spike/piercing pin
Flange
Drop orifice
Drip chamber

Tubing (long for primary; short for secondary)
Clamp
Injection ports (primary sets only)

Volume-control sets have a calibrated chamber within a primary set.

Blood Sets

Y or straight
Built-in, 170-micron filter

Peripheral Infusion Devices

1. **Scalp vein needles:** Used for short-term therapy
2. **Over-the-needle catheters:** Used for long-term peripheral therapy; composed of Teflon, vialon, or aquavene
3. **Inside-the-needle catheters:** Rarely used today; catheter is threaded through large-bore needle

Central Infusion Devices

1. **PICC:** Inserted peripherally and threaded to midclavicular or superior vena cava site; considered centrally placed. Used for therapy lasting no more than 3 months. Physicians, nurses, and nurse practitioners can insert.
2. **Hickman-Broviac catheter:** Long-term indwelling catheter placed surgically and tunneled into place with a Dacron cuff. Physicians only may insert.
3. **Groshong catheter:** Long-term indwelling catheter placed surgically and tunneled. Has two-way valve at end to prevent blood return.

Filters

Membrane screen filters: 0.22-micron filter is air-venting as well as bacteria-retentive filter.

Optimal Filter Characteristics

- Automatically vents air
- Retains bacteria, fungi, and endotoxins
- Is nonbinding to drugs
- Allows high-gravity flow rates
- Is pressure tolerant to withstand the psi of the infusion pump

169

Blood Filters

1. **Microaggregate:** This supplemental filter can be added to an in-use blood administration set, thereby permitting infusion of blood and easy replacement of the filter for delivery of multiple units.
2. **Leukocyte-poor:** This filter is used to remove leukocytes from red blood cells.

Regulation Devices

1. **Controller:** Used in 80 percent of situations requiring rate-control device; is gravity dependent. Most models are nonvolumetric although a few volumetric types are available with peristaltic action. Calibrated in drops per minute.
2. **Volumetric pumps:** Calibrated in mL per hour, these pumps require a special cassette or cartridge to be used with the machine. Very accurate, used in delivery of high-potency drugs or when accuracy is imperative.
3. **Peristaltic pumps:** Calibrated in mL per hour, these pumps are used primarily for delivery of enteral feedings; they use a rotary disk or rollers to compress tubing.

Patient-Controlled Analgesia

PCA pumps are designed for delivery of pain medication at certain intervals. The patient, nurse, or significant other uses a remote control bolus device to administer the medication when he or she chooses. PCA pumps are available in the bedside pole mount and as small ambulatory pumps.

Accessory Equipment

1. **Fluid warmers:** Used for warming blood; coils attach to blood set; blood circulates through warm water via the coil tubing.
2. **prn device:** Accessory that attaches to hub of catheter and converts the cannula to an intermittent device, usually with a Luer lock or Luer slip connection. Also referred to as saline or heparin locks.
3. **I.V. loop:** May be a J or U loop, connected to hub of catheter to turn tubing in different direction. Often attached to catheter placed in patient's hand.
4. **Extension tubing:** Add-on set to extend tubing.
5. **Needle protector system:** New devices to protect against needle sticks.

Activity Journal

1. You are asked to set up an I.V. piggyback of 100 mL of 5% dextrose and water and 20 mEq of KCl. What type of rate-regulation device would you use?

2. In setting up the regulation infusion device for the potassium piggyback, you find that the facility in which you are working uses a regulation pump you have never used. What are your options for solving this problem?

3. At the beginning of your shift you walk into a room to check on a unit of packed cells. You find the packed cells being pumped via a volumetric pump and the bag of packed cells placed in a wash basin of warm water. Is the rate-control device appropriate for the administration of blood? Is the warm-water bath appropriate?

4. You are asked to add an inline (0.22-micron) filter to an I.V. line that is connected to an infusion pump. What do you have to do before adding the filter?

5. The skilled nursing facility where you work uses a closed glass system for delivery of I.V. fluids. What type of administration set must you use?

Quality Assessment Model

Instructions: Use this quality assessment model to conduct retrospective audits of charts, establish quality control standards, or develop outcome criteria for quality assurance. Refer to Chapter 2 for details on quality assessment.

STRUCTURE

(Resources that affect outcome)
Material Resource: Equipment
↓

PROCESS

(Actual giving and receiving of care)
Therapist activities related to quality and integrity of equipment are:

1. To change primary tubing every 48 to 72 hours, based on agency policy.
2. To check infusate containers for clarity, integrity, and expiration dates.
3. To check cannula for integrity before use.
4. To change intermittent secondary sets every 24 hours, based on standards of care.
5. To use rate-infusion devices following manufacturer's recommended practice.
↓

OUTCOME STANDARDS

(Effects of care)
Documentation will reflect integrity of equipment and standards of practice:

1. Evidence of documented tubing changes according to standards of practice.
2. Evidence of accuracy in flow rates.
3. Evidence of documented use of adjunct equipment to I.V. therapy and its appropriate use according to agency policy and procedure.

Post-test, Chapter 6

Match the definition in column 2 to the correct term in column 1.

Column 1

1. _____ Filter
2. _____ Drip chamber
3. _____ Infusate
4. _____ Lumen
5. _____ Hub
6. _____ Microdrip
7. _____ Macrodrip
8. _____ Port
9. _____ Coring
10. _____ Gauge

Column 2

A. A point of entry

B. Size of cannula opening

C. Visible, as well as microscopic particles of rubber dung displaced by the spike during piercing.

D. Porous device used to prevent the passage of undesirable substances.

E. Area of the I.V. tubing usually found under the spike where the solution drips and collects

F. I.V. solution

G. The space within an artery, vein, or catheter

H. Small drop factor—60 drops/mL

I. Standard drop factor ranges from 10 to 20 drops/mL

J. Female connection point of I.V. cannula where tubing or other equipment will attach

11. List the three types of infusate containers.
    A. _____
    B. _____
    C. _____

12. In using a flexible plastic system, which type of administration set should you choose?
    A. Vented
    B. Nonvented
    C. Vented or nonvented; does not matter, as both will work with this system

13. Advantages of the ONC include all except which of the following:
    A. Is patent longer than scalp vein needle
    B. Is radiopaque
    C. Has decreased infiltration risks
    D. Has low incidence of mechanical phlebitis

Match the venous access device in column 1 to its correct description in column 2.

Column 1

14. _____ PICC

15. _____ Hickman

16. _____ Groshong

17. _____ Implanted port

Column 2

A. Long-term catheter inserted surgically via an incision in the deltopectoral groove terminating near the right atrium

B. Surgically implanted catheter with two-way valve adjacent to the closed tip

C. Completely closed system, placed in a subcutaneous pocket, with a self-sealing septum

D. Long-term peripheral catheter, inserted in peripheral vein and threaded to midclavicular or superior vena cava site

18. A 0.22-micron filter should be used when:
   A. An additive has been combined with the solution.
   B. The patient is susceptible to infusion phlebitis.
   C. Infusion is delivered by the central route.
   D. All of the above.

19. The standard blood administration set has a clot filter of _____ microns.
   A. 170
   B. 40
   C. 20
   D. 0.22

20. Microaggregate filters are used for administration of:
   A. Protein solutions
   B. Whole blood and packed cells stored more than 5 days
   C. Isotonic saline solutions
   D. Cryoprecipitate

True-False

21. **T F** Controllers are gravity dependent.

22. **T F** Volumetric pumps require special cassette tubing.

23. **T F** Peristaltic pumps are primarily used for delivery of enteral feedings.

24. **T F** Syringe pumps are useful in delivery of large volumes.

25. **T F** According to INS standards of practice, intermittent administration sets should be changed every 24 hours.

26. Fluid warmers are used primarily for:
   A. Administration of hyperalimentation
   B. Administration of solutions to the pediatric patient
   C. Administration of blood
   D. Administration of solutions to the geriatric patient

27. Locking devices must be monitored every 4 hours and kept patent with:
    A. Saline flushes only
    B. Heparin flushes
    C. Medication administration
    D. Saline or heparin, based on hospital policy and physician preference

28. Needle protector systems are now being marketed to:
    A. Decrease risk of needle-stick injuries
    B. Protect the I.V. line's integrity
    C. Decrease tubing changes
    D. Enable quicker blood draws

29. Disadvantages of glass systems are that they:
    A. Are breakable and difficult to store
    B. React with some solutions and medications
    C. Make it difficult to read fluid levels
    D. May develop leaks

30. INS standards of practice recommend that primary peripheral sets be changed:
    A. Every 48 hours
    B. Every 24 hours
    C. Only when needed

Post-test answers, Chapter 6

1. D	15. A
2. E	16. B
3. F	17. C
4. G	18. D
5. J	19. A
6. H	20. B
7. I	21. T
8. A	22. T
9. C	23. T
10. B	24. F
11. A. Open glass	25. T
B. Closed glass	26. C
C. Plastic	27. D
12. C	28. A
13. D	29. A
14. D	30. A

References

Ausman, R.K. (1984). *Intravascular infusion systems: Principles and practices.* Massachusetts: MTP Press Limited.

Burrows, C.W. (1984). Take a step toward making better I.V. needle selection. *Nursing 84, 12,* 32–34.

Centers for Disease Control. (1981). *Guideline for prevention of intravenous therapy-related infections.* US Department of Health and Human Services, Atlanta, GA.

Chrystal, C. (1985). Selecting an IV tubing system. *Infection Control, 6*(7), 484–485.

Crocker, K.S., Devereaux, G.B., Ashmore, D.L., & Coker, M.H. (1990). Clinical evaluation of elastometric hydrogel peripheral catheters during home infusion therapy. *Journal of Intravenous Nursing, 13*(2), 89–97.

Delaney, C.W., & Lauer, M.L. (1988). *Intravenous therapy: A guide to quality care.* Philadelphia: J.B. Lippincott.

Engler, M.M., & Engler, M.B. (1986). Comparative evaluation of I.V. regulating devices. *Heart and Lung, 15*(3), 262–267.

Falchuk, K.H., Peterson, L., & McNeil, B.J. (1985). Microparticulate-induced phlebitis. *New England Journal of Medicine, 1*(10), 78–81.

Gurevich, I. (1984). I.V. filters: A standard of care. *NITA, 7*(5), 393–396.

Gurevich, I. (1986). Are I.V. in-line filters worth the price? *Nursing 86,* 42–43.

Hadaway, L.C. (1990). A midline alternative to central and peripheral venous access. *Caring Magazine,* 45–50.

Hershey, D.O., Tomford, J.W., & McLaren, C.E. (1984). The natural history of intravenous catheter associated phlebitis. *Arch Internal Medicine, 144,* 1374–1375.

Intravenous Nursing. (1990). *Standards of practice.* Philadelphia: J.B. Lippincott.

Larson, E., Lunche, S., & Tran, J.T. (1984). Correlates of I.V. phlebitis. *National Intravenous Therapy Association, 7,* 203–205.

McKee, J.M., Shell, J.A., Warren, T.A., & Campbell, V.P. (1989). Complications of intravenous therapy: A randomized perspective study — Vialon vs Teflon. *Journal of Intravenous Therapy, 12*(5), 288.

Menlo Care 1989. *Landmark catheters.* Palo Alto: Menlo Care, Inc.

Millam, D.A. (1990). Controlling the flow: Electronic infusion devices. *Nursing 90,* 65–68.

Moorhatch, P., & Chiou, W.L. (1974). Interactions between drugs and plastic intravenous fluid bags. *American Journal of Hospital Pharmacy, 31,* 149–152.

Pall Biomedical Corporation (1990). *Pall PC 50 and RC 100 leukocyte removal filters. Product brochure.* New York: Pall Biomedical Products Corporation.

Plumer, A.L., & Cosentino, F. (1987). *Principles and practices of intravenous therapy.* Boston: Little, Brown.

Stewart, R.D., & Sanislow, G.A. (1961). Silastic intravenous catheter. *New England Journal of Medicine, 265,* 1238–1285.

Bibliography

Beaumont, E. (1987). I.V. infusion pumps. *Nursing Management, 18*(9), 27–32.

Jackson, B.S., Egan, A., & Sullivan, M. (1985). Choosing products: An in-house test of 3 types of clamps. *Nursing Management, 16*(11), 39–43.

Jones, S. (1985). New I.V. catheters that can do it all. *RN, 2,* 20–21.

Koch, P. (1984). What's new in infusion pumps and how they provide more effective I.V. therapy. *Nursing Life, 3,* 54–59.

Koszuta, L.E. (1984). Choosing the right infusion control device for your patient. *Nursing 84 (3),* 55–56.

Nursing Management. (1987). *Infusion system guide.* 95–101.

Ritter, H.T. (1987). Evaluating and selecting general-purpose infusion pumps. *13*(3), 156–161.

Sherman, J.E., & Sherman, R.H. (1989). I.V. therapy that clicks. *Nursing 89, 5,* 50–51.

Steele, J. (1988). *Practical I.V. therapy.* Springhouse, PA: Springhouse Corporation.

Storc, R. (1984). Current concepts in flow ocntrol. *NITA, 7*(5), 517–520.

CHAPTER 7

Techniques for Peripheral Intravenous Therapy

CHAPTER CONTENTS

178

Glossary

Antimicrobial: An agent that destroys or prevents development of microorganisms

Bevel: Slanted edge on opening of a needle or cannula device

Cannula: A hollow tube made of plastic that is used for accessing the vascular system

Distal: Farthest from the heart; farthest from point of attachment (below previous site of cannulation)

Endothelial lining: A thin layer of cells lining the blood vessels and heart

Gauge: Size of a cannula (catheter) opening; gradual measurements of the outside diameter of a cannula (e.g., 14, 16, 18, 20, 22, 24)

Microabrasions: Superficial breaks in skin integrity that may predispose the patient to infection

OSHA: Occupational Safety and Health Administration

Palpation: Examination by touch

Prime: To fill the administration set with infusate for the first time

Proximal: Nearest to the heart; closest point to attachment (*above previous site of cannulation*)

Spike: To insert the administration set into the infusate container

---

LEARNING OBJECTIVES

Upon completion of this chapter, the reader will be able to:

☐ Define the terminology related to peripheral veins.
☐ Recall the anatomy and physiology related to the venous system.
☐ Identify the five tissue structures the therapist must penetrate for a successful venipuncture.
☐ Identify the peripheral veins appropriate for venipuncture.
☐ List the factors affecting site selection.
☐ Document the initiation of intravenous therapy.
☐ Demonstrate the Phillips 15-step approach for initiating intravenous therapy.
☐ List the sites appropriate for labeling.
☐ State the Intravenous Nursing Standards of Practice for site management.
☐ Recall the steps in performing a heparin lock flush.
☐ Describe the advantages and disadvantages of prn locking devices.
☐ Contrast the advantages and disadvantages of saline lock flush versus heparin lock flush.
☐ Identify the use of lidocaine in the initiation of intravenous therapy.
☐ Calculate drops per minute, using varied drop factor tubing.
☐ Determine the nursing diagnosis appropriate for the patient experiencing peripheral intravenous therapy.

Pre-test, Chapter 7

Instructions: The pre-test is to review prior knowledge of the theory related to initiation of intravenous therapy. Each question in the pre-test is based on the learning objectives of the chapter.

1. The three layers of a vein are the:
    A. Tunica center, tunica media, and facia
    B. Tunica intima, tunica media, and tunica adventitia
    C. Tunica intima, epidermis, and dermis

Match the definition in column 2 to the correct term in column 1.

Column 1

2. _____ Cannula

3. _____ Bevel

4. _____ Gauge

5. _____ Proximal

6. _____ Distal

Column 2

A. Farthest from the heart

B. Size of cannula opening

C. Slanted edge on opening of a cannula device

D. Nearest to the heart

E. Catheter

7. A physician's verbal order must be validated by a written order within _____ hours.
   A. 24
   B. 48
   C. 72

8. The first step in heparin flush of a prn device is to:
   A. Flush with sodium chloride
   B. Check for patency of the catheter
   C. Flush with heparin

9. According to the Intravenous Nursing Society standards of practice, intravenous sites should be rotated every _____ hours.
   A. 24
   B. 36
   C. 48
   D. 72

10. What peripheral vein is appropriate for antibiotic therapy?
    A. Cephalic vein
    B. Dorsal metacarpal vein
    C. Digital vein
    D. Median antecubital vein

11. The calculation of drop rate depends on the:
    A. Tubing length
    B. Filter size
    C. Drop factor of tubing
    D. mL/hour

12. Labels should be applied to the:
    A. Catheter site
    B. Tubing
    C. Solution container
    D. All of the above

13. What factors affect site selection?
    A. Type of solution
    B. Condition of vein
    C. Duration of therapy
    D. Presence of disease, shunts, or grafts in extremity
    E. All of the above

14. The purpose of a prn device is to:
    A. Prevent phlebitis
    B. Provide access to vascular system without administration of solutions
    C. Administer solutions at a more rapid rate
    D. Prevent infiltration

ANSWERS TO PRE-TEST, Chapter 7

1. B   2. E   3. C   4. B   5. D   6. A   7. A   8. B   9. C
10. A   11. C   12. D   13. E   14. B

ANATOMY AND PHYSIOLOGY RELATED TO INTRAVENOUS PRACTICE

To perform intravenous (I.V.) therapy as a knowledgeable therapist, the nurse must be cognizant of the anatomy of the skin and veins prior to venipuncture. A review of the anatomy and physiology of the skin and venous system, along with the physiologic response of a vein to heat, cold, and stress, will provide a knowledge base for the clinical specialty of I.V. therapy.

Skin

The skin is the first barrier to a successful venipuncture. Familiarity with skin thickness and consistency at various venipuncture sites aids the practitioner in successful needle sticks (Table 7–1). The skin consists of two main layers—the epidermis and the dermis—overlying the superficial fascia. The epidermis, which is composed of squamous cells that are less sensitive than underlying structures, is the first line of defense against infections. The epidermis is thickest on the palms of the hands and soles of the feet and thinnest on the inner surfaces of the extremities. Thickness varies with age and exposure to the elements, such as wind and sun.

The dermis, a much thicker layer, is located directly below the epidermis. As with the epidermis, the thickness of the dermis varies with age and physical condition. This layer consists of blood vessels, hair follicles, sweat glands, se-

Table 7–1 □ **FIVE LAYERS TO PENETRATE FOR SUCCESSFUL VENIPUNCTURE**

1. Epidermis
2. Dermis
3. Tunica adventitia
4. Tunica media
5. Tunica intima

baceous glands, small muscles, and nerves. The skin being a special sense of touch organ, the dermis reacts quickly to painful stimuli, as well as to temperature changes and pressure sensation. This is the most painful layer during a venipuncture because of the large amount of blood vessels and nerves contained in this sheath.

The fascia lies below the epidermis and dermis and provides a covering for blood vessels. This connective tissue layer varies in thickness and is found over the entire body surface. This superficial tissue layer connects with deeper fascia. The superficial fascia consists of subcutaneous fibroareolar connective tissue.

✎ **Note:** To decrease pain during venipuncture, get quickly through these layers.

✎ **Note:** Any infection in this tissue spreads easily throughout the body. An infection in the superficial fascia is called cellulitis. Use strict aseptic technique for insertion of infusion devices (Channell, 1987).

Venous System

The body transport mechanism is the circulatory system, which has two main subdivisions—the cardiopulmonary and the systemic systems. The systemic circulation, particularly the peripheral veins, is used in I.V. therapy.

The venous system is analogous to the arterial system (Table 7–2). Walls of veins are thinner and less muscular than those of arteries. The wall of a vein is only 10 percent of the total diameter of the vessel, whereas the wall of an artery constitutes 25 percent of the vessel's diameter. Because the vein is thin and less muscular it can distend easily, allowing for storage of large volumes of blood in the veins under low pressure. Approximately 75 percent of the total blood volume is contained in the veins; thus, veins are referred to as capacitance vessels.

Some veins, usually those that transport blood against gravity (e.g., in the lower extremities), have valves. Valves are composed of endothelial leaflets and are one way to prevent the distal reflux of blood. Valves occur at points of branching and have a noticeable bulge (Brunner & Suddarth, 1988, pp 659–661).

Arteries and veins have three layers of tissue that form the wall (Fig. 7–1).

Table 7–2 □ **COMPARISON OF ARTERY AND VEIN**

Artery*	Vein*
Thick walled	Thin walled
25% of arterial wall	10% of vein wall
Valveless	Greater distensibility
Pulsates	Valves present approximately every 3 in

*Has three tissue layers.

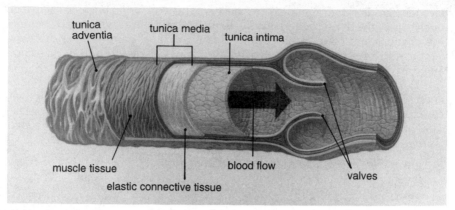

Figure 7–1 □ Anatomy of a vein. (Reprinted by permission of Medical Economics Publishing/ Benjamin Goode.)

Tunica Adventitia

The outermost layer, called the tunica adventitia, consists of connective tissue that surrounds and supports the vessel. Sometimes during venipuncture you can feel a "pop" as the needle enters the tunica adventitia. The blood supply of this layer, which nourishes the tunica media and adventitia layers, is called the vasa vasorum.

Tunica Media

The middle layer, called the tunica media, is composed of muscular and elastic tissue with nerve fibers for vasoconstriction and vasodilation. The middle layer is not as strong and rigid in a vein as it is in an artery, so it tends to collapse or distend as pressure falls or rises. Stimulation by change in temperature or by mechanical or chemical irritation can produce a response in this layer. Cold blood or infusants can produce spasms that impede blood flow and cause pain. Application of heat promotes dilation, which can relieve a spasm or improve blood flow (Plumer & Cosentino, 1987, p 60).

✎ **Note:** During venipuncture, if the tip of the catheter has nicked the tunica adventitia or is placed in the tunica media layer, a small amount of blood will appear in the catheter; however, the catheter will not thread because it is trapped between layers. If you cannot get a steady backflow of blood the needle might be in this layer, so advance the stylet of the cannula slightly before advancing the catheter.

Tunica Intima

The tunica intima is the innermost layer; it has one thin layer of cells which are referred to as the **endothelial lining**. The surface is smooth, allowing blood to flow through vessels easily. Any roughening of this bed of cells during venipuncture, while the catheter is in place, or upon discontinuing the system encourages the process of thrombosis (Chapter 8) whereby cells and platelets adhere to vessel wall.

184

Digital Veins

Location

The digital veins of the hands are located along the lateral and dorsal portions of the fingers.

Catheter Choice

A small-**gauge cannula** (22 gauge) can be inserted and securely anchored in this area—primarily in the thumb.

Considerations

A padded tongue blade can be used to splint the cannula. Only solutions that are isotonic without additives should be used in this location because of the risk of infiltration.

Metacarpal Veins

Location

There are three dorsal metacarpal veins, located on the dorsum of the hand and formed by union of digital veins between the knuckles (Fig. 7–2).

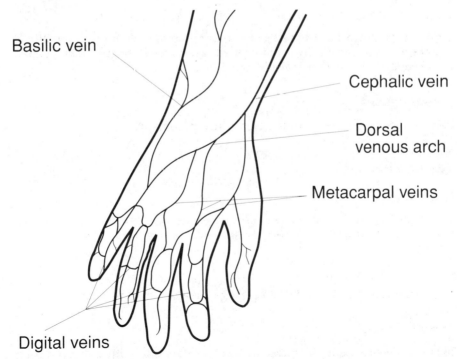

Basilic vein

Cephalic vein

Dorsal venous arch

Metacarpal veins

Digital veins

Figure 7–2 ☐ Superficial veins of the dorsum of the hand. (Courtesy of Becton Dickinson, Deseret Division, Sandy, Utah.)

Catheter Choice

A 20- to 22-gauge cannula is appropriate for these veins. An 18-gauge catheter for blood administration is too large for most metacarpal veins. Use a short 3/4-in or 1-in long cannula for this site. If a longer catheter is used for hand veins the tip placement would end at the joint flexion of the wrist and create difficulty in infusing the solution.

Considerations

This is a good site to begin I.V. therapy in order to place in subsequent venipunctures **proximal** to the last venipuncture. However, if you are infusing antibiotics, potassium chloride, or chemotherapeutic agents, begin therapy in a larger vein in the forearm. Veins in the metacarpal area are too small for chemically irritating agents.

Cephalic Vein

Location

The cephalic vein originates from the metacarpal vein and the radial portion of the lower arm. This network runs along the radial bone of the forearm (Fig. 7–3).

Catheter Choice

Cannulas ranging from 18 to 22 gauge are appropriate for this location. Blood transfusions and chemically irritating medications can be delivered in this vein with reduced risk of chemical phlebitis.

Considerations

Start in the lowest, best site to begin infusion therapy.

Basilic Vein

Location

The basilic vein is formed from the metacarpal veins on the ulnar aspect of the lower arm and runs up the ulnar bone.

Catheter Choice

As for the cephalic vein, 18- to 22-gauge catheters may be used.

Considerations

This vein moves easily; therefore, it must be stabilized with traction during venipuncture. This site is a difficult area in which to perform venipuncture. If

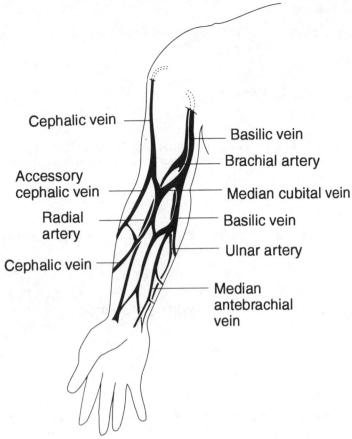

Figure 7 – 3 ☐ Superficial veins of the forearm. (Courtesy of Becton Dickinson, Deseret Division, Sandy, Utah.)

possible, have the patient roll onto the side and place the extremity on the hip for easier access.

Accessory Cephalic Vein

Location

The accessory cephalic vein branches off the cephalic vein along the radial bone. This site does not impair mobility.

Catheter Choice

As for the cephalic vein, 18- to 22-gauge catheters may be used.

Considerations

This site is difficult to palpate in patients with excessive adipose tissue. Vein selection in this area varies from person to person.

Upper Cephalic Vein

Location

The upper cephalic vein is located on the radial aspect of the upper arm, above the elbow. It is an excellent vein to use for long-term therapy with irritating medications.

Catheter Choice

Because of the large size of this vein, all sizes (16 to 20 gauge) may be used.

Considerations

Experience is needed to gain access to this vein, owing to inability to visualize the vein. This site is excellent to use in confused patients who tend to pull at their I.V. sites.

Median Veins

Location

Median veins arise from the palm of the hand. The three veins that extend up the front of the forearm form the median antecubital veins. These veins are well supported in the musculature.

> Median antebrachial
> Median basilic
> Median cubital

Catheter Choice

Catheters from 18 to 22 gauge may be used.

Considerations

The median antebrachial vein is located near many nerve endings and should be avoided. Infiltration occurs easily in this area.

The median basilic vein, located on the ulnar portion of the forearm, is a good site for I.V. therapy.

The median cubital vein is located on the radial side of the forearm. This vein crosses in front of the brachial artery at the antecubital space and is formed from the median antebrachial vein.

Antecubital Veins

Location

The antecubital space, in the bend of the elbow, originates from the palm of the hand.

Catheter Choice

All sizes are acceptable, especially 16 to 18 gauge. This site should be reserved for blood draws for laboratory analysis only, unless in an emergency.

Considerations

This site is usually uncomfortable for the patient, because the arm must extend unnaturally. This area is difficult to splint with an armboard. If this area is accessed in an emergency situation, the site should be changed within 24 hours.

Worksheet No. 1: Fill in Superficial Veins of Upper Extremities

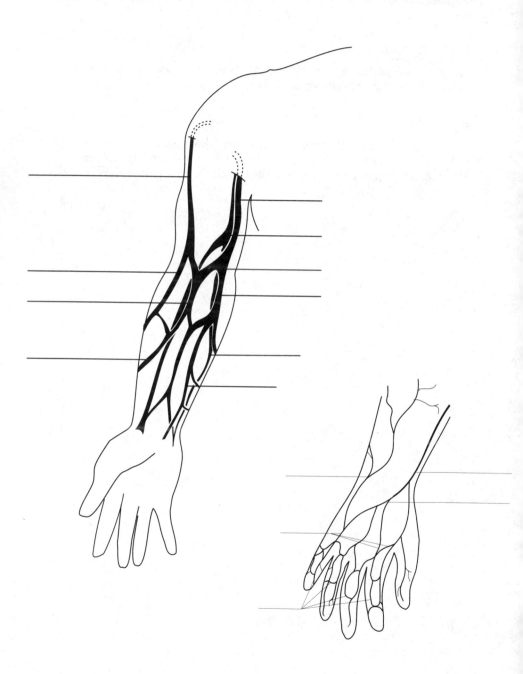

PHILLIPS 15-STEP APPROACH TO VENIPUNCTURE

Precannulation

1. Checking physician's order
2. Handwashing procedure
3. Equipment preparation
4. Patient assessment and psychologic preparation
5. Site selection and vein dilation

Cannulation

6. Needle selection
7. Gloving and site preparation
8. Vein entry, direct versus indirect
9. Catheter stabilization
10. Dressing management

Postcannulation

11. Labeling
12. Equipment disposal
13. Patient instructions
14. Rate calculations
15. Charting

PRECANNULATION

Step 1: Checking Physician's Order

A physician's order is necessary to initiate I.V. therapy. A physician's order should be clear, concise, legible, and complete. The physician's order should include:

Solution
Medication (if an additive is needed)
Dosage
Volume
Rate
Frequency
Route

Verbal orders must be written in the medical record within 24 hours (Hogan, 1986).

Step 2: Handwashing Procedure

Handwashing has been shown to decrease significantly the potential risk of contamination and cross contamination. Touch contamination is a common cause of transfer of pathogens. Soap and water is adequate for handwashing prior to insertion of peripheral cannulas; however, an antiseptic solution containing iodine or chlorhexidine is recommended prior to manipulation of central cannulas. Wash hands for 15 to 20 seconds before equipment preparation and before catheter insertion. Do not apply hand lotion after handwashing (Delaney & Lauer, 1988). The agent that you use for washing affects efficiency. Bar, powdered, leaflet, or liquid soaps that do not contain an antibacterial agent are unacceptable for surgical scrubs (Larson, 1984). Agents recommended for handwashing are antiseptic soaps containing chemicals of:

Iodine
Chlorhexidine

✎ **Note:** Avoid wearing false fingernails, which can increase the number of hand-carried microorganisms (National Intravenous Therapy Association, 1985).

Step 3: Equipment Preparation

Inspect the infusate container at the nurse's station, in the clean utility, or in the medication room. In modern practice two systems are available:

Glass system (open or closed)
Plastic system (rigid or soft)

To check the glass system, hold the container up to the light to inspect for cracks as evidenced by flashes of light. Rotate the container and look for particulate contamination and cloudiness. Inspect the seal and check the expiration date.

✎ **Note:** Glass systems are crystal clear.

In checking a plastic system, squeeze the soft plastic infusate container to assess for breaks in the integrity of the plastic; pinholes are detectable only by squeezing the container. Observe for any particulate contamination and check the expiration date. Plastic systems are not crystal clear. The outer wrap of the soft plastic systems should be dry.

✎ **Note:** All I.V. solutions should be checked against the physician's order.

Selection of Tubing

Tubing sets may be primary or secondary.

Primary Tubing Sets

Long tubing sets with medicinal ports are used for initial therapy. Primary sets are available with vented and nonvented tubing (Fig. 7–4).

Vented

Vented administration sets are needed for closed glass systems because air is required to displace the solution. These sets may be used for all systems.

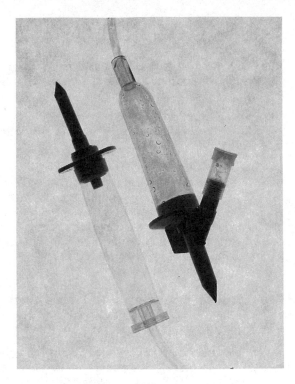

Figure 7–4 ☐ Vented and non-vented sets.

Nonvented

Nonvented administration sets may be used on all containers that have access to displacement of the fluid (e.g., plastic systems by bag collapsing and open glass systems by the straw to outside air).

Secondary Tubing Sets

Secondary tubing sets are short and are used for piggyback medication delivery. This tubing also is available in vented and nonvented sets, and does not have medicinal ports.

Administration sets may have microdrip or macrodrip chambers. Microdrip chambers are used for drip rates of less than 50 mL/hour as with pediatric patients and in medication delivery. Macrodrip tubing, used most frequently, is appropriate for rates higher than 50 mL/hour.

✎ **Note:** It is wise to **spike** the solution container and **prime** the administration set at the nurses' station in order to detect defective equipment.

✎ **Note:** Be sure to choose the correct tubing to match the solution container. Closed glass systems use vented tubing sets only. Plastic or open glass systems may use vented or nonvented sets.

193

Step 4: Patient Assessment and Psychologic Preparation

The first part of patient assessment is to provide privacy. Explain the procedure to the patient to decrease anxiety. Instruct the patient regarding the following:

Purpose of the I.V. therapy
Procedure
What the physician has ordered in the infusate, and why
Limitations

Evaluate the patient's psychologic preparedness for the I.V. by talking with the patient before actually assessing the vein. The therapist should consider aspects such as autonomy, independence, and invasion of personal space when I.V. placement is necessary.

Often the patient has a fear of the pain associated with venipuncture because he or she does not understand the necessity of the therapy (Delaney & Lauer, 1988, p 112).

Step 5: Site Selection and Vein Dilation

Factors Affecting Site Selection

Several factors should be considered before a venipuncture is attempted (Table 7-3). These factors allow the therapist to make a competent choice of location for the infusion. They also represent the therapist's rationale upon which to base sound professional choices.

1. **Type of solution:** Fluids that are hypertonic, more than 340 mOms, such as antibiotics and potassium chloride, are irritating to vein walls. Select a large vein in the forearm to initiate this therapy. Remember to start at the best, lowest vein.
2. **Condition of vein:** A soft, straight vein is the ideal choice for venipuncture. **Palpate** the vein by moving the tips of the fingers down the vein to observe how it refills. Using the dorsal metacarpal veins in elderly patients is a poor choice because blood extravasation (hematoma) occurs more readily in small thin veins. When a patient is hypovolemic, peripheral veins collapse more quickly than larger ones (Plumer, 1987, p 174).

Table 7-3 □ **FACTORS AFFECTING SITE SELECTION**

1. Type of solution
2. Condition of vein
3. Duration of therapy
4. Cannula size
5. Patient age
6. Patient preference
7. Patient activity
8. Presence of disease or prior surgery
9. Presence of shunt or graft

Avoid:

Bruised veins
Red swollen veins
Veins near a previously infected area
Sites near previously discontinued site (Steele, 1988)

3. **Duration of therapy:** Choose a vein that will support I.V. therapy for at least 72 hours. Start at the best, lowest vein. Start at the hand only if a nonirritating solution is being infused. The need for long courses of infusion therapy makes preservation of veins essential. Perform venipuncture **distally** with each subsequent puncture proximal to previous puncture and on alternate arms.

Avoid:

A joint flexion
A vein too small for cannula size

4. **Cannula size:** Hemodilution is important. The gauge of the cannula should be as small as possible. When performing transfusion therapy an 18-gauge catheter is preferred so the cellular portion of blood will not be damaged during infusion.
5. **Patient age:** Infants do not have the accessible sites that older children and adults have owing to increased fat. Veins in the hands, feet, and antecubital region may be the only accessible sites. Veins in the elderly are usually fragile. Approach venipuncture gently and evaluate the need for a tourniquet.

✎ **Note:** Fragile veins can be penetrated with less extravasation of blood if a tourniquet is not used.

6. **Patient preference:** Consider the patient's personal feelings when determining a site for catheter placement. Evaluate the extremities, taking into account the dominant hand.
7. **Patient activity:** Ambulatory patients using crutches or a walker will need cannula placement above the wrist so the hand can still be used.
8. **Presence of disease or prior surgery:** Patients with vascular disease or dehydration may have limited venous access. Avoid phlebitis sites, previously infiltrated sites, or a site of infection. If the patient has a condition with poor vascular venous return, the affected side *must be avoided*; examples include:

Cerebrovascular accident
Mastectomy
Amputation
Orthopedic surgery of hand or arm
Plastic surgery of hand or arm

9. **Presence of shunt or graft:** *Do not* use a patient's hand or arm that has a patent graft or shunt site for dialysis.

Vein Dilation

There are many ways to increase the flow of blood in the upper extremities. Factors affecting the capacity for dilation are:

Blood pressure
Valves
Sclerotic veins
Multiple previous I.V. sites

Ways in which veins can be dilated are:

1. **Gravity:** Position the extremity lower than the heart for several minutes.
2. **Fist clenching:** Instruct the patient to open and close the fist; having him or her squeeze a rubber ball or rolled washcloth works well.
3. **Tapping:** Using thumb and second digit, flick the vein; this releases histamines beneath the skin and causes dilation.
4. **Warm compresses:** Apply warm towels to the extremity for 10 minutes. Do not use a microwave to heat towels; the temperature can become too hot and cause a burn.
5. **Blood pressure cuff:** This is an excellent choice for vein dilation. Pump the cuff up to the point between the systolic and diastolic pressures (e.g., if blood pressure is 120/80, cuff pressure should be 100). This method prevents constriction of the arterial system.
6. **Tourniquet:** A Velcro strap or rubber tubing can be used. Apply the tourniquet 6 to 8 in above the venipuncture site if the blood pressure is within normal range. If the patient is hypertensive, the tourniquet should be placed high on the extremity; occasionally the tourniquet is not needed with severely hypertensive patients. With hypotensive patients, move the tourniquet as close as possible to the venipuncture site without contamination of prepared area.

✎ **Note:** Use the tourniquet only once; using the same tourniquet on multiple patients leads to cross contamination (Intravenous Nursing Society [INS], 1990, S34).

Troubleshooting interventions for difficult veins are listed in Table 7-4.

Table 7-4 □ **TROUBLESHOOTING DIFFICULT VEINS**

Problem	Intervention
Paper-thin transparent skin	Use smallest catheter possible for this type of therapy (preferably 22 gauge); use direct entry; decrease angle of entry to 15 degrees; apply minimal tourniquet pressure
In obese patient, when unable to palpate or see veins	Create a visual image of venous anatomy; select a longer catheter (preferably 2 in)
Vein rolls when venipuncture attempted	Apply traction to vein with thumb during venipuncture; leave tourniquet on to promote venous distention; use a blood pressure cuff for better filling of the vein; use 16- or 18-gauge catheter

CANNULATION

Step 6: Needle Selection

Infusions may be delivered with a plastic or steel cannula (see Chapter 6 for needle choice and sizes). The choice of catheter depends on the purpose of the infusion and the condition and availability of the veins. Catheters are made of polyethylene, Teflon, Silastic, and Vialon. Radiopaque over-the-needle catheters (ONCs) are the state of the art. Most hospitals, clinics, and home care agencies have policies and procedures for selection of catheters. Recommended are:

18 to 20 gauge for infusion of hypertonic solutions or isotonic solutions with additives

18 gauge for blood administration, although 2 U of packed cells may be infused through a 20-gauge ONC.

22 to 24 gauge for pediatric patients

22 gauge for fragile veins in the elderly, if unable to place a 20-gauge catheter

It is recommended to attempt venipuncture twice only because multiple unsuccessful attempts cause unnecessary trauma to the patient and limit vascular access (INS, 1990, S38).

✎ **Note:** When aseptic technique is compromised (as in an emergency situation) the cannula is also considered compromised and a new catheter should be placed within 24 hours (INS, 1990, S37).

Step 7: Gloving and Site Preparation

Gloves must be worn during the venipuncture procedure, and the gloves should be put on at this step. Cleansing the insertion site reduces the potential for infection. The following **antimicrobial** solutions may be used to prepare the cannula site:

Tincture of iodine 1 to 2%
Iodophors (povidone iodine)
70% isopropyl alcohol
Chlorhexidine

In preparing the site use a vigorous circular motion, working from the center outward to a diameter of 2 to 3 in, for *20 seconds*. The solutions should be allowed to air dry. Use 70% alcohol as a defatting agent before applying the povidone iodine (Betadine). If the patient is allergic to iodine, use 70% alcohol with friction for at least *30 seconds*.

Hair removal is not recommended; instead hair should be clipped with scissors. Shaving is not recommended because of the potential for **microabrasions**, which increase the risk of infection (INS, 1990, S35).

✎ **Note:** Aqueous benzalkoniumlike compounds and hexachlorophene should not be used as preparation solutions prior to venipuncture.

197

Step 8: Vein Entry, Direct versus Indirect

Gloves should be in place before venipuncture and kept on until after the cannula is stabilized. Although most practitioners have difficulty working with transparent dressings with gloves on, the gloves can be removed only *after* the risk of exposure to body fluids has been eliminated.

PROCEDURE FOR VENIPUNCTURE
1. Pull skin below puncture site to stabilize the skin and avoid rolling the vein.
2. Grasp flashback chamber.
3. Insert the needle of choice **bevel**-up at a 45-degree angle.
4. Insert the needle using direct or indirect method (see below).
5. When the needle enters the vein, you should get a *steady* backflow of blood, which indicates a successful entry.

✎ **Note:** Remember, the catheter is shorter than the needle; therefore, backflow may occur before the catheter tip is fully in the vein.

6. Once the vein is entered, cautiously move the cannula up the lumen, threading it into the vein. Hold the catheter hub with thumb and middle finger and use the index finger to advance the catheter.
7. While the needle (stylet) is still partially inside the catheter, release the tourniquet.
8. Remove the needle.
9. Connect the adaptor on the administration set to the hub of the catheter.

✎ **Note:** Blood may ooze from the catheter, depending on the brand of needle chosen. If there is absence of blood, the catheter may not be placed correctly or may possibly have penetrated the vein wall. If this is the case, remove the catheter and restart with a sterile cannula.

Direct Method: One Step	Indirect Method: Two Step
Appropriate for small gauge needles, fragile hand veins, or rolling veins	Appropriate for all venipunctures
✓ Cannula inserted directly over the vein at a 30- to 45-degree angle	✓ Cannula inserted at a 30- to 45-degree angle to the skin alongside the vein; cannula gently inserted distal to the point where needle will enter vein
✓ All layers of the vein penetrated with one motion	✓ Parallel alignment maintained and cannula advanced through subcutaneous tissue
Increases the chance of hematoma formation	✓ Vein then relocated and angle of cannula decreased and vein entered

✎ **Note:** If the vein has sustained a thorough puncture as evidenced by a hematoma, the catheter should immediately be removed and direct pressure applied to the site.

✎ **Note:** Do not reapply a tourniquet to an extremity immediately after the venipuncture, as a hematoma will form (Plumer & Cosentino, 1987, p 181).

Step 9: Catheter Stabilization

The catheter should be stabilized in a manner that does not interfere with assessment of the site. Stabilization reduces the risk of complications related to I.V. therapy such as phlebitis, infiltration, sepsis, and cannula migration. Junctions should be secured to aid in the reduction of complications (INS, 1990, S39).

There are three methods appropriate for stabilization of the catheter hub. The U method, the H method, and the Chevron method (page 200).

✎ **Note:** On the last piece of tape you apply be sure to include the date, time of insertion, gauge and length of needle or catheter, and your initials.

Step 10: Dressing Management

There are two methods for dressing management. One is the use of a gauze dressing secured with tape; the other is the use of a transparent semipermeable membrane (TSM) dressing (Table 7–5).

1. **Gauze:** A sterile gauze dressing can be applied aseptically with edges secured with tape. Gauze dressings should be changed every 48 hours on peripheral sites or when integrity of the dressing is compromised.
2. **TSM:** These transparent dressings should be applied aseptically and changed every 48 to 72 hours, depending on the standard of practice within the facility. The dressing and catheter should be replaced together, unless the integrity of the dressing is impaired; then removal of the dressing with replacement of a new sterile TSM dressing is required. Do not use ointment of any kind under a TSM dressing. Adhesive-coated semipermeable film is available from many manufacturers. The TSM dressing should be applied only to the cannula hub and wings.

ADVANTAGES OF TSM DRESSINGS
Continuous observation of site
Effective protection against infection
Cost-effectiveness (Byers, 1985; Katich, 1985)

✎ **Note:** The use of an adhesive bandage in place of a gauze dressing is *not* recommended because it does not adequately cover and protect the site.

199

U Method	H Method	Chevron Method
Use for Winged Set	**_Use for Winged Set_**	**_Use for All Sets_**
1. Cut three strips of 1/2-in tape. With sticky side up, place one strip under tubing.	1. Cut three strips of 1-in tape.	1. Cover the venipuncture with transparent dressing or 2 × 2 gauze dressing.
2. Bring each side of the tape up, folding it over the wings of the needle. Press it down, parallel to the tubing.	2. Place one strip of tape over each wing, keeping the tape parallel to the needle.	2. Cut a long (5- to 6-in) strip of 1/2-in tape. Place one strip sticky side under hub, parallel to the dressing.
3. Cover venipuncture site with a sterile gauze pad or transparent dressing.	3. Place another strip of tape perpendicular to the first two. Place over the wings to stabilize wings and hub.	3. Cross the end of the tape over the opposite side of the needle so the tape sticks to the patient's skin.
4. Loop the tubing and secure it with a piece of 1-in tape.	4. Cover the venipuncture site with a sterile gauze pad or transparent dressing.	4. Apply a piece of 1-in tape across the wings of the chevron. Loop the tubing and secure with another piece of 1-in tape.

Table 7–5 □ **SUMMARY OF STABILIZATION AND TRANSPARENT DRESSING MANAGEMENT***

1. Cleanse area of any excess moisture after venipuncture before applying tape.
2. Secure cannula hub by stabilization with use of the H-, U-, or chevron method of taping.
3. Center transparent dressing over cannula site and partially over the hub.
4. Press dressing down, sealing catheter site.

*Do not put any tape over the transparent film, as tape causes difficulty in removing the transparent film when the dressing needs to be changed.

POSTCANNULATION

Step 11: Labeling

The I.V. setup should be labeled in three spots. The insertion site, the tubing, and the solution container should be time-stripped.

1. The venipuncture site should be labeled on the side of the transparent dressing or across the hub. Do not place the label over the site, as this obstructs visualization of the site. Include on the label:
   ✓ Date and time
   ✓ Type and length of catheter (e.g., 20-gauge; 1-in)
   ✓ Initials of nurse
2. Label the tubing following agency policy and procedure so that practitioners on subsequent shifts will be aware when the tubing must be changed.

INS RECOMMENDATIONS (INS, 1990, S54)
   ✓ Peripheral and central primary sets should be changed every 48 hours.
   ✓ Peripheral and central secondary sets should be changed every 48 hours.
   ✓ Primary intermittent administration sets should be changed every 24 hours.
   ✓ Administration sets used for total parenteral nutrition (TPN) must be changed every 24 hours.

CENTERS FOR DISEASE CONTROL RECOMMENDATIONS
   ✓ I.V. administration tubing, including piggyback tubing, should be routinely changed every 48 hours (category I).
   ✓ Tubing used for hyperalimentation should be routinely changed every 24 to 48 hours (category II).
   ✓ Tubing should be changed after the administration of blood, blood products, or lipid emulsions (category III) (Centers for Disease Control [CDC], 1981).

201

Note: A study by Maki and colleagues (1987) supported the practice of leaving primary peripheral sets for 72 hours. This is a common standard of practice owing to the understanding that changing catheter, dressing, and tubing together decreases the manipulation of the entire system.

3. Time-strip the solution container with name of the solution, additives, initials of nurse, and the time solution was started. Time strips are used to assess if the solution is on schedule.

Use of Armboards

The practice of using an armboard to stabilize the catheter site is not usually necessary with ONCs. Because frequent patient position changes can cause erratic flow rate, it may be necessary to use a disposable lightweight armboard. The armboard may be covered with a washcloth or a paper cover, usually provided with armboards, to absorb perspiration. Secure the armboard with two to three pieces of double-backed tape to protect the patient's skin. Avoid taping over the site and leave the patient's fingers free for movement (Millam, 1987).

Step 12: Equipment Disposal

Recapping needles increases the risk of needle-stick injuries to the practitioner. Needles and stylets should be disposed of in nonpermeable tamper-proof containers. Needles and stylets should not be recapped, broken, or bent, in accordance with the Occupational Safety and Health Administration (**OSHA**) and the Joint Commission on Accreditation of Healthcare Organizations (JCAHO) (CDC, 1987). After venipuncture is complete, dispose of all paper and plastic equipment in a container suitable for burning.

Step 13: Patient Instructions

After completion of the stabilization, dressing application, and labeling of the I.V. fluid:

✓ Inform the patient of any limitations.
✓ Explain all alarms if an electronic control device is used.
✓ Instruct the patient to call for assistance if the venipuncture site becomes tender or sore, or if redness or swelling develops.
✓ The venipuncture site will be checked frequently by the nurse.

Step 14: Rate Calculations

Nurses now have the advantage of unit dose systems, but situational I.V. therapy requires skilled rate calculation. Because many clinical environments require delivery of I.V. medications or unusual rates, the I.V. therapist must be capable of accurate mathematic calculations. Calculating the proper I.V. rate for medication and solution delivery can be time-intensive for a busy professional individual.

The drop factor is listed on the side, front, or back of the administration package. In calculation of drip rates, one must know two key components before using the formula:

1. Drop factor of the I.V. administration set to be used
2. Amount of solution to be infused over 1 hour

Administration sets are provided as follows:

PRIMARY SETS
    10 drops = 1 mL
    15 drops = 1 mL
    20 drops = 1 mL

} Macrodrip sets

SECONDARY SETS
    10 drops = 1 mL
    15 drops = 1 mL
    20 drops = 1 mL

PEDIATRIC SETS
    60 drops = 1 mL   Microdrip set

BLOOD SETS
    10 drops = 1 mL

✎ **Note:** Be sure to check manufacturer for the correct drop factor (drops/mL).

The physician orders the amount to be infused. There are two ways in which orders are written — in total amount over a specific length of time (e.g., 1000 mL over 8 hours) or in amount to be delivered per hour (e.g., 125 mL/hour).

FORMULA

$$\frac{\text{Drops mL (drop factor)}}{60 \text{ (minutes in an hour)}} \times \text{mL per hour} = \text{Drops minute}$$

The health care provider must calculate the drops per minute under the circumstances when an electronic rate control device is not being used or when an electronic controller is used that does not have a mechanism to dial in mL/hour.

Example

Physician orders are for 125 mL/hour and primary tubing is available that has a drop factor of 15.

Step 1 $\dfrac{15 \times 125 \text{ mL}}{60} = \text{Drops per minute}$

Step 2 $\dfrac{1 \times 125 \text{ mL}}{4} = \dfrac{125}{4} = 31 \text{ drops per minute}$

203

When using microdrip (pediatric tubing) that is 60 drops per mL, the $\frac{60}{60} = 1$, so the drops per minute equal the mL per hour.

Example

The physician orders 35 mL of solution per hour on a 2-year-old girl. You would set up your rate calculation as follows:

Step 1 $\dfrac{60 \times 35 \text{ mL}}{60} = \text{Drops per minute}$

Step 2 $1 \times 35 \text{ mL} = 35$ drops per minute

✎ **Note:** Use the following conversion chart to assist in rate calculation.

Try the practice problems in Worksheet No. 2 to test your comprehension of rate calculation.

CONVERSION CHART: RATE CALCULATION

Order: mL/hour	Drop Factors			
	10 drops/mL	15 drops/mL	20 drops/mL	60 drops/mL
10	2	3	3	10
15	3	4	5	15
20	3	5	7	20
30	5	8	10	30
50	8*	13	17	50
75	13	19	25	N/A
80	13	20	27	N/A
100	17	25	33	N/A
120	20	30	40	N/A
125	21	31	42	N/A
150	25	38	50	N/A
166	27	42	55	N/A
175	29	44	58	N/A
200	33	50	67	N/A
250	42	63	83	N/A
300	50	75	100	N/A

*The italicized rates are common in infusion therapy. Microdrip tubing is not appropriate for rates over 50 mL/hour.

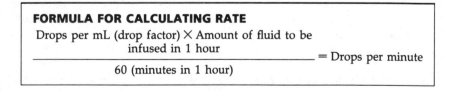

FORMULA FOR CALCULATING RATE

$$\frac{\text{Drops per mL (drop factor)} \times \text{Amount of fluid to be infused in 1 hour}}{60 \text{ (minutes in 1 hour)}} = \text{Drops per minute}$$

Step 15: Charting

Documentation of I.V. therapy usually includes:

Date of insertion
Location

Gauge and length of cannula
Name of person inserting the device

Patient teaching is lacking in most charting audits; therefore, documentation of patient response to the procedure needs to be included in the charting format. This needs to be addressed in narrative charting or in a checkoff format, which includes:

Status of patient
Reason for restart
Procedure
Comments

SUMMARY OF STEPS IN INITIATING INTRAVENOUS THERAPY

PRECANNULATION
1. Check physician order; check all parts of the order for accuracy.
2. Wash hands for 15 to 20 seconds using bactericidal soap.
3. Prepare equipment: check for breaks in integrity and check expiration date. Spike and prime the infusion system.
4. Provide privacy. Explain procedure to patient. Evaluate patient psychologic preparation of I.V. therapy.
5. Selection of site and vein dilation: Assess both arms, keeping in mind the factors for vein selection. Decide whether to use blood pressure cuff or tourniquet for dilation. Use other methods for venous distension, such as warm packs, gravity, and tapping, if necessary.

CANNULATION
6. Needle selection: choose appropriate catheter for duration of infusion and type of infusate, based on facility policy and procedure. Rewash hands.
7. Glove. Prepare site by using 70% alcohol to cleanse site, followed by a 20-second scrub with povidone iodine. Leave the povidone iodine to air dry. Do not remove. If patient is allergic to iodine, substitute alcohol in a 30-second vigorous scrub. Do not retouch. Put on gloves before venipuncture.
8. Insert ONC via the direct or indirect method. Thread the catheter while removing the stylet needle. Connect the catheter hub to I.V. tubing or insert a locking (prn) device.
9. Stabilize the catheter hub with the chevron taping method.
10. Dressing management:

    Gauze: 2 × 2 gauze with all edges taped; change every 48 hours
    TSM: Transparent film applied with aseptic technique and changed every 48 to 72 hours or if integrity of dressing is compromised

POSTCANNULATION
11. Labeling of insertion site with cannula size, date, time, and initials; labeling of the tubing with date, and time-stripping of the solution.
12. Equipment disposal: Use OSHA and JCAHO standards for needle disposal.

13. Patient instructions: Explain to patients their limitations, equipment in use, and observations of the site.
14. Rate calculations: If a roller clamp or electronic controller is used, the drops per minute will need to be calculated based on the drop factor.
15. Charting: Document the procedure, how patient tolerated the venipuncture, and patient instructions.

Discontinuation of Intravenous Cannula

I.V. therapy should be discontinued if the integrity of the cannula is compromised or the physician orders therapy to be discontinued.

Procedure

To discontinue therapy:

1. Wear gloves for this procedure.
2. Use a dry 2 × 2 gauze (alcohol stings and promotes bleeding).
3. Loosen the tape and apply loosely the 2 × 2 over the site.
4. Remove the cannula and transparent dressing as one unit, without pressure over the site.
5. Once the catheter is removed, apply direct pressure with the sterile 2 × 2 gauze over site.

An adhesive bandage may be applied to the venipuncture site after bleeding is controlled. Document in the chart the site appearance, how the patient tolerated the procedure, and the intactness of the cannula.

TIPS
✓ A suitable vein should feel relatively smooth and pliable, with valves well spaced.
✓ Veins are difficult to stabilize in a patient who has recently lost weight.
✓ Debilitated patients and those taking corticosteroids will have fragile veins that bruise easily.
✓ Sclerotic veins are common among intravenous drug users.
✓ Sclerotic veins are common in elderly patients.
✓ Patients who receive dialysis usually know which veins are good for venipuncture.
✓ Start with distal veins and work proximally.
✓ Veins that feel bumpy, like running your finger over a cat's tail, are usually thrombosed or extremely valvular.

Worksheet No. 2: Rate Calculations*

1. The physician orders 1000 mL of 5% dextrose and water at 100 mL/hour. You have available 20 drop-factor tubing. Calculate the drops per minute.

2. The physician orders 1000 mL of 5% dextrose and 0.45% sodium chloride at 150 mL/hour. You have available 15 drop-factor tubing. Calculate the drops per minute.

3. The physician orders 250 mL (1 U) of packed cells over 2 hours. Remember, blood tubing is always 10 drop factor. Calculate the drops per minute.

4. The physician orders 45 mL/hour of 0.45% sodium chloride fluid on an 8-month-old baby. Calculate the drops per minute using 60-drop factor administration set.

*Answers to rate calculations are on p. 222.

5. The physician orders 3000 mL of a multiple electrolyte fluid over 24 hours. Calculate the drops per minute using 20 drop-factor tubing.

6. The physician orders 500 mL of whole blood cells to be administered over 4 hours. Calculate the drops per minute using 10-drop factor tubing.

7. The physician orders 500 mL of 5% dextrose/0.25% sodium chloride to be administered at 75 mL/hour. You have available 15 drop-factor tubing.

8. Calculate problem 7 using 20 drop-factor tubing.

9. A physician orders 50 mL/hour of 5% dextrose and water to rehydrate an 85-year-old woman. You assess the patient and find her cardiovascular status compromised. What tubing do you choose? Microdrip or macrodrip, and why? Calculate the drops per minute using 20-drop factor tubing and 60-drop factor tubing.

10. The physician orders a fluid challenge of 250 mL of 0.45% sodium chloride over 45 minutes. You have 20 drop-factor tubing available. Calculate the drops per minute in order to accurately deliver the 250 mL over 45 minutes.

prn DEVICES (LATEX RESEALABLE LOCKS)

Locking devices, available from several companies, are capped resealable latex diaphragms. Originally, heparin locks were used only for pediatric and geriatric patients.

ADVANTAGES
✓ Provide access to the vascular system, allowing for more flexibility than hanging keep vein open (KVO) I.V. fluids
✓ Allow for reduced volume of fluid administered, which can be important in a cardiac patient
✓ Can be used in collection of blood samples for glucose tolerance tests, eliminating multiple puncture sites
✓ Provide access for delivery of emergency medications

DISADVANTAGES
✓ Occlusion or blood clotting within the lock
✓ Possibility of speed shock and damage resulting from drug being too rapidly introduced into the circulation (Turco, 1982)

HEPARIN FLUSH VERSUS SALINE FLUSH

Heparin Lock Flush

Heparin inhibits reactions that lead to blood coagulation and the formation of fibrin clots in vitro and in vivo. Heparin's anticoagulant effect is almost immediate. Heparin acts indirectly by means of a plasma cofactor, thereby neutralizing several activated clotting factors. Because of these properties it can be used therapeutically as a flushing agent.

Current INS recommendation is the use of 1 mL of heparin lock flush solution containing heparin sodium, 10 or 100 U, to maintain patency of indwelling venipuncture devices. This solution is injected into the diaphragm (hub) of the device after each use or every 8 hours if not in use. The procedure for heparin lock flush is presented in Table 7–6.

The use of heparinized saline has been successful for many years and is a recognized standard of practice in the medical community (Cole, 1989).

ADVANTAGES
✓ Reduced risk of phlebitis
✓ Low incidence of side effects when properly used
✓ Low risk of tort liability with heparin flushing practices (Cole, 1989)

The literature contains well-documented studies supporting the use of heparin in small amounts as an effective way to maintain the locking device (Hanson, Grant, & Majors, 1976; Epperson, 1984; Hamilton, Plis, Clay, & Sylvan, 1988).

One dose of heparin solution maintains anticoagulation in the lumen of the prn device for up to 4 hours. Omission of heparin is thought to allow the formation and accumulation of fibrin material within the lumen of the needle or catheter or both, causing loss of patency and leading to the development of phlebitis (INS, 1990, S77).

DISADVANTAGES
✓ Must be used with caution in patients with known hypersensitivity to pork and beef

---

Table 7–6 □ **PROCEDURE FOR HEPARIN LOCK FLUSH***

1. Check patency of lock.
2. Flush lock with 1 mL of saline to clear lock of any bioincompatibility.
3. Administer medication.
4. Flush with saline again to clear lock of any bioincompatibility.
5. Heparinize with 10 to 100 U of heparin in 1 mL of saline to reseal lock.
6. Positive pressure within the lumen of the catheter must be maintained during and after the administration of the flush solution to prevent reflux of blood into the cannula lumen.

*This is the SASH method: saline-administration-saline-heparin.

✓ Has one extra step
✓ Means increased cost to patient (Dunn & Lenihan, 1987)
✓ Complications, including hemorrhage and thrombocytopenia
✓ Has bioincompatibilities

✎ **Note:** Heparinized saline flushing of an intermittent I.V. device is the accepted practice to maintain patency of the devices. It is recommended that the lowest possible concentration of heparin be used (INS, 1990, S77).

Saline Lock Flush

Because of the increase in diagnostic related groups (DRGs), evaluating cost is a factor influencing the choices of practice in today's health care field. Evaluation of saline to maintain heparin locks has been investigated. At present, data supporting the proposition that 0.9% sodium chloride may be as effective as heparinized saline in maintaining patency of intermittent I.V. devices are inconclusive (Cole, 1989). Despite pressures to reduce costs, hospitals legally and ethically should only support policies that benefit, or at least have no adverse effects on, the patient (Cole, 1989).

ADVANTAGES
✓ Fewer steps
✓ Lower cost
✓ Takes 2 minutes for a nurse to administer and document a flush (eliminating two thirds of the flushes per year saves nursing time) (Dunn & Lenihan, 1987).
✓ Epperson study (1984) show no statistically significant difference in the rate of site loss among the patients who received normal saline flushes and those who received heparin flushes

DISADVANTAGES
✓ Further controlled studies in larger numbers of patients needed to confirm results that heparin and saline are equally effective (Epperson, 1984)
✓ Flushing with saline possibly not adequate method for ensuring device patency (clots may be embolized during medication administration or subsequent flushing) (Lawson, 1984).

✎ Positive pressure within the lumen of the catheter must be maintained during and after the administration of the flush solution to prevent reflux of blood into the cannula lumen.

Table 7–7 □ **PROCEDURE FOR SALINE LOCK FLUSH**

1. Check patency of catheter.
2. Flush with 1 mL of 0.9% sodium chloride.
3. Administer medication.
4. Flush with 0.9% sodium chloride, 1 mL.

CONTROVERSIAL PRACTICES

Use of Xylocaine Hydrochloride Prior to Venipuncture

Lidocaine, used in clinical practice since 1948, is one of the safest anesthetics. Lidocaine is an amide that works by stopping impulses at the neural membrane. The anesthetized site is numb to pain, but the patient perceives touch and pressure and control of muscles. The anesthetic becomes effective within 15 to 30 seconds and lasts 30 to 45 minutes (Millam & Warren, 1985).

The use of lidocaine (Xylocaine Hydrochloride) is a simple process. A tuberculin syringe with a 27-gauge needle is used to draw up 0.1 to 0.2 mL of 1% lidocaine. The vein site is selected and the skin prepared after the tourniquet is tightened. The lidocaine is then injected intradermally to the side of the vein. A wheal of lidocaine is injected closely parallel to the vein and directed toward the vein but is not injected into the vein wall. It is also important that the vein be fully dilated, pulled taut by stretching, and stabilized while the local anesthetic is administered.

✎ **Note:** Local anesthetics should not be injected into the vein because of the possibility of an undesirable systemic effect. The local anesthetic will not "freeze" the venipuncture site if it is injected into the vein.

✎ **Note:** INS does not advocate the routine use of lidocaine for insertion of a cannula. INS recognizes this as a controversial practice. Some clinicians believe that lidocaine prior to catheter insertion increases patient comfort and decreases anxiety. However, its use may expose the patient to complications which include, but are not limited to:

> Allergic reaction
> Anaphylaxis
> Inadvertent injection of the drug into the vascular system
> Obliteration of the vein

The nurse must have knowledge of the actions and side effects associated with this medication. A history of previous allergies precludes the administration of lidocaine (INS, 1990, S81).

Use of Nitroglycerine as Topical Agent Prior to Venipuncture

The use of 1 to 2 mg of nitroglycerine rubbed topically into the skin area has been studied as a method to dilate veins before venipuncture. This technique has been studied in Australia by Hecker, Lewis, and Stanley (1983). The study, which needs replication, found that the use of topical Nitrobid distended the veins without the need for other adjuncts such as tapping, swabbing, or clenching the fist. The use of nitroglycerine as a topical agent is currently not advocated by the INS as a method of vein distension (Pauley, 1985).

PHYSICAL ASSESSMENT

Insertion Techniques

The nurse must use a systems approach to assess for problems associated with the insertion of an I.V. line and the maintenance of the infusion. The nursing assessment should include infusion rate, intake and output, and an awareness of agency policy and procedure to prevent complications associated with I.V. therapy (see Chapter 8 for complications). The following body systems should be assessed at the beginning of each shift and as needed to monitor the patient's reactions to infusions. Symptoms listed with each system may indicate problems.

NEUROMUSCULAR
Complaints of pain
Tremors
Paresthesia of the extremities

CARDIOVASCULAR
Bleeding from the site

INTEGUMENTARY
Edema at or near insertion site
Change in skin color
Sensation of heat at or near insertion site
Red line visible above venipuncture site
Bruising around or near insertion site
Tender cordlike vein

NURSING DIAGNOSES RELATED TO INTRAVENOUS INSERTION SITES

1. Anxiety (mild, moderate, or severe) related to threat to or change in health status; misconceptions regarding therapy
2. Fear related to insertion of catheter (fear of "needles")
3. Knowledge deficit related to new procedure and maintaining I.V. therapy
4. Impaired physical mobility related to pain or discomfort resulting from placement and maintenance of I.V. catheter
5. Impaired skin integrity related to I.V. catheter; I.V. solution
6. Pain related to physical trauma (e.g., catheter insertion)
7. Risk of infection related to broken skin or traumatized tissue

---

SUMMARY OF CHAPTER 7

TECHNIQUES FOR PERIPHERAL INTRAVENOUS THERAPY

The first step is an understanding of the anatomy and physiology of the venous system. The five layers in the approach to successful venipuncture are:

Epidermis
Dermis
Tunica adventitia
Tunica media
Tunica intima

A working knowledge of the veins in the hand and forearm is vital so the practitioner can successfully locate an acceptable vein for venipuncture and cannula placement.

The factors affecting vein selection are:

Type of solution
Condition of vein
Duration of therapy
Patient age
Patient preference
Patient activity
Presence of disease or prior surgery
Presence of shunts or grafts

The 15 steps in placing a catheter that can support I.V. therapy for 48 to 72 hours follow.

PRECANNULATION
Step 1: Checking physician's order
Step 2: Handwashing procedure
Step 3: Equipment preparation
Step 4: Patient assessment and psychologic preparation
Step 5: Site selection and vein dilation

CANNULATION
Step 6: Needle selection
Step 7: Gloving and site preparation
Step 8: Vein entry, direct versus indirect
Step 9: Catheter stabilization
Step 10: Dressing management

POSTCANNULATION
Step 11: Labeling
Step 12: Equipment disposal
Step 13: Patient instructions
Step 14: Rate calculations
Step 15: Charting

The choice of using heparin or saline to maintain latex injection ports (locks) is made based on the agency's policies and procedures and the physician's order. Check these before using the heparin or saline lock flush.

HEPARIN LOCK FLUSH
1. Check for patency.
2. Flush lock with sodium chloride, 1 mL.
3. Administer medication.
4. Flush lock with sodium chloride, 1 mL.
5. Inject 1 mL of 10 to 100 U of heparin with positive pressure to fill the lock.
6. Positive pressure within the lumen of the catheter must be maintained during and after the administration of the flush solution to prevent reflux of blood into the cannula lumen.

✎ **Note:** Locks must be flushed every 8 hours if not being used for medication administration.

SALINE LOCK FLUSH

1. Check patency.
2. Flush with 1 mL of 0.9% sodium chloride.
3. Administer medication.
4. Flush with 1 mL of 0.9% sodium chloride.

SUMMARY OF INS GUIDELINES
Cannula replacement every 48 hours
Administration set replacement every 48 hours
Intermittent secondary administration set replacement every 24 hours

✎ **Note:** Standards of practice within the health care system accept the policy of cannula replacement and primary set replacement every 72 hours. (Maki, Botticelli, LeRoy & Thielke, 1987).

Activity Journal

1. Check the policy and procedure manual at your facility to check the procedure for:

   Flushing a prn device:

   Recommendations for tubing changes:

   Recommendations for catheter replacement:

2. Do you feel checking for patency is necessary prior to flush procedure? Why?

3. Check the infusion practices at your facility for correct labeling practices. What did you find?

4. Identify techniques that you have observed that might contribute to contamination of an I.V. site.

Quality Assessment Model

Instructions: Use this quality assessment model to conduct retrospective audits of charts, establish quality control standards, or develop outcome criteria for quality assurance. Refer to Chapter 2 for details on quality assessment.

STRUCTURE

(Resource that affects outcome)
Material Resource: Technical Equipment
↓

PROCESS

(Actual giving and receiving of care)
Therapist activities related to quality and integrity of equipment are:

1. Change primary tubing every 48 to 72 hours based on agency policy.
2. Check solution containers for integrity before administration.
3. Check administration sets for integrity.
4. Change cannula sites every 48 to 72 hours, based on agency policy.
5. Change intermittent secondary sets every 24 hours.
6. Check cannula for manufacturer defects before insertion.
7. Label site, tubing, and solution container with initials, date, and time.
↓

OUTCOME STANDARDS

(Effects of care)
Documentation reflects standards of care for administering peripheral I.V. therapy:

1. Evidence of documented site rotation after 48 or 72 hours, based on agency policy.
2. Evidence of labels in three sites on all I.V. therapy.
3. Evidence of charting consistent with standards of practice per shift.

Post-test, Chapter 7

1. List the five layers that must be penetrated during a venipuncture.

   A. _____

   B. _____

   C. _____

   D. _____

   E. _____

2. List three of the nine factors that affect site selection.

   A. _____

   B. _____

   C. _____

Match the definition in column 2 to the correct term in column 1.

Column 1

3. _____ Antimicrobial

4. _____ Cannula

5. _____ Bevel

6. _____ Priming

7. _____ Spiking

Column 2

A. Hollow tube made of plastic or Teflon to access the vascular system

B. Slanted portion of cannula device

C. Filling the administration set with infusate

D. Inserting the administration set into the infusate container

E. An agent that destroys or prevents development of microorganisms

8. List the five steps in a heparin flush of a prn device.

   A. _____

   B. _____

   C. _____

   D. _____

   E. _____

9. List the 15-step approach in initiating I.V. therapy.

   Precannulation

   Step 1: _____

   Step 2: _____
   (How?)

   Step 3: _____
   (List what to check.)

   Step 4: _____

   Step 5: _____

219

Cannulation

Step 6: _____

Step 7: _____
       (How?)

Step 8: _____

Step 9: _____
       (With what?)

Step 10: _____

Postcannulation

Step 11: _____
       (What three sites?)

Step 12: _____

Step 13: _____

Step 14: _____

Step 15: _____

10. INS Standards of Practice state:

    A. Primary tubing should be changed every _____ hours.

    B. Catheter sites should be changed every _____ hours.

    C. Dressings over venipuncture sites should be changed every _____ hours, or _____ if integrity of site is compromised.

11. State one controversial practice:

    _____

12. Handwashing for _____ to _____ seconds with an antimicrobial soap is recommended before equipment setup and venipuncture.
    A. 10 to 30
    B. 15 to 20
    C. 30 to 60
    D. 45 to 60

13. Labels should be on the:
    A. Catheter site, tubing, and solution container
    B. Tubing, solution container, and chart
    C. Solution container, catheter site, and patient's armband

Answers to Post-test, Chapter 7

1. A. Epidermis
   B. Dermis
   C. Tunica adventitia
   D. Tunica media
   E. Tunica intima
2. A. Type of solution
   B. Condition of vein
   C. Duration of therapy
   D. Cannula size
   E. Patient size
   F. Patient preference
   G. Patient activity
   H. Presence of disease or prior surgery
   I. Presence of shunts or grafts
3. E
4. A
5. B
6. C
7. D
8. A. Check for patency
   B. Flush with saline
   C. Administer medication
   D. Flush with saline
   E. Heparin 10 to 100 U to fill the lock

9. **Precannulation**
   Step 1: Checking physician's order
   Step 2: Washing hands for 15 to 20 seconds with antimicrobial soap.
   Step 3: Preparing equipment: checking for clarity, expiration date, and integrity of glass or plastic
   Step 4: Assessing and psychologically preparing patient
   Step 5: Selecting site and dilating vein

   Cannulation
   Step 6: Selecting needle
   Step 7: Preparing site for 20 seconds with povidone iodine, using circular motion from inside out
   Step 8: Directly or indirectly entering
   Step 9: Stabilizing catheter
   Step 10: Managing dressing

   Postcannulation
   Step 11: Site, tubing, and solution container labeling
   Step 12: Disposing of equipment
   Step 13: Instructing patient
   Step 14: Calculating rate
   Step 15: Charting
10. 48 hours, 48 hours, 48 hours, promptly
11. Use of lidocaine or nitroglycerine ointment before venipuncture
12. B
13. A

Answers to Worksheet #2, Rate Calculations

1. $\dfrac{20 \times 100 \text{ mL}}{60 \text{ minutes}} = \text{drops per minute}$

   $\dfrac{2000 \text{ mL}}{60 \text{ minutes}} = \textbf{33 drops per minute}$

2. $\dfrac{15 \times 150 \text{ mL}}{60 \text{ minutes}} = \text{drops per minute}$

   $\dfrac{2250 \text{ mL}}{60 \text{ minutes}} = \textbf{38 drops per minute}$

3. The first step in this problem is to find out how many mL per hour the patient must receive. Divide the total amount ordered by the number of hours to deliver the fluid.

   250 mL ÷ 2 hours = 125 mL/h

   Then proceed with the formula:

   $\dfrac{10 \times 125 \text{ mL}}{60 \text{ minutes}} = \text{drops per minute}$

   $\dfrac{1250 \text{ mL}}{60 \text{ minutes}} = \textbf{21 drops per minute}$

4. $\dfrac{60 \times 45 \text{ mL}}{60 \text{ minutes}} = \text{drops per minute}$

   $\dfrac{2700 \text{ mL}}{60 \text{ minutes}} = \textbf{45 drops per minute}$

✎ **Note:** When using microdrip or pediatric administration sets, the mL per hour are the same as the drops per minute.

5. In this problem the hourly volume must be determined by dividing the total mL in 24 hours by 24.

   3000 mL ÷ 24 hours = 125 mL/h

   $\dfrac{20 \times 125 \text{ mL}}{60 \text{ minutes}} = \text{drops per minute}$

   $\dfrac{2500 \text{ mL}}{60 \text{ minutes}} = \textbf{42 drops per minute}$

6. In this problem the total whole blood volume, 500 mL, must be divided by the amount of time the infusion will be administered over.

500 mL ÷ by 4 hours = 125 mL/h

$$\frac{10 \times 125 \text{ mL}}{60 \text{ minutes}} = \text{drops per minute}$$

$$\frac{1250 \text{ mL}}{60 \text{ minutes}} = \textbf{21} \text{ drops per minute}$$

7. $\dfrac{15 \times 75 \text{ mL}}{60 \text{ minutes}} = \text{drops per minute}$

$$\frac{1125}{60 \text{ minutes}} = \textbf{19} \text{ drops per minute}$$

8. $\dfrac{20 \times 75 \text{ mL}}{60 \text{ minutes}} = \text{drops per minute}$

$$\frac{1500 \text{ mL}}{60 \text{ minutes}} = \textbf{25} \text{ drops per minute}$$

9. A. $\dfrac{20 \times 50 \text{ mL}}{60 \text{ minutes}} = \text{drops per minute}$

$$\frac{1000}{60 \text{ minutes}} = \textbf{17} \text{ drops per minute}$$

B. $\dfrac{60 \times 50 \text{ mL}}{60 \text{ minutes}} = \text{drops per minute}$

$$\frac{3000 \text{ mL}}{60 \text{ minutes}} = \textbf{50} \text{ drops per minute}$$

10. This is a unique problem in that the amount of time to infuse the fluid is less than 60 minutes. Therefore 45 minutes must be substituted for the 60 minutes in order to work the problem.

$$\frac{20 \times 250 \text{ mL}}{45 \text{ minutes}} = \text{drops per minute}$$

$$\frac{5000}{45 \text{ minutes}} = \textbf{111} \text{ drops per minute}$$

References

Brunner, L.S., & Suddarth, D.S. (1988). *Textbook of medical-surgical nursing* (6th ed.) Philadelphia: J.B. Lippincott.

Byers, P.H. (1986). Comparison of application factors among three brands of transparent semipermeable films for peripheral I.V.'s. *National Intravenous Therapy Association, 8*(4), 315–318.

Centers for Disease Control. (1981). *Guidelines for prevention of intravascular infections.* US Department of Health and Human Services.

Channell, S.R. (1987). *Manual for IV therapy procedures.* Oradell, NJ: Medical Economics Books.

Cole, M.G. (1989). Flushing heparin locks: Is saline flushing really cost effective? *Journal Intravenous Nursing Supplement*, 12(1), S23–S29.

Delaney, C.W., & Lauer, M.L. (1988). *Intravenous therapy—A guide to quality care.* Philadelphia: J.B. Lippincott.

Dunn, D.L., & Lenihan, S.F. (1987). The case of the saline flush. *American Journal of Nursing, 6,* 798–799.

Epperson, E.L. (1984). Efficacy of 0.9% sodium chloride injection with and without heparin for maintaining indwelling intermittent injection sites. *Clinical Pharmacology, 3,* 626–629.

Hamilton, R., Plis, J., Clay, C., & Sylvan, L., (1988). Heparin sodium versus 0.9% sodium chloride injection for maintaining patency of indwelling intermittent infusion devices. *Clinical Pharmacology, 7,* 439–443.

Hanson, R., Grant, A., & Majors, K. (1976). Heparin-lock maintenance with ten units of sodium heparin in one milliliter of normal saline solution. *Surgical Gynecology and Obstetrics, 142,* 373–376.

Hecker, J.F., Lewis, G.B., & Stanley, H. (1983). Nitroglycerine ointment as an aide to venipuncture, *Lancet, 2,* 332–333.

Hogan, G.F. (1986). Signature requirements for drug orders in medical records. *American Journal Hospital Pharmacy, 43*(5), 1152

Intravenous Nursing Society. (1990). *Standards of practice,* Revised. Philadelphia: J.B. Lippincott.

Katich (1985). Local infection of the intravenous-cannula wound associated with transparent dressings. *Journal of Infectious Disease, 151*(5), 971–972.

Larson, E. (1984). Current handwashing issues. *Infection Control, 5*(1), 15–17.

Lawson, M. (1984). The clot thickens. *Nursing Life,* Nov/Dec.

Maki, D.G., Botticelli, J.T., LeRoy, L.L., & Thielke, T.S. (1987). Prospective study of replacing administration sets for intravenous therapy at 48 vs 72 hour intervals. 72 hours is safe and cost effective. *JAMA, 258*(13), 1777–1781.

Millam D.A. (1987). Tips for improving your venipuncture technique. *Nursing 87, 6,* 46–49.

Millam, D.A., & Warren, J. (1985). Using local anesthetic for I.V. insertion: Pro and con. *Nursing Life,* 1.

National Intravenous Therapy Association (editorial). (1985). Infection traced to false fingernails. *JIN, 6*(6), 6.

Pauley, S. (1985). Nitro vein dilation. *National Intravenous Therapy Association, 6*(2), 5.

Plumer & Cosentino, (1987). Principles and Practices of I.V. Therapy. (4th ed.). Boston: Little, Brown.

Steele, J. (1988). *Practical I.V. therapy.* Springhouse, PA: Springhouse Corporation.

Turco, S.J. (1982). Editorial: Heparin locks. *Infusion, 4,* 123–124.

Bibliography

Boykoff, S.L., & Boxwell, J.J. (1988). Six ways to clear the air from an I.V. line. *Nursing 88, 2,* 46–48.

Cyganski, J.M., Donahue, J.M., & Heaton, J.S. (1987). The case for the heparin flush. *American Journal of Nursing, 6,* 796–797.

Newton, G.A. (1988). A better way to chart IV therapy, *RN, 7,* 26–27.

Paduano, M. (1984). Calculate I.V. drip rates with ease. *RN, 47,* 59–60.

Peck, N. (1985). Perfecting your IV therapy techniques. Part I. *Nursing 85, 5,* 36–43.

Peck, N. (1985). Perfecting your IV therapy techniques. Part II. *Nursing 85, 6,* 48–51.

Peck, N. (1985). Perfecting your IV therapy techniques. Part III. *Nursing 85, 7,* 32–35.

Rutala, W.A. (1984). Antiseptics and disinfectants safe and effective? *Infection Control, 5*(4), 215–217.

Schulmeister, L. (1987). A comparison of skin preparation procedures for accessing implanted ports. *National Intravenous Therapy Association, 10*(1), 45–47.

Thompson, D.R., Jowett, N.I., & Folwell, A.M. (1989). A trial of povidone-iodine antiseptic solutions for prevention of cannula related thrombophlebitis. *Journal of Intravenous Therapy, 12*(2), 99–102.

Weinstein, S.M. (1990). Math calculations for intravenous nurses. *Journal of Intravenous Nursing, 13*(4), 231–236.

Winskunas, C.A. (1990). A creative approach to comprehensive IV therapy documentation. *Journal of Intravenous Therapy, 13*(2), 115–118.

CHAPTER 8

Complications of Intravenous Therapy

CHAPTER CONTENTS

PHYSICAL ASSESSMENT

NURSING DIAGNOSES RELATED
  TO COMPLICATIONS OF
  INTRAVENOUS THERAPY

INTRAVENOUS NURSING
  STANDARDS OF PRACTICE
  (1990)

CENTERS FOR DISEASE
  CONTROL

RECOMMENDATIONS, BY
  CATEGORY (1981)

SUMMARY OF CHAPTER 8

ACTIVITY JOURNAL

QUALITY ASSESSMENT MODEL

POST-TEST, CHAPTER 8

Glossary

Circulatory overload: An excess in the extracellular fluid volume.

Colonization: Forming compact groups, or colonies, of the same type of microorganism

Ecchymosis: Bruise; "black-and-blue spot" on the skin caused by escape of blood from injured vessels

Embolism: Sudden obstruction of a blood vessel by a clot or foreign material formed or introduced elsewhere in circulatory system and carried to that point by the bloodstream

Extravasation: Escape of fluid from a vessel into the surrounding tissue

Hematoma: Localized mass of blood outside of the blood vessel, usually found in a partially clotted state

Hemodilution: Increase in the plasma content of the blood, with resulting decrease in the concentration of red blood cells

Infiltration: Process of seepage or diffusion into tissue of intravenous infusate

Phlebitis: Inflammation of the intima of a vein

Septicemia: Systemic disease caused by the presence of pathogenic microorganisms in the body

Speed shock: Systemic reaction that occurs when a substance foreign to the body is rapidly introduced into the circulation

Thrombophlebitis: Inflammation of a vein associated with thrombus formation.

Thrombosis: Formation or presence of a blood clot; venous thrombosis (or phlebemphraxis), arrest of circulation in the vein by a blood clot

Venous spasm: Contraction of the muscular coats of the blood vessels; also called angiospasm

Vesicant: Any agent that produces blisters

LEARNING OBJECTIVES

Upon completion of this chapter, the reader will be able to:

☐ Define terms related to the hazards associated with intravenous therapy.
☐ Differentiate between local and systemic complications.
☐ Identify prompt treatment for each local and systemic complication.
☐ Describe the signs and symptoms for seven local complications.
☐ List three factors that increase the risk of phlebitis.
☐ Identify and rate postinfusion phlebitis using the phlebitis criteria chart.
☐ Compare erratic flow rates as they relate to intravenous therapy.
☐ Identify organisms responsible for most cases of septicemia related to infusion therapy.
☐ Identify prevention techniques for the six systemic complications.
☐ Contrast the recommendations of the Centers for Disease Control against those of the Intravenous Nursing Society Standards for Practice in prevention of complications related to intravenous therapy.
☐ Determine nursing diagnoses appropriate for the patient experiencing complications associated with intravenous therapy.

Pre-test, Chapter 8

Instructions: The pre-test is to review prior knowledge of the theory related to local and systemic complications. Each question in the pre-test is based on the learning objectives of the chapter.
Match the definition in column 2 to the correct term in column 1.

Column 1

1. _____ Colonization
2. _____ Extravasation
3. _____ Phlebitis
4. _____ Septicemia
5. _____ Hematoma

Column 2

A. A localized mass of blood outside of the blood vessel

B. Forming a compact group, or colony, of the same organism

C. Systemic disease caused by the presence of pathogenic microorganisms

D. Inflammation of the intima of a vein

E. Escape of fluid from a vessel into the surrounding tissue

Match the type of complication (local or systemic) in column 2 to the correct complication in column 1.

Column 1

6. _____ Thrombosis
7. _____ Septicemia
8. _____ Speed shock
9. _____ Catheter embolism

Column 2

A. Local

B. Systemic

10. _____ Phlebitis

11. _____ Vasospasm

12. _____ Thrombophlebitis

13. _____ Hematoma

14. The risk of phlebitis is increased in which of the following patient populations?
   A. Patients receiving total parenteral nutrition
   B. Immunosuppressed patients
   C. Patients with burns
   D. Patients who have multiple intravenous manipulations
   E. All of the above

15. The recommended treatment of phlebitis stage 2+ is to:
   A. Discontinue the cannula and apply heat to site
   B. Watch the site and document observations
   C. Leave cannula in place and apply heat to site
   D. Flush cannula with normal saline

16. The first symptom of venous vasospasm is:
   A. Sharp pain extending from the site of infusion
   B. Redness along vein
   C. Increased temperature
   D. Cold feeling in extremity

17. The organism responsible for most cases of septicemia related to infusion is:
   A. *Proteus*
   B. *Escherichia coli*
   C. *Staphylococcus aureus*
   D. *Pseudomonas*

True-False

18. **T F** Intravenous push drugs should be administered over at least 1 minute to prevent speed shock

19. **T F** Use of hypertonic solutions increases the risk of phlebitis.

20. **T F** The phlebitis criteria, according to the Intravenous Nursing Society, have three stages.

21. **T F** To prevent local complication it is necessary to use a good aseptic technique when starting or maintaining an infusion.

ANSWERS TO PRE-TEST, Chapter 8

1. B   2. E   3. D   4. C   5. A   6. A   7. B   8. B   9. B

10. A   11. A   12. A   13. A   14. E   15. A   16. A   17. C

18. T   19. T   20. T   21. T

Since the nursing profession assumed the role of providing intravenous (I.V.) care in the 1940s, a large body of knowledge has been gathered about I.V. therapy. Complications such as embolism, catheter dislodgment or perforation, metabolic imbalance, hypervolemia, and nosocomial infection have been documented. The fact that 80 percent of hospitalized patients receive I.V. fluids and medications puts patients at risk for developing complications associated with this form of therapy (Feldstein, 1986).

LOCAL COMPLICATIONS

Local complications of I.V. therapy occur as adverse reactions or trauma to the surrounding venipuncture site (Table 8 – 1). Local complications are rarely serious. These complications can be recognized early by objective assessment. Assessing and monitoring are the key components in early intervention. Venipuncture technique is the main factor related to the prevention of most local complications associated with I.V. therapy.

Hematoma

The formation of a **hematoma** at the venipuncture site is usually related to nursing venipuncture technique. Patients who bruise easily can develop a hematoma when large cannulas are used to initiate I.V. therapy, owing to trauma to the vein during insertion. Hematomas are most often related to:

1. Nicking the vein during an unsuccessful venipuncture attempt
2. Discontinuing of I.V. cannula or needle without pressure held over site after removal of needle
3. Applying a tourniquet too tightly above a previously attempted venipuncture site

Signs and symptoms of hematoma are:

Discoloration of the skin surrounding the venipuncture (**ecchymosis**)
Site swelling and discomfort

Prevention

Techniques for prevention of hematoma formation include:

1. Use an indirect method for starting an I.V. until technique is perfected for direct needle sticks. This will decrease the chance of piercing

Table 8 – 1 □ **LOCAL COMPLICATIONS**

1. Hematoma
2. Thrombosis
3. Phlebitis: mechanical and chemical
4. Thrombophlebitis
5. Extravasation (infiltration)
6. Local infection
7. Venous spasm

through the vein, causing seepage of blood into the subcutaneous tissue (see Chapter 5 for techniques of venipuncture).

2. Apply the tourniquet just before venipuncture.

Treatment

1. Apply direct pressure with sterile 2 × 2 gauze over site, after catheter or needle is removed.
2. Have patient elevate the extremity over head or on pillow to maximize venous return.

Charting

Chart observable symptoms. Be sure to document the nursing interventions you used for care of the site.

✎ **Note:** For elderly patients, patients on corticosteroids, or patients with paper-thin skin, use a small needle or catheter, preferably 20 or 22 gauge. Use a blood pressure cuff instead of rubber tourniquet to fill the vein so you have better control of the pressure exerted on the vein. Be very gentle in your venipuncture technique.

Thrombosis

Trauma to the endothelial cells of the venous wall causes platelets to adhere to the vein wall and may cause a clot to form. The **thrombosis** usually occludes the circulation of blood. Signs that a thrombus has formed are manifested in changes in flow of the I.V. solution: the drip rate slows, or the line does not flush easily and resistance is felt, especially in a locking device. The I.V. site may appear healthy. In assessing for thrombosis, first, be careful not to propel the clot into the bloodstream with pressure from a syringe, and second, remember that a thrombus within a vein traps bacteria.

The causes of thrombosis formation are:

1. Blood backing up in the system of a hypertensive patient
2. Low flow rate, which limits fluid movement to maintain patency
3. Location of the I.V. cannula (catheters placed in a flexor area may occlude when position is changed)
4. Flow rate obstruction due to patient compressing
5. I.V. line remaining dry for an extended time
6. Cannula traumatizing wall of the vein during venipuncture

Thrombosis, along with thrombophlebitis, can lead to a systemic embolism.

✎ **Note:** The therapist must avoid:

✓ Injuring the vein wall
✓ Multiple punctures
✓ Through-and-through punctures

Prevention

Techniques for the prevention of a thrombosis include:

1. Use pumps and controllers for managing rate control. Rate control devices prevent blood from backing up in the tubing and alarm when the I.V. line is dry.
2. Choose microdrip tubing, 60 drops/mL, when gravity flow I.V. rates are below 50 mL/hour. Remember, more drops means more movement.
3. Avoid flexion areas for placement of I.V. cannulas.

Treatment

1. Discontinue the I.V. and restart the cannula in a new vein.

 Note: In managing an occluded catheter, follow the steps in Table 8–2.

Do not irrigate. Irrigation of an occluded line with saline can propel the clot into the circulatory system and cause an embolism.

Urokinase, a fibrinolytic drug, is being studied to remove occlusions from catheters and maintain patency. One study using urokinase in 1600 occluded central venous catheters had a success rate of 98.6 percent with no adverse reaction reported. Urokinase works by lysing blood clots, but it does not work instantly. Often the urokinase must be left in the catheter 15 minutes or longer

Table 8–2 □ **STEPS IN CHECKING SLOWED INFUSION**

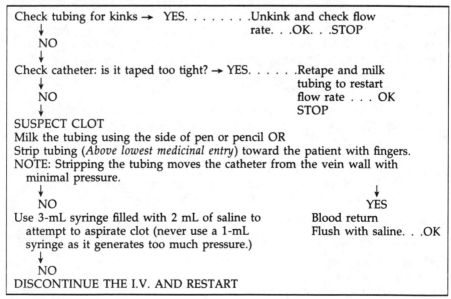

```
Check tubing for kinks → YES. . . . . . .Unkink and check flow
        ↓                          rate. . .OK. . .STOP
       NO
        ↓
Check catheter: is it taped too tight? → YES. . . . . .Retape and milk
        ↓                                    tubing to restart
       NO                                    flow rate . . . OK
        ↓                                    STOP
SUSPECT CLOT
Milk the tubing using the side of pen or pencil OR
Strip tubing (Above lowest medicinal entry) toward the patient with fingers.
NOTE: Stripping the tubing moves the catheter from the vein wall with
  minimal pressure.
        ↓                                         ↓
       NO                                        YES
Use 3-mL syringe filled with 2 mL of saline to     Blood return
  attempt to aspirate clot (never use a 1-mL       Flush with saline. . .OK
  syringe as it generates too much pressure.)
        ↓
       NO
DISCONTINUE THE I.V. AND RESTART
```

before aspirating. Check your hospital protocol for specific directions (Barrus & Danek, 1987).

Charting

Chart the change of infusion rate, the steps taken to solve the problem, and the end result. Be sure to chart the new I.V. site, its patency, and the size of the catheter used for restart. Document appearance of the occluded site.

Phlebitis

Phlebitis is a commonly reported complication of I.V. therapy. The fact that 20 to 80 percent of patients receiving I.V. therapy develop some stage of phlebitis makes this local complication one of the most common hazards associated with over-the-needle catheters (ONCs) in modern practice (Ervin, 1987). Phlebitis is an inflammation of the vein when the endothelial cells of the venous wall become irritated and cells roughen, allowing platelets to adhere and predispose the vein to inflammation-induced phlebitis (Harrigan, 1984). The site is tender to touch and can be very painful. At the first sign of redness or complaint of tenderness, the I.V. site should be checked. This complication can prolong hospitalization unless treated early (Falchuk, Peterson, & McNeil, 1985).

Signs and symptoms associated with phlebitis are:

Redness
Site warm to touch
Local swelling
Palpable cord along the vein
Sluggish infusion rate
Increase in basal temperature

The process of phlebitis formation involves an increase in capillary permeability, which allows proteins and fluids to leak into the interstitial space. The traumatized tissue continues to be irritated mechanically or chemically. The immune system causes leukocytes to gather at the inflamed site. When leukocytes are released, pyrogens stimulate the hypothalamus to raise the body temperature. Pyrogens also stimulate bone marrow to release more leukocytes. Redness and tenderness increase with each step of the phlebitis (Millam, 1988). According to Hecker (1988), when local inflammation was viewed under a microscope, histologic changes were marked, showing a loss of endothelial cells, edema, and presence of neutrophils in the vein wall.

Factors Affecting Phlebitis Formation

Factors that influence the development of phlebitis include but are not limited to:

Insertion techniques
Condition of patient
Vein condition
Compatibility

Table 8-3 □ CRITERIA FOR RATING INFUSION PHLEBITIS

Rating	Signs and Symptoms
1+	Pain at site, erythema and/or edema, no streak, no palpable cord
2+	Pain at site, erythema and/or edema, streak formation, no palpable cord
3+	Pain at site, erythema and/or edema, streak formation, palpable cord

Source: From *Standards of Practice* by the Intravenous Neurology Society, 1990, Philadelphia: J.B. Lippincott Company. Copyright 1990 by J.B. Lippincott Company. Reprinted by permission.

Type and pH of medication or solution
Ineffective filtration
Gauge, size, length, and material of cannula

The phlebitis scale (Table 8-3) is recommended to establish a uniform standard for measuring degrees of phlebitis. This inflammation of the vein is usually because of chemical or mechanical irritation. Risk factors for phlebitis are listed in Table 8-4.

Mechanical irritation of the vein can be attributed to using too large a cannula, in a small vein. The smaller the space used by the cannula, the better. Large veins with thick walls hold up better during an infusion. Veins higher on the forearm are less likely to develop phlebitis. The other cause of mechanical phlebitis is improper taping. The catheter tip rubs the vein wall, damaging the endothelial cells. Manipulation of the catheter during infusion causes irritation of the vein wall. Securely affix catheter hub and tubing, using the chevron method, to prevent wiggling of the catheter.

 Avoid use of hand veins for long-term therapy with antibiotics and potassium infusions.

Chemical irritation is caused by increased acidity of the I.V. fluid. The more acidic the fluid, the greater the risk of chemical phlebitis. The I.V. fluids have a pH range from 3 to 6. This helps prevent solutions from caramelizing during sterilization and maintains stability. Dextrose solutions have a pH of 4.5 or lower, whereas saline solutions have a pH of 5.5. The pH also falls further with storage; in date-expired 5% glucose solutions, pH values of 3.4 have been found (Hecker, 1988). Additives such as vitamin C, Adriamycin, and cimetidine can further decrease the pH. Some drugs, such as heparin with a pH of 5 to 7.5, can raise the pH. Hypertonic fluids having a tonicity of greater than 340,

Table 8-4 □ RISK FACTORS FOR PHLEBITIS

1. Patients receiving total parenteral nutrition
2. Immunosuppressed patients, those with burn wounds, valvular heart disease, cardiac or major orthopedic prosthesis, and neonates.
3. High risk: ICU patients with multiple I.V.s and manipulations; infusions with multiple drug additives

Source: From "Phlebitis, Infections, and Filtration" by P. Jemison-Smith and L.D. Thrupp, 1982, *Journal of Intravenous Therapy, 5,* pp. 328-335. Copyright 1982. Reprinted by permission.

such as 10% dextrose, increase the hazards of phlebitis. An increase in electro-lytes also adds to the tonicity of the solution.

✎ **Note:** Heparin infusions rarely cause phlebitis (Millam, 1988).

Potassium chloride (KCl) is the most common medication added to I.V. fluids (Gong & King, 1983). An association between KCl and infusion phlebitis has been reported. Jones (1982) found that phlebitis developed in 27.2 percent of patients who received continuous infusion of KCl in addition to intermittent medications. Patients who receive greater than 30 mEq of KCl/liter of solution have a greater risk of phlebitis.

Another factor in development of chemical phlebitis is particulate matter in a solution. Longe (1980) demonstrated that there was a mean total of 269 particles in a parenteral fluid containing 40 mEq of KCl. Most particles were 10 to 24 microns and capillaries were approximately 10 to 12 microns in diameter. Hence, a particle larger than that may lodge and lead to occlusion. Addition-ally, increasing exposure of the vein lumen to irritating particles may increase the incidence of infusion phlebitis by as much as 50 to 60 percent (Ervin, 1987). Drug particles that do not fully dissolve during mixing may not be visible to the eye. Use of a 0.22-micron inline or final filter removes not only air and bacteria but also harmful particles from the solution (DeLuca, Rapp, Bivins, McKean, & Griffen, 1975); Jemison-Smith & Thrupp, 1982).

Intermittent infusions with heparin locks cause less irritation to the vein wall over time than do continuous infusions. The slower the rate, the less irri-tating the solution will be to the vein wall, because cells of the vein are exposed for a shorter period of time to solutions with less than normal pH. The fact that heparin is used to maintain the lock might have further significance in the re-duction of phlebitis rates.

Bacterial Phlebitis

Bacterial phlebitis, also referred to as septic phlebitis, can be prevented by pre-paring solutions aseptically under a laminar flow hood. To prevent bacterial phlebitis, all solution containers should be inspected carefully before hanging, in addition to washing hands and preparing skin carefully.

Prevention

Techniques for prevention of phlebitis include:

1. Use larger veins for hypertonic solutions.
2. Use central lines or long-arm catheters for long-term hypertonic solutions.
3. Choose the smallest I.V. catheter appropriate for the infusate.
4. Rotate I.V. site every 72 hours, a practice that has been shown to de-crease risk of phlebitis significantly.
5. Stabilize the catheter to prevent mechanical irritation.
6. Use a 0.22-micron inline final filter, which will remove air and bacteria as well as harmful particulates (Millam, 1988).

The nurse must be aware that:

✓ Phlebitis risk factors in I.V. therapy increase after 24 hours.

Table 8–5 ☐ **FREQUENTLY ADMINISTERED INTRAVENOUS DRUGS, THEIR pH VALUES, AND RECOMMENDED DILUTION RATES**

Drug	pH Range	Minimal Dilution Rate (mL)
Amikacin (Amikin)	4.5	150
Amphotericin B (Fungizone)	5–7	100
Cimetidine (Tagamet)	3.8–6	150
Doxycycline (Vibramycin)	2.6	200
Dopamine (Dopastat)	3.0–4.5	200
Cefazolin (Ancef)	4.5–5.5	150
Gentamicin (Garamycin)	3.0–5.5	150
Morphine	3.0–6.0	150
Nafcillin (Unipen)	6.0–6.5	100
Norepinephrine (Levophed)	3.0–4.5	200

Source: From "A Cost-Effective Guide for the Prevention of Chemical Phlebitis Caused by the pH of Pharmaceutical Agents" by C.A. Harrigan, 1984, *Journal of Intravenous Therapy, 7,* pp. 478–482. Copyright 1984. Adapted by permission.

✓ All peripheral I.V.'s should be changed every 48 to 72 hours.
✓ A 3+ phlebitis takes from 10 days to 3 weeks to heal.
✓ Dextrose solutions, KCl, antibiotics, and vitamin C have a lower pH; patients receiving these are at higher risk for phlebitis (Jones, 1982).

✏ **Note:** Use of inline final filters decreases phlebitis by two thirds, according to *Nurse's Drug Alert* (1985).

Prevention of chemically induced phlebitis presents a problem in I.V. therapy. The use of 0.9% sodium chloride or 5% dextrose and water is usually recommended for admixtures. A study on admixtures and dilution rates by Harrigan (1984) concluded that increasing dilution rates decreased the amount of chemically induced phlebitis. It was also noted that the amount of diluant must be increased when multiple medication therapy is administered. Harrigan suggested diluting irritating drugs in the following manner: drugs with a pH of 5 to 10 should be diluted in 100 mL of solution; drugs with a pH of 3.5 to 6 should be diluted in 150 mL of solution; and drugs with a pH of 2.6 to 5.5 should be diluted in 200 to 250 mL of solution. Refer to Table 8–5 for frequently administered I.V. drugs, their pH values, and recommended dilution rates.

Thrombophlebitis

Thrombophlebitis denotes a twofold injury: thrombosis and inflammation. A painful inflamed vein develops from the point of thrombosis and causes the patient discomfort. The vein becomes progressively hard, tortuous, tender, and painful. Sluggish flow rates accompany the progressive process (Plumer & Cosentino, 1987, p 270). Chemical or mechanical phlebitis can precipitate thrombophlebitis.

✏ **Note:** If the inflammation is the result of bacterial phlebitis, a much more serious condition leading to septicemia may occur if not treated promptly.

Signs and symptoms of thrombophlebitis are:

Sluggish flow rate
Edema in limb
Vein tender and cordlike
Site warm to touch
Red line visible above venipuncture site

Prevention

Techniques to prevent thrombophlebitis include:

1. Use veins in forearm and avoid hands when infusing any medication.
2. Do not use veins in joint flexion areas.
3. Check the infusion site at least every 4 hours in an adult and every 2 hours in pediatric patients for signs and symptoms of redness, swelling, or pain at the site.
4. Anchor the cannula securely to prevent manipulation of catheter tip.
5. Infuse solutions at prescribed rate. Do not play "catch up."
6. Use the smallest size catheter that meets the patient's needs.
7. Dilute irritating medications.

Septic thrombophlebitis can be prevented with:

1. Appropriate skin preparation
2. Aseptic technique in maintenance of infusion
3. *Good handwashing*

✎ **Note:** Thrombophlebitis can lead to a potential embolism owing to thrombus formation in the vein wall.

Treatment

1. Remove entire I.V. catheter and restart with fresh equipment in opposite extremity.
2. Notify the physician.
3. Apply moist warm compresses for 20 minutes to provide comfort.

✎ **Note:** You must discontinue the infusion and restart the infusion; otherwise, the signs and symptoms of thrombophlebitis will only continue to progress.

Charting

Chart all observable symptoms and the patient's subjective complaints (e.g., "feels tender to touch, hurts"). State the actions you took to resolve the problem and what time you notified the physician. State the site where you restarted I.V. therapy.

Infiltration

Infiltration is the seepage of solution or medication into surrounding tissue. The term **extravasation** is used to refer to infiltration of a **vesicant** medication. Infiltration occurs from the dislodgment of the cannula from the intima of the

237

Table 8-6 ☐ **RISKS FOR EXTRAVASATION INJURY**

1. *Age related*
   Neonates
   Geriatric patients
2. *Condition related*
   Oncology patient
   Comatose patient
   Anesthetized patient
   Patients with peripheral or cardiovascular disease
   Diabetic patient
3. *Equipment related*
   High-pressure infusion pumps

vein. Infiltration can occur also from phlebitis, causing the veins to become threadlike and the lumen along the cannula shaft to narrow so that fluid leaks from the site where the cannula enters the vein wall (Hecker, 1988). Table 8-6 lists risks for extravasation injury. Drugs known to cause extravasation injury are listed in Table 8-7.

Signs and symptoms of infiltration are:

Coolness of skin around site
Taut skin
Dependent edema
Backflow of blood absent, or a "pinkish" blood return
Solution rate slowing but continuing to infuse

Prevention

Techniques to prevent infiltration include:

1. Monitor I.V. site for edema.
2. Choose veins that avoid the dorsum of the hand, wrist, and digits. Avoid the median basilic vein above the elbow, which is too close to artery and nerves.
3. Avoid the use of high-pressure infusion pumps when administering highly vesicant drugs. Pumps continue infusing solutions when infil-

Table 8-7 ☐ **DRUGS KNOWN TO CAUSE INJURY TO TISSUE**

Dextrose 10%
Norepinephrine
Dopamine
Radiopaque contrast media: Renografin 30, 60, 76
Cytoxic agents
Dilantin

Source: From "Extravasation" by C.D. Ford, 1990. Paper presented at the Annual Meeting of the Intravenous Nurse's Society, Reno, Nevada. Reprinted by permission.

tration is present until occlusion pressure is reached and an alarm goes off.
4. Dilute all medications as indicated in the literature.
5. Avoid areas of multiple venipunctures.
6. Secure cannula so site is visible.
7. Check for patency before flushing with saline.
8. Educate the patient to report any feelings of burning (Ford, 1990).
9. Avoid using the antecubital area for administration of vesicant drugs.

Treatment

The best treatment is prevention.

INFILTRATION
1. Discontinue the infusion.
2. Elevate the extremity.
3. Apply warm compresses to aid in the reabsorption of the solution.

IF EXTRAVASATION IS SUSPECTED
1. Stop I.V. flow and remove the needle.
2. Notify the physician (request a plastic surgery consultation if a vesicant drug has infiltrated).
3. Administer prescribed antidote, which cannot be delayed (Table 8–8).
4. Elevate the extremity.
5. Apply ice for 20 minutes every 4 hours when indicated (Ford, 1990).

✎ **Note:** Soft tissue damage from extravasation can lead to:
  Prolonged healing
  Potential infections
  Necrosis
  Multiple debridement surgeries
  Cosmetic disfiguration
  Loss of limb function
  Amputation

✎ **Note:** Older pumps have a higher pressure than 20 lb of pressure (Millam, 1988).

✎ **Note:** To recognize early edema at site with infusion running, apply pressure 3 in above catheter site in front of catheter tip. If infusion continues to run, suspect infiltration. When the vein is compressed and catheter is in proper alignment in the vein, the I.V. solution will stop owing to occlusion.

Antidotes

Antidotes fall into four categories—those that:

1. Alter local pH
2. Alter DNA binding
3. Chemically neutralize
4. Dilute extravasated drug (Ford, 1990)

Table 8–8 □ **ANTIDOTE CHART FOR EXTRAVASATED DRUGS***

Extravasated Drug	Antidote and Dose	Nursing Tips	Side Effect of Antidote
Protein Enzyme			
Calcium solutions Contrast media 10%, 20%, 50% dextrose Nafcillin Hyperalimentation solutions Potassium solutions Vinblastine (Velban) Vincristine (Oncovin) Vindesine (Eldisine)	Hyaluronidase (Wydase) 150 U/mL. Inject 1–6 mL in divided doses into extravasated site. (This agent reduces venous spasm).	Use 27-to 25-gauge needle. Use moist *warm* compresses and elevate extremity.	Rash, urticaria
Adrenergic Blocker			
Dobutamine (Dobutrex) Dopamine (Dopastat) Epinephrine Metaraminol biturtrate (Aramine) Norepinephrine	Phentolamine mesylate (Regitine) 5–10 mg SC diluted in 10–15 mL sodium chloride.	Treatment must start immediately with this group of vesicants. Use *warm* compresses.	CV†: Hypotension, tachycardia, flushing GI†: Nausea and vomiting

240

Alkalization Agent		
Mechlorethamine (Nitrogen Mustard) Sodium nitroprusside (Nipride)	Sodium thiosulfate. Dilute 4 mL with 6 mL *sterile water* for injection. Administer 10 mL I.V. push over 10 min through existing line and SC into extravasated area.	Use *ice* compresses.	Rash Hypersensitivity

Glucocorticoid Steroid		
Doxorubicin (Adriamycin) Vincristine (Oncovin) Daunorubicin (Cerubidine) Dacarbazine (DTIC) Dactinomycin (Actinomycin) Plicamycin (Mithracin)	Hydrocortisone sodium succinate (100 mg/mL) and Dexamethasone (long-acting) 4 mg/mL. Inject 0.5 mL SC into existing line and 0.5 mL SC into extravasated site.	After long-acting steroid given. Apply 1% topical hydrocortisone cream. Use *cool* moist compresses.	Delayed wound healing Various skin eruptions

*If you work with high-risk patients, copy this chart to be used in medication area for quick reference.

†SC = subcutaneous; CV = central venous; GI = gastrointestinal.

Data from: Gahart, B. (1991). *Intravenous medications.* (7th ed.). St. Louis: Mosby Year Book and Oncology Nursing Society (1988). *Cancer chemotherapy guidelines module V: Recommendations for the management of extravasation and anaphylaxis.* Evansville: Bristol-Myers, Oncology Division.

If you are going to instill an antidote, do so via the existing I.V. catheter. The other method is with a 1-mL tuberculin syringe, injecting small amounts subcutaneously in a circle around the infiltrated area.

Local Infection

The 1962 edition of American Hospital Association's *Control of Infections in Hospitals* provides no mention that infections due to I.V. therapy may be hazardous (Lenox, 1990). I.V.-related infections consist of those related to microbial contamination of the cannula or infusate. Cannula contamination is the most common source of local infections. Local infections are preventable by maintaining aseptic technique and following guidelines established by the Intravenous Nursing Society (INS) or Centers for Disease Control (CDC) for duration of infusion, length of time of catheter placement, and tubing change criteria. Local infections are difficult to control in the immunosuppressed patient.

Signs and symptoms of local infection include:

Redness at site
Swelling at site
Possible exudate of purulent material
Increased white blood cells
Elevated temperature (chills not associated with local infection)

Local infections are one of the most frequent complications of I.V. therapy, second only to phlebitis. Occult I.V. site, the most common cannula-related infection, is a broadly defined term used to describe infections that characteristically do not produce pus or inflammation at the I.V. site (Goldmann et al., 1973).

The ways in which a catheter tip may acquire bacteria are

During introduction or venipuncture
During removal of stylet
Colonization from skin
Contaminated I.V. fluids

Prevention

Techniques to prevent local infections include:

1. Inspect all solution containers for cracks and leaks before hanging.
2. Change fluid containers every 24 hours.

Risk of local infection is affected by choice and preparation of site. The venipuncture site should be scrubbed with 70% alcohol to remove blood or dirt, which can interfere with disinfectant preparing solution. Then, a 20-second circular preparation with povidone iodine, allowing the site to dry, has excellent bactericidal capability. If patient is allergic to iodine, 70% alcohol should be used for a 1-minute *vigorous* scrub.

I.V. cannulas contaminated during time of insertion by microorganisms on the hands of hospital personnel contribute significantly to local infections.

Table 8–9 □ **MOST COMMON BACTERIA DETECTED ON CANNULA TIP**

Staphylococcus aureus (highest)
Staphylococcus epidermidis
Klebsiella
Enterococci
Pseudomonas
Proteus
Candida

Almost half of personnel randomly sampled carry gram-negative bacilli on their hands, two thirds carry *Staphylococcus aureus*. Refer to Table 8–9 for common bacteria detected on cannula tips. Washing hands with soap and water with mechanical friction for at least 15 seconds removes most transient acquired bacteria (Steere & Mallison, 1975).

✎ **Note:** Handwashing, the strict no-touch technique, thorough cleansing of insertion site, and site rotation help to significantly decrease I.V.-related infections (Lonsway, 1987).

✎ **Note:** Three-way stopcocks within the infusion system have been shown to become contaminated with microorganisms from hands of personnel owing to frequency of manipulations. Syringes used to flush or draw blood specimens become contaminated easily because the stopcock is not treated with aseptic technique (Kaye, 1982). Fifty-one percent of all stopcocks are contaminated (Brosnan, Parham, Rutledge, Baker, & Redding, 1988).

The most common microorganisms found in I.V. fluids are listed in Table 8–10.

✎ **Note:** Thrombus formation appears to be related to the presence of microorganisms on a catheter tip (Stratton, 1982). Presence of phlebitis connotes an 18-fold increased risk of sepsis compared with absence of phlebitis (Jemison-Smith & Thrupp, 1982). Risk factors for device-related infections decrease with use of steel needles over plastic catheters.

Table 8–10 □ **MOST COMMON MICROORGANISMS FOUND IN INTRAVENOUS FLUIDS**

5% dextrose and water:
Klebsiella
Enterobacter
Serratia marcescens
Pseudomonas
Hypertonic glucose solutions:
Candida

Nursing Procedure: Steps in Catheter Culturing

EQUIPMENT
Sterile scissors
Sterile gloves
70% alcohol swab
Sterile specimen container
Label

STEPS
1. Explain procedure to patient.
2. Remove dressing over I.V. site.
3. Wash hands and put on sterile gloves.
4. Wipe skin around puncture site with 70% alcohol to cleanse area of any blood or antimicrobial ointment.
5. Withdraw catheter carefully. Be sure to direct the removed portion of the catheter upward to keep it away from patient's skin.
6. Hold over specimen container and with sterile scissor cut half the length of catheter and drop it in the container.
7. Close container and label.

✎ **Note:** Culture any purulent drainage from site. If the I.V. solution is the suspected source of infection, send the fluid container and tubing to laboratory for analysis (Castle, 1983, p 190).

Venous Spasm

Venous spasm can occur suddenly and for a variety of reasons. The spasm usually results from the administration of a cold infusate, irritating solutions, or viscous solutions such as blood products, or to a too rapid administration of an I.V. solution.

Signs and symptoms include:

Sharp pain at I.V. site traveling up the arm, owing to piercing stream of fluid that irritates or shocks the vein wall
Slowing of infusion

Prevention

Techniques to prevent venous spasm include:

1. Dilute medication additive adequately.
2. Keep I.V. solution at room temperature.
3. Wrap extremity with warm compresses during infusion.

Treatment

1. Apply warm compresses to warm the extremity and decrease flow rate until spasm subsides.
2. Restart the I.V. infusion if venous spasm continues.

✎ **Note:** If a rapid infusion rate is desired, use a larger cannula.

244

KEY TIPS—PREVENT LOCAL COMPLICATIONS

1. Maintain guidelines from INS 1990 on tubing Δ every 48 hours (72 hours acceptable practice) and cannula Δ every 48 hours (72 hours acceptable practice).
2. Follow aseptic technique in skin preparation and venipuncture techniques.
3. *Wash hands.*
4. Choose transparent dressing.
5. Secure tubing and cannula with good taping technique.
6. Use 0.22-micron inline filter as extra safeguard.
7. Keep solutions at prescribed rate.
8. Document observed I.V. site every 4 hours for adults and every 2 hours for infants and children.

Summary Worksheet No. 1: Local Complications

Complication	Signs and Symptoms	Treatment
Hematoma		
Thrombosis		
Phlebitis		
Thrombophlebitis		
Infiltration		
Local infection		
Venous spasm		

SYSTEMIC COMPLICATIONS

The following systemic complications are discussed in this chapter:

1. Septicemia
2. Circulatory overload

3. Pulmonary edema
4. Air embolism
5. Speed shock
6. Catheter embolism

Septicemia

In 1986, approximately 70 percent of the 40 million patients hospitalized in the United States received some form of infusion therapy. This therapy was assumed to be responsible for 30 percent of all hospital-associated bacteremias. Neither the intravascular device nor the infusate are cultured in most of these infections; consequently, the source remains unknown (Crow, 1987). **Septicemia** can occur when microorganisms migrate into the bloodstream. Scalp vein needles produce lower rates of infection than do plastic catheters. However, plastic catheters provide a more stable access and are therefore used more frequently (Kaye, 1982). The nurse must be aware of risk factors, prevention techniques, and the presence of an infected catheter tip because bacteremia, fungemia, or septicemia could occur (Stratton, 1982).

Septicemia is related to poor aseptic techniques and contaminated equipment during manufacturing and storage or use. In addition, peripheral I.V. infusions are contaminated less frequently than are infusions used for central venous access or total parenteral nutrition. Infusions from intensive care unit (ICU) patients with both peripheral and central venous lines are more frequently contaminated than are infusions from patients on medical-surgical units (Maki, 1986). Irrigation of clogged I.V. catheters can propel a clot, which is a significant source of bacterial contamination, into the systemic circulation. Microbial pathogens associated with infusion-related septicemia (Stratton, 1982; Simmons, Stover, & Rhame, 1982) are:

Staphylococcus aureus (greater than 50 percent)
Staphylococcus epidermis
Enterococcus
Klebsiella
Enterobacter
Serratia

Signs and symptoms of septicemia are:

Fluctuating fever—tremors, teeth chattering
Profuse cold sweat
Nausea and vomiting
Diarrhea, sudden and explosive

Organism growth can lead to overwhelming infection, which in turn leads to:

Hypotension
Vascular collapse
Shock and death

247

Prevention

Techniques to prevent septicemia include:

1. Parenteral fluids should be carefully inspected for abnormal cloudiness, cracks, and pinholes.
2. Use only freshly opened fluids.
3. Protein fluids, such as albumin and protein hydrolysates, must be used as soon as the seal is broken.
4. Handwashing and sterile technique are imperative to minimize the risk of technique-induced septicemia.
5. Iodine-containing antiseptics have a superior spectrum of antimicrobial activity. They are inexpensive, well tolerated, and highly reliable.
6. Infusion sites should be covered with a sterile dressing.
7. Inspection of the site and assessment of the patient are important nursing measures for early recognition of symptoms.

✎ **Note:** The best key to prevention is staff education.

Treatment

It is sometimes difficult to distinguish infusion-associated sepsis from septicemia of other causes, unless the condition is associated with phlebitis (Goldmann et al., 1973). Steps in treating suspected septicemia based on patient signs and symptoms are

1. Notify physician.
2. Restart new I.V. system in opposite extremity.
3. Obtain cultures from:

   Administration set
   Container
   Catheter tip
   Site
   Blood

4. Initiate antimicrobial therapy as ordered.
5. Monitor the patient closely.
6. Determine whether the patient's condition requires transfer to ICU.

Charting

Document the signs and symptoms assessed, the time you notified the physician, and all treatments instituted. Document the time of transfer to ICU, the time the new I.V. system was inserted, and how the patient is tolerating interventions.

✎ **Note:** Parenteral fluids temporarily discontinued to administer blood components should be discarded and fresh fluid containers restarted after transfusion is terminated.

Circulatory Overload

Circulatory overload is caused by infusing excessive amounts of sodium chloride solution too rapidly, failure to monitor the I.V. infusion, or infusing any fluid too rapidly in a patient compromised by cardiopulmonary or renal disease.

Signs and symptoms of circulatory overload include:

Weight gain
Edema
Puffy eyelids
Hypertension
Rise in blood pressure
Wide variance between intake and output (I & O)
Rise in central venous pressure (CVP)
Shortness of breath and rales (crackles)
Distended neck veins

Prevention

Techniques to prevent circulatory overload include:

1. Monitor the infusion, especially sodium chloride, and know the solution's physiologic effects on the circulatory system. This technique, in particular, is key to prevention of circulatory overload.
2. Maintain flow at prescribed rate.
3. Do not play "catch up" with I.V. solutions.
4. Monitor I & O on all patients receiving I.V. fluids.
5. Know the patient's cardiovascular history.

Treatment

Notify the physician if you suspect circulatory overload.

1. Decrease I.V. flow to keep vein open (KVO) rate.
2. Raise the head of the bed.
3. Keep the patient warm to promote peripheral circulation.
4. Monitor vital signs.
5. Administer oxygen as ordered.

Pulmonary Edema

Circulatory overload leads to pulmonary edema. Fluids too rapidly infused increase venous pressure, leading to pulmonary edema. Pulmonary edema is an abnormal accumulation of fluid in the lungs. In pulmonary edema, fluids leak through the capillary wall and fill the interstitium and alveoli. "The pulmonary vascular bed has received more blood from the right ventricle than the left can accommodate and remove. The slightest imbalance between inflow on the right side and outflow on the left side may have drastic consequences"

(Smeltzer & Bare, 1992, p 686). It is important to identify patients at risk for pulmonary edema and provide nursing care that decreases the heart's workload. Patients at risk for pulmonary edema are those with cardiovascular disease, with renal disease, and who are elderly. Sodium chloride given to correct profound sodium deficits can lead to pulmonary overload and must be monitored closely (Metheny, 1984, p 328).

Prevention

Techniques to prevent pulmonary edema include:

1. Prevention techniques for circulatory overload.
2. Monitor lung sounds for crackles.

Treatment

Same as for circulatory overload.

Air Embolism

Air **embolism** is a rare but lethal complication, especially involving subclavian central lines. This problem is treatable with prompt recognition, but prevention is the key.

The causes of air embolism include:

Solution container allowed to run dry
Air in tubing, which gets infused into patient
Loose connections allowing air to enter system
Poor technique in dressing and tubing changes for central lines

Initial signs and symptoms of air embolism include:

Hypoxia
Hypotension
Respiratory distress
Changes in cardiac and neurologic status

These signs and symptoms lead to the following if left untreated:

Hemiplegia
Aphasia
Generalized seizures
Coma
Cardiac arrest

Prevention

Techniques to prevent air embolism include:

1. Wrap tubing around a pencil to force air bubbles upward into infusion drip chamber.
2. Use a clamp on the patient side of an injection port if air is removed by a needle at the injection port (Fig. 8–1, Table 8–11).

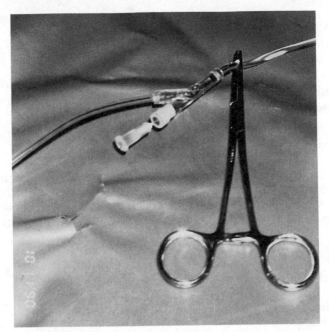

Figure 8–1 ☐ Removal of air from primary set.

3. Use a 0.22-micron air-eliminating filter.
4. Tape all connectors, especially on central lines.
5. Follow protocol for dressing and tubing changes of central lines.
6. Start a new I.V. fluid before the previous solution runs completely dry.
7. Attach piggyback medications to high injection ports, so the check valve will prevent air from being drawn into the line after infusion of medication.
8. Use Luer lock connectors whenever possible.

 Do not bypass "pump housing" of electric volumetric pump.

Treatment

1. Call for help.
2. Place patient in Trendelenburg's position on left side, head down. This

Table 8–11 ☐ REMOVAL OF AIR FROM PRIMARY SET

1. Clamp tubing to patient, distal to lowest medicinal entry. (This prevents air from entering patient.)
2. Swab medicinal port with alcohol.
3. Insert 20-gauge 1-in needle without syringe into medicinal entry. This will vent all air out of primary line.
4. When all air has been removed, remove needle, then unclamp.

causes the air to rise in the right atrium, preventing it from entering the pulmonary artery (Plumer & Cosentino, 1987, p 275).
3. Administer oxygen.
4. Monitor vital signs.

✎ **Note:** A common sign of air embolism is the "cog wheel" sound connoting a heart murmur secondary to right ventricular outflow tract obstruction (Coppa, Gouge, & Hofstetter, 1980).

Speed Shock

Speed shock occurs when a foreign substance, usually a medication, is rapidly introduced into the circulation. Rapid injection permits the concentration of medication in the plasma to reach toxic proportions, flooding the organs rich in blood — the heart and the brain. Syncope, shock, and cardiac arrest may result.

Prevention

1. Reduce the size of drops; use microdrip sets for medication delivery.
2. Use an electronic flow control for high-risk drugs.
3. Monitor the infusion rate for accuracy before piggybacking in the medication.
4. Be careful not to manipulate the catheter, as cannula movement could speed up flow rate.

✎ **Note:** Prevention is the key. When giving I.V. push drugs, give *slowly* and according to manufacturer's recommendations.

Treatment

1. *Get help*
2. Give antidote or resuscitation medications as needed.
3. If giving I.V. narcotics, have naloxone (Narcan) available on the unit.

✎ **Note:** Refer to Chapter 11 for steps in delivery of I.V. push medications.

Catheter Embolism

Catheter embolism is an infrequent systemic complication of plastic catheters. The signs and symptoms include:

Sharp sudden pain at I.V. site
Minimal blood return
Short, rough, and uneven catheter noted on removal
Cyanosis
Chest pain
Tachycardia
Hypotension

Catheter embolus may migrate to the chest and lodge in the pulmonary artery or the right ventricle. This could cause pulmonary embolism, cardiac dysrhythmia, sepsis, endocarditis, thrombosis, and death (Feldstein, 1986).

Prevention

Techniques to prevent catheter embolism include:

1. Never reinsert a needle in an ONC after removal.
2. Avoid inserting the catheter over joint flexion where movement causes catheter to bend back and forth.
3. Splint arm if the patient is restless.

✎ **Note:** Always use radiopaque catheters. That way, the catheter will be detectable on x-ray examination.

Treatment

Have the patient apply digital pressure on the vein above the insertion site, if the patient is cooperative. This may prevent the catheter from migrating.

1. Apply tourniquet above elbow.
2. Contact physician and radiolog.
3. Start a new I.V. infusion.
4. Prepare patient for x-ray examination.
5. Measure remainder of the catheter tip to know the length of embolized tip.

Charting

Document the patient's subjective complaints in quotes. Document discontinuation of catheter, technique, and length of catheter removed. State the nursing interventions and the time the physician was notified.

✎ **Note:** Be sure to watch circulation of extremity while tourniquet is on arm.

Summary Worksheet No. 2: Systemic Complications

Complication	Signs and Symptoms	Treatment
Septicemia		
Circulatory overload		
Pulmonary edema		

Air embolus

Speed shock

Catheter embolism

PROBLEMS OF ERRATIC FLOW RATES

There are many factors to consider in determining flow rate (Table 8–12). These include body size, fluid type, patient's age and condition, physiologic responses as reflected by urinary output, pulmonary status, and specific drugs being infused. The very young and the very old need a slow rate and small volumes. Patients with cardiac or renal disease may also have problems tolerating

255

Table 8–12 □ **FACTORS IN FLOW RATE CONTROL**

Patient Related	*Vein Related*
Patient or family intervention	Infiltration
Patient blood pressure	Phlebitis
Tubing Related	Venous spasm
"Cold flow" of plastic tubing	*Clot formation*
Drop formation rate	Needle or catheter position
Final inline filters kinked or pinched	*Other*
tubing	Height of I.V. standard
Rate of fluid flow	Bed position
Slipping of roller clamp	

Source: From "Too Fast or Too Slow: The Erratic I.V." by J. Steele, 1983, *American Journal of Nursing, 6,* pp. 898–900. Copyright 1983 by American Journal of Nursing. Adapted by permission.

large fluid volumes or fast rates. Flow rate is critical and inaccuracies are unacceptable in nursing care of the patient receiving I.V. therapy (Steel, 1983). Poorly regulated flow can have serious consequences. Accurate flow rate is imperative when a drug level must be kept constant.

If the rate is too *slow*:

- The patient is not receiving the desired amount of drug or solution.
- A too-slow rate can lead to clogged I.V. needle or catheter and perhaps the loss of a premium vein.

If the rate is too *fast*:

- Hypotonic solutions can lead to pulmonary edema or congestive heart failure.
- Rapid infusion of hypertonic glucose can result in osmotic diuresis, leading to dehydration.
- Hypertonic solutions are also irritating and can result in phlebitis.

✎ **Note:** *A fast rate is considered more dangerous than a rate that is too slow.*

✎ **Note:** Following a hypertonic solution with an isotonic solution will help to cleanse the vein of irritating solutions.

PHYSICAL ASSESSMENT

The nurse must use a systems approach to assess for both local and systemic complications associated with an I.V. insertion line and maintenance of the infusion. The nursing assessment should include infusion rate, I & O, and an awareness of agency policy and procedures to prevent complications associated with I.V. therapy. The following body systems should be assessed at the beginning of each shift and as needed to monitor the patient's reactions to infusions. Symptoms listed with each system may indicate local problems or life-threatening systemic complications. All laboratory findings should be monitored.

NEUROMUSCULAR
Change in level of consciousness

Confusion
Complaints of pain

Tremors
Paresthesia of the extremities
Paralysis of the extremities
Muscle weakness
Seizures

CARDIOVASCULAR
Increased or decreased blood pressure
Increased heart rate
Extra cardiac sounds
Distended neck veins
Bleeding from the site

RESPIRATORY
Shortness of breath
Hypoxia
Cyanosis
Respiratory distress

GASTROINTESTINAL
Nausea
Vomiting
Diarrhea

RENAL
Decreased urinary output
Variance between I & O

INTEGUMENTARY
Fever
Profuse sweating
Edema at or near insertion site
Change in skin color
Sensation of heat at or near insertion site
Red line visible above venipuncture site
Tender, cordlike vein
Bruising around or near insertion site
Sluggish flow rate
Back flow absent
Coolness of the skin
Taut skin around venipuncture site

BODY WEIGHT
Rapid weight gain

NURSING DIAGNOSES RELATED TO COMPLICATIONS OF INTRAVENOUS THERAPY

1. Altered thought processes related to impaired circulation to the brain.
2. Anxiety (mild, moderate, severe) related to threat to or change in health status; misconceptions regarding therapy.
3. Altered tissue perfusion (peripheral) related to infiltration of vesicant medication.
4. Decreased cardiac output related to sepsis, contamination; infusion of isotonic or hypertonic solutions.
5. Fear related to insertion of catheter; fear of "needles."
6. Hyperthermia related to increased metabolic rate; illness; dehydration.
7. Impaired gas exchange related to ventilation perfusion imbalance; embolism.
8. Impaired skin integrity related to I.V. catheter; irritating I.V. solution; inflammation; infection; infiltration.
9. Impaired tissue integrity related to altered circulation; fluid deficit or excess; irritating I.V. solution; inflammation; infection; infiltration.
10. Impaired physical mobility related to pain or discomfort resulting from placement and maintenance of I.V. infusion.
11. Pain related to physical trauma (e.g., catheter insertion).
12. Risk of infection related to broken skin or traumatized tissue.

INTRAVENOUS NURSING STANDARDS OF PRACTICE (1990)

Peripheral Venous Cannula

1. A peripheral insertion site should be aseptically cleansed with an antimicrobial solution before cannula placement. Antimicrobial solutions may include tincture of iodine 1 to 2%, iodophors, 70% isopropyl alcohol, or chlorhexidine. The solution should completely air dry. The application of 70% isopropyl alcohol after an iodophor preparation should not be done, as alcohol negates the effect of the iodophor (S35).
2. A peripheral venous cannula should be removed every 48 hours and immediately upon suspected contamination or complication (S46).
3. Peripheral and central primary sets should be changed every 48 hours and immediately upon suspected contamination or when the integrity of the product has been compromised (S54).
4. Peripheral and central secondary sets shall be changed every 48 hours and immediately upon suspected contamination or when the integrity of the product has been compromised (S54).
5. Primary intermittent administration sets shall be changed every 24 hours (S54).
6. Gauze dressing must be securely taped at all edges. Gauze dressings shall be changed routinely every 48 hours on peripheral and central cannula sites in conjunction with the administration set change (S40).
7. Transparent semipermeable membrane dressings shall be changed every 48 hours in conjunction with cannula and administration set change (S41).
8. A 0.22-micron bacteria-retentive filter shall be routinely used for the delivery of I.V. therapy (S56).

CENTERS FOR DISEASE CONTROL RECOMMENDATIONS, BY CATEGORY (1981)

Category I: Strongly recommended

Category II: Moderately recommended for adoption

Category III: Weakly recommended for adoption

1. Cannulas should be replaced every 48–72 hours. Category II.
2. Site preparation: Tincture of iodine (1 to 2%) is preferred, but chlorhexidine, iodophors, or 70% alcohol can be used. The antiseptic should be applied liberally and allowed to remain in contact for at least 30 seconds before venipuncture. Category I.
3. Peripheral venous cannulas should be changed and a new cannula inserted every 48 to 72 hours. Category I.
4. Piggyback tubing should be routinely changed every 48 hours. Category I.
5. Tubing should be changed after the administration of blood, blood products, or lipids. Category III.
6. The use of I.V. inline filters is not recommended as a routine infection control measure. Category II.

SUMMARY OF CHAPTER 8

COMPLICATIONS OF INTRAVENOUS THERAPY

After reading this chapter you have increased your awareness about the risks to the patient who is receiving I.V. therapy. Remember, you have observation skills to assess for local complications, as well as cognitive skills to assess for systemic complications.

Local Complications

Hematoma

Observe the skin for swelling and discoloration. Prevent a hematoma by using the indirect method of venipuncture, applying a tourniquet just before venipuncture, and using microdrip tubing with rates of less than 50 mL.

Thrombosis

Observe for slowed drip rate or resistance when attempting to flush the catheter with sodium chloride. Prevent thrombosis by use of pump or controller.

Phlebitis

Observe the I.V. site for warmth, increased temperature, redness, and sluggish flow rate or a palpable cord. Prevent phlebitis by using large veins, changing I.V. site every 72 hours, and documenting observations at every shift.

Thrombophlebitis

Observations are the same as for phlebitis, with the addition of observing for a red line above venipuncture site, edema of the limb, and increased basal temperature. Prevention of thrombophlebitis includes the use of a 0.22-micron filter, site checks, dilution of irritating medication, and good handwashing technique.

Infiltration

Observe the venipuncture site for coolness of the skin, taut skin, dependent edema, and backflow of blood. Prevent by early recognition, use of appropriate veins, and checking for patency before administering drug. Extravasation may occur with vesicant drugs. Care must be taken to observe for a patent I.V. with vesicant materials and know the antidote if extravasation should occur.

Local Infection

Observe the site for redness and exudate. Monitor the white blood cell level and vital signs. Prevent local infection with good aseptic technique, handwashing, and safe standards of practice. Inspect all solutions for cracks, leaks, or discoloration.

Venous Spasm

Observe for slowed I.V. rate. The patient may complain of a sharp pain at site and traveling up the arm. Prevent venous spasm by infusing solutions at room temperature and administrating solution at the prescribed rate.

Systemic Complications

Septicemia

Observe for signs and symptoms of septicemia, including fluctuating fever, profuse sweating, nausea and vomiting, diarrhea, and decreasing blood pressure. Prevent septicemia by inspecting all solutions, using aseptic techniques, and following proper standards of practice for site care.

Circulatory Overload

Signs and symptoms of circulatory overload include weight gain, edema, puffy eyes, increased blood pressure, and variance in I & O records. Know the cardiovascular history of your patient. Prevent circulatory overload by taking time to know your patient and keeping the I.V. rate at the prescribed rate.

Pulmonary Edema

In addition to assessing for signs and symptoms of circulatory overload, assess for pulmonary edema by listening to your patient's lungs for rales. Prevent pulmonary edema by using extreme caution when giving hypertonic solutions such as 5% dextrose/0.9% saline and isotonic saline. Use less fluid volume with patients with congestive heart failure.

Air Embolism

Observe for signs of hypoxia, hypotension, and respiratory distress. Prevent this complication by using a 0.22-micron air-venting filter, using Luer lock connectors, and maintaining drip rate.

Speed Shock

Observe for signs and symptoms of syncope, shock, and cardiac arrest. Prevention is the key. Give all I.V. drugs according to manufacturer's recommendation for administration.

Catheter Embolism

Observe for patient reporting of sudden pain. Check catheter for signs of a blood return. Upon removal of a catheter, if the end is rough and uneven, report findings to the physician. Prevent catheter embolism by *never* reinserting the needle of an ONC after it has been removed. Do *not* apply pressure over the site during catheter removal.

Activity Journal

1. Check the policy and procedure manual in the facility in which you are working. Is there a policy that addresses:

   a. Length of time I.V. catheter is to be left in patient?
   b. Frequency of tubing changes?
   c. Type of solution used for preparing site before venipuncture?

2. Do you feel that more attention should be paid to the quality management of the I.V.s in your hospital, extended care facility, or home care setting? Why?

   If yes, how can you contribute to safer I.V. therapy?

3. During a given shift, note how many times nurses on your unit wash their hands.

4. Have you ever detected a phlebitis caused by an infusion? If so, describe.

Quality Assessment Model

Instructions: Use this quality assessment model to conduct retrospective audits of charts, establish quality control standards, or develop outcome criteria for quality assurance. Refer to Chapter 2 for details on quality assessment.

STRUCTURE

(Resource that affects outcome)
Human Resource: Nurse I.V. Therapist
↓

PROCESS STANDARD

(Actual giving and receiving of care)
Therapist activities related to following standards of practice are:

1. Use good handwashing techniques.
2. Pay attention to venipuncture techniques.
3. Inspect all equipment before use.
4. Keep I.V. solutions at prescribed rates.
5. Change tubing every 48 to 72 hours.
6. Change catheter location every 48 to 72 hours.
7. Follow safety steps in removing air from tubing.
8. Assess adults every 4 hours, pediatric patients every 2 hours.
↓

OUTCOME STANDARD

(Effects of care on outcome)
Documentation will reflect standards of practice:

1. Patient will be free of local and systemic complications associated with I.V. therapy.
2. Documentation in the chart at every shift will reflect assessment and standards of care.

Post-test, Chapter 8

Match the definition in column 2 with the correct term in column 1.

Column 1

1. _____ Vasospasm
2. _____ Ecchymosis
3. _____ Thrombosis
4. _____ Extravasation
5. _____ Speed shock

Column 2

A. Foreign substance injected into body too rapidly

B. Escape of fluid from vessel

C. Contraction of muscular coat of the blood vessels

D. Formation or presence of blood clot

E. Bruise

6. Which of the following are local complications associated with I.V. therapy?
   A. Speed shock, septicemia, and venous spasm
   B. Phlebitis, venous spasm, and hematoma
   C. Septicemia, thrombophlebitis, and hematoma
   D. Phlebitis, pulmonary edema, and speed shock

7. The nurse can avoid a thrombosis formation by:
   A. Avoiding injury to the vein wall
   B. Avoiding multiple punctures
   C. Avoiding through-and-through punctures
   D. All of the above

8. Mr. Jenkins states his I.V. site is sore. You assess the site and note redness and swelling but no signs of a palpable cord or streak. Using the criteria for rating infusion phlebitis, what is the severity of this phlebitis?
   A. +3
   B. +1
   C. +2
   D. 0

9. The highest risk for phlebitis is among patients who are:
   A. Immunosuppressed
   B. Neonates
   C. Receiving total parenteral nutrition
   D. Receiving medications by multiple lines
   E. All of the above

10. Mrs. Clark has fluctuating fever, profuse sweating, and nausea, and her blood pressure is lower than normal. You would suspect:
    A. Local infection
    B. Septicemia
    C. Venous spasm
    D. Circulatory overload

11. The I.V. container runs dry and you superimpose a new solution. There is air in the tubing. How would you safely remove the air from the tubing? Give four steps.
    A. _____

B. _____

C. _____

D. _____

12. List two of the four ways a catheter tip may acquire bacteria.

A. _____

B. _____

13. List two of the three prevention techniques for avoiding phlebitis.

A. _____

B. _____

14. The infusion slows on your patient. What is the first step in checking on or managing this situation?

_____

15. Phlebitis is caused by two mechanisms. Name them.

A. _____

B. _____

16. Mrs. Clark, age 75, needs an I.V. for rehydration. You attempt an I.V. with a 20-gauge catheter but are unsuccessful. A large hematoma forms over the puncture site. Give two treatments for this tissue injury.

A. _____

B. _____

17. In the foregoing situation, what nursing tip could be used to decrease the risk of hematoma formation?

18. Of the six causes of thrombosis formation, list two.

A. _____

B. _____

19. While a solution is infusing, what treatment can be given for venous spasm?

20. What is the initial treatment for a suspected air embolism?

Answers to Post-test, Chapter 8

1. C
2. E
3. D
4. B
5. A
6. B
7. D
8. B
9. E
10. B
11. A. Clamp tubing.
    B. Swab lowest Y port with alcohol.
    C. Insert 20-gauge 1-in needle and turn on roller clamp.
    D. When all air is vented, remove needle and then unclamp.
12. A. During venipuncture
    B. Colonization from skin
    C. Contaminated I.V. solution
    D. During removal of catheter
13. A. Use larger veins for hypertonic solutions.
    B. Rotate sites every 72 hours
    C. Use 0.22-micron filter
14. Check tubing for kinks.
15. A. Chemical
    B. Mechanical
16. A. Apply direct pressure with 2 × 2 gauze and elevate extremity.
    B. Use small-gauge needle for elderly patients or other patients with thin skin.
17. Use blood pressure cuff instead of tourniquet.
18. A. Blood backing up system in a hypertensive patient.
    B. Not enough fluid movement to maintain patency.
    C. I.V. site in flexor area.
    D. I.V. solution runs dry.
    E. Cannula traumatizes wall of the obstructed vein.
    F. Flow rate due to patient compressing.
19. Wrap extremity with warm compress.
20. Place patient in Trendelenburg's position and on left side, administer oxygen, monitor vitals, and *get help.*

References

Barrus, D.H., & Danek, G. (1987). Should you irrigate an occluded I.V. line. *Nursing 87, 3*, 63–64.

Brosnan, K.M., Parham, A.M., Rutledge, B., Baker, D., & Redding, J.S. (1988). Stopcock contamination. *American Journal of Nursing, 3*, 320–324.

Castle, M. (1983). Intravenous catheter cultures. In *Procedures.* Nurse's Reference Library. Springhouse, PA: Intermed Communications.

Centers for Disease Control. (1981). *Guideline for prevention of intravascular infections.* Atlanta: US Department of Health and Human Services.

Coppa, G.F., Gouge, T.H., & Hofstetter, S.R. (1980). Air embolism: A lethal but preventable complication of subclavian vein catheterization. *Journal of Parenteral and Enteral Nutrition, 5*(2), 166–168.

Crow, S. (1987). Infection risks in I.V. therapy. *National Intravenous Therapy Association, 10*(2), 101–105.

DeLuca, P.P., Rapp, R.P., Bivins, B., McKean, H.E., & Griffen, W.O. (1975). Filtration and infusion phlebitis: A double blind prospective clinical study. *American Journal Hospital Pharmacy, 32*, 1001–1007.

Ervin, S.M. (1987). The association of potassium chloride and particulate matter with the development of phlebitis. *National Intravenous Therapy Association, 10*(2), 145–149.

Falchuk, K.H., Peterson, L., & McNail, B.J. (1985). Micro particulate-induced phlebitis: Its prevention by in-line filtration. *New England Journal of Medicine,* (1), 78–82.

Feldstein, A. (1986). Detect phlebitis and infiltration before they harm your patient. *Nursing 86*, (1), 44–46.

Ford, C.D. (1990) *Extravasation*. Paper presented at the Intravenous Nursing Society Annual Meeting, Reno, Nevada.

Gahart, B. (1991). *Intravenous medications*. (7th ed.). St. Louis: Mosby Year Book.

Goldmann, D.A., Maki, D.G., Rhame, F.S., Kaiser, A.B., Tenney, J.H., & Bennett, J.V. (1973). Guidelines for infection control in intravenous therapy. *Annals of Internal Medicine, 79,* 848–850.

Gong, H., & King, C. (1983). Inadequate drug mixing: A potential hazard in continuous intravenous administration. *Heart Lung, 12,* 528–532.

Harrigan, C.A. (1984). A cost-effective guide for the prevention of chemical phlebitis caused by the pH of the pharmaceutical agent. *Journal of Intravenous Therapy, 7,* 478–482.

Oncology Nursing Society. (1988). *Cancer chemotherapy guidelines module V: Recommendations for management of extravasation and anaphylaxis*. Evansville: Bristol-Myers, Oncology Division.

Smeltzer, S.C., & Bare, B.G. (1992). *Brunner and Suddarth's textbook of medical-surgical nursing*. (7th ed.). Philadelphia: J.B. Lippincott.

Hecker, J. (1988). Improved technique in I.V. therapy. *Nursing Times, 84*(34), 28–33.

Inline filters can prevent much infusion-related phlebitis. (1985). *American Journal of Nursing, Nurse's Drug Alert, 85*(4), 27–28.

Intravenous Nursing Society. (1990). *Standards of practice*. Philadelphia: JB Lippincott.

Jemison-Smith & Thrupp, L.D. (1982). Phlebitis, infections and filtration. *Journal of Intravenous Therapy, 5*(4), 328–335.

Jones, E. (1982). Relationship between pH of intravenous medications and phlebitis: An experimental study. *National Intravenous Therapy Association, 5*(4), 273.

Kaye, W. (1982). Catheter and infusion-related sepsis: The nature of the problem and its prevention. *Heart & Lung, 11*(3), 221–227.

Lenox, A.C. (1990). I.V. therapy reducing the risk of infection. *Nursing 90, 3,* 60–61.

Longe, R. (1980). Particulate contamination in selected parenteral drugs. *Canadian Anaesthetists Society Journal 27,* 62–64.

Lonsway, R.A. (1987). Research, standards and infection control: The impact on I.V. nursing. *National Intravenous Therapy Association, 10*(2), 106–109.

Maki, D.G. (1985). Infections due to infusion therapy. In *Hospital infections* (2nd ed.). Boston: Little, Brown.

Maki, D.G. (1986). Skin as a source of nosocomial infection: Directions for future research. *Infection Control, 7*(2), 113–115.

Metheny, N.M. (1984). *Quick reference to fluid balance*. Philadelphia: J.B. Lippincott.

Millam, D.A. (1988). Managing complications of I.V. therapy. *Nursing 88, 18*(3), 34–42.

Nelson, R., & Miller, H. (1986). Keeping air out of I.V. lines. *Nursing 86, 3,* 57–59.

Plumer, A.L., & Cosentino, F. (1987). *Principles and practice of intravenous therapy* (4th ed.). Boston: Little, Brown.

Steel, J. (1983). Too fast or too slow: The erratic I.V. *American Journal of Nursing, 6,* 898–900.

Steere, A.C., & Mallison, G.F. (1975). Handwashing practices for the prevention of nosocomial infections. *Annals of Internal Medicine, 83,* 683.

Simmons, B.P., Stover, B.H., & Rhame, F.S. (1982). The CDC intravenous guidelines: Comments and clarification. *Conversations in Infection Control, 3*(3), 1–12.

Stratton, C.W. (1982). Infection related to intravenous infusion. *Heart & Lung, 11*(2) 123–137.

270

CHAPTER 9

Intravenous Therapy: Special Problems

CHAPTER 9

Intravenous Therapy: Special Problems

CHAPTER CONTENTS

Glossary

Body surface area: Surface area of the body determined through use of a nomogram

Caloric method: Calculation of metabolic expenditure of energy

Catabolism: Breakdown of chemical compounds into more elementary principles by the body; an energy-producing metabolic process

Ecchymoses: Bruising, caused by escape of blood from injured vessels into the surrounding tissue

Infant: Child from the end of the first month to age 1 year

Intraosseous infusion: Infusion within the bone marrow cavity

Meter square method: Use of nomogram to determine surface areas of a patient

Neonate: Child in the period of extrauterine life up to the first 28 days after birth

Oncotic: Within the tissue; tissue pressure

Purpura: Condition in which spontaneous bleeding occurs in the subcutaneous tissue, causing purple patches to appear on skin

Tangential lighting: Light touching a curve; indirect lighting

Weight method: Formula based on weight in kilograms to estimate fluid needs

LEARNING OBJECTIVES

Upon completion of this chapter, the reader will be able to:

☐ Describe terms related to delivery of intravenous therapy to pediatric and geriatric patients

☐ Identify physiologic characteristics of neonates, infants, children, and geriatric patients related to venous structure

☐ Locate common sites for venipuncture in the neonate and infant

☐ Identify common reasons for neonate and infant infusions

☐ List the formulas available for calculating fluid needs of an infant

☐ Contrast the stages of development and fears through the lifespan as related to performance of invasive procedures

☐ Identify types of needles and catheters available for the pediatric patient

☐ Describe special considerations for successful venipuncture of neonates, infants, and geriatric patients

☐ Describe the use of intraosseous infusions in the pediatric patient

☐ Identify the complications related to intraosseous infusions

☐ List the risk factors associated with pediatric and geriatric infusions
☐ Describe techniques for venipuncture in patients with sclerotic veins, alterations in skin integrity, obesity, and edema

Pre-test, Chapter 9

Instructions: The pre-test is to review prior knowledge of the theory related to care of the patient with special problems in intravenous therapy. Each question in the pre-test is based on the learning objectives of the chapter.

Match the definition in column 2 to the correct term in column 1.

Column 1

1. _____ Ecchymosis
2. _____ Intraosseous
3. _____ Weight method
4. _____ Caloric method
5. _____ Neonate
6. _____ Body surface area

Column 2

A. Infant in the first 28 days of life

B. Calculation of metabolic expenditure of energy

C. Bruise

D. Within the bone marrow cavity

E. Formula based on kilograms of weight

F. Surface area determined through use of nomogram

7. Risk factors affecting the need for infusion therapy in the neonate include:
   A. Prematurity
   B. Catabolic disease
   C. Hypothermia
   D. Acid-base imbalance
   E. All of the above

8. Identify the three methods for assessment of 24-hour fluid needs in the infant:
   A. Meter square, diaper weight, and urinary output
   B. Meter square, weight, and caloric
   C. Meter square, specific gravity, and head circumference

9. *Common* sites for venipuncture in infants less than 9 months of age include:
   A. Antecubital space, dorsum of the foot, and scalp veins
   B. Dorsum of the foot, external jugular vein, and saphenous vein
   C. Dorsum of the hand, dorsum of the foot, and external jugular vein
   D. Scalp veins, antecubital space, and external jugular vein

10. Intraosseous infusions are useful for:
    A. Emergency delivery of medication and fluids
    B. Long-term nutritional support
    C. Home antibiotic therapy

11. Disadvantages of intraosseous infusions include:
    A. Potential osteomyelitis
    B. Potential cellulitis
    C. Potential damage to epiphyseal plate
    D. All of the above

12. The physiologic changes in the geriatric patient that affect intravenous placement include:
    A. Arteriosclerosis
    B. Increased density and amount of collagen in vessel walls
    C. Loss of subcutaneous fat
    D. Thinning of the skin
    E. All of the above

13. How many superficial veins in the infant's head are accessible for venipuncture?
    A. 1
    B. 2
    C. 4
    D. 6

14. To perform an intravenous infusion on a preschool child, the nurse should:
    A. Explain the procedure in simple terms
    B. Explain the procedure completely
    C. Restrain the child to perform the venipuncture
    D. Provide reading materials before performing venipuncture

15. To perform a venipuncture on a toddler, it is helpful if the nurse:
    A. Provides pictures to color during the procedure
    B. Provides a doll or stuffed animal in which to start the intravenous infusion prior to venipuncture
    C. Has assistance for the venipuncture
    D. Has parents assist with procedure

16. Tangential lighting should be used with patients who have:
    A. Alterations in skin surfaces
    B. Burned skin surfaces
    C. Edematous tissue
    D. Easily palpable and visible veins

17. The use of multiple tourniquets can be helpful with
    A. Pediatric patients
    B. Frail geriatric patients, to distend veins
    C. Patients with sclerosed veins
    D. Patients with dark skin

True-False

18. **T F** Digital pressure to displace edematous fluid allows for visualization of the veins.

19. **T F** Minor trauma can easily cause bruising in the frail geriatric patient.

20. **T F** Hard sclerosed veins are found in patients in renal failure, who have sickle cell anemia, and who are intravenous drug abusers.

SPECIAL CONSIDERATIONS OF THE PEDIATRIC PATIENT

Intravenous (I.V.) therapy related to the pediatric patient has unique problems. The practitioner must be aware of the special assessments (Table 9–1), the body composition of an **infant**, and the homeostatic differences between children and adults in order to provide safe therapeutic care to these patients.

Physiologic Characteristics

The nurse must understand the normal physiologic state of the infant in order to meet the goals of replenishing losses and promoting the child's growth and development. A **neonate** is defined as a child in the period of extrauterine life up to the first 28 days after birth. Low-birth-weight and premature infants have decreased energy stores and increased metabolic requirements, compared with those of a full-term, average-weight newborn.

The premature infant's body is approximately 90 percent water; the newborn infant's 70 to 80 percent, and the adult's about 60 percent. Infants have proportionately more water in the extracellular compartment than do adults. Therefore, any depletion in these water stores may lead to dehydration. As the infant becomes older, the ratio of extracellular to intracellular fluid volume decreases.

Although infants have a relatively greater total body water content, this does not protect them from excessive fluid loss. Infants are more vulnerable than adults to fluid volume deficit because they ingest and excrete a relatively greater daily water volume than adults (Metheny, 1987, p 332). Any condition that interferes with normal water and electrolyte intake or that produces ex-

Table 9–1 □ **COMPONENTS OF A PEDIATRIC PHYSICAL ASSESSMENT**

Measurement of head circumference (up to 1 year)
Height or length
Weight
Vital signs
Skin turgor
Presence of tears
Moistness and color of mucous membranes
Urinary output
Characteristics of fontanelles
Level of child's activity as related to growth and development

cessive water and electrolyte losses will produce a more rapid depletion of water and electrolyte stores in the infant than it will in the adult.

Other factors influence metabolic demands as well, such as illness, increased muscular activity, thermal stress, congenital disorders, and respiratory distress syndrome (Teitell, 1984). The metabolic demand of an infant is two times higher per unit of weight than that of adults.

In most cases 100 to 120 calories/kg per day will maintain the normal infant and provide sufficient calories for growth. For high-risk infants who require increased handling for procedures the calorie requirement is up to 100 percent more than the normal newborn requirement. Heat production increases calorie expenditure by 7 percent per degree of temperature elevation. The infant and young child cannot store protein as well as adults; therefore, preventive nutritional support is needed.

Young children have immature homeostatic regulating mechanisms that need to be considered when water and electrolyte replacement is needed. Renal functioning, acid-base balance, **body surface area** differences, and electrolyte concentrations all must be taken into consideration when planning fluid needs.

The newborn's renal function is not yet completely developed. The infant's kidneys appear to become mature by the end of the neonate period. An infant's kidneys have a limited concentrating ability and require more water to excrete a given amount of solutes. The infant is less likely to be able to regulate fluid intake and output.

The buffering capacity to regulate acid-base balance is less in the newborn than in older children. Neonates, with an average pH of 7.0 to 7.38, are slightly more acidotic than adults (Maxwell & Kleeman, 1980, p 1560). This base bicarbonate deficit is thought to be related to high metabolic acid production and to renal immaturity.

The integumentary system in the neonate is an important route of fluid loss, especially in illness. This must be considered when determining fluid balance in infants and young children, as their body surface area is greater than those of older children and adults. Any condition that produces a decrease in intake or output of water and electrolytes affects the body fluid stores of the infant. Because the gastrointestinal membranes are an extension of the body surface area, relatively greater losses occur from the gastrointestinal tract in the sick infant.

Plasma electrolyte concentrations do not vary strikingly among infants, small children, and adults. The plasma sodium concentration changes little from birth to adulthood. The potassium and chloride concentrations are higher in the first few months of life than at any other time.

Magnesium and calcium are both low in the first 24 hours after birth. The serum phosphate level is elevated in the early months of infancy, which contributes to a low calcium level. The newborn infant is vulnerable to disrupted calcium homeostasis when stressed by illness or by an excess phosphate load. Hypocalcemia is a risk in the neonate (Metheny, 1987, pp 332–333) Table 9–2 provides normal serum electrolyte levels of the newborn.

Risk factors that must be considered during the assessment phase prior to I.V. therapy include:

Prematurity
Catabolic disease state

Table 9–2 □ **NORMAL LABORATORY VALUES FOR INFANTS**

Laboratory Value	Neonate	Infant	2–5 years	6–12 years	Adolescent
Blood Count					
Red blood cells		2.7–5.4	4.27	4.31	4.60
White blood cells		6–17,500	5500–15,500	4500–13,500	4500–11,000
Platelet count	84,000–478,000	150,000–400,000--------all remaining ages			
Partial thromboplastin time		<17 s	18–22 s----------all remaining ages		
Prothrombin time					
Hemoglobin	14.5–22.5	9.0–14.0		11.5–15.5	Male 13–16 Female 12–16
Serum Electrolytes					
Sodium		139–146	138–145	136–146	136–146
Potassium		4.1–5.3		3.4–4.7	3.5–5.1
Magnesium	1.4–1.9 mEq/L------------all remaining ages				
Calcium	7.5–11 mg/dL	8.8–10.8----------all remaining ages		8.4–10.8 mg/dL	
Chloride	98–106------------all remaining ages				
Phosphorus	4.0–10.5 mg/dL	5.0–7.8 mg/dL------all remaining ages			

Hypothermia
Hyperthermia
Metabolic or respiratory alkalosis or acidosis
Other metabolic derangements

CANDIDATES FOR NEONATAL INTRAVENOUS THERAPY
1. Children with congenital cardiac disorders
2. Children with gastrointestinal defects
3. Children with neurologic defects

CANDIDATES FOR INFANT INTRAVENOUS THERAPY
1. Fluid volume deficit (dehydration)
2. Electrolyte imbalance (diarrhea)
3. Antibiotic therapy for treatment of serious infections
4. Nutritional support when maintenance of growth and development is needed
5. Antineoplastic therapy for treatment of cancer

Assessment of Fluid Needs

There are three different methods for assessment of 24-hour maintenance of fluids: the meter square, weight, and caloric methods.

Meter Square Method

The nomogram (Appendix A) is used to determine surface area of the patient. To use a nomogram in the **meter square method**, draw a straight line between the point representing patient's height on the left vertical scale to the point representing the patient's weight on the right vertical scale. The point where the line intersects height and weight indicates the body surface area in square meters (Weinstein, 1990).

ADVANTAGES
Provides calculation of body surface area to help determine the amount of fluid and electrolytes to be infused and assists with computing rate of infusion
Helps calculate adult and pediatric dosages of I.V. medications
Is simple to calculate

DISADVANTAGE
Accessibility to visual nomogram

To calculate the maintenance fluid requirements, use the following:

FORMULA

$$1500 \text{ mL per m}^2 \text{ per 24 hours}$$

Example

If child's surface area is 0.5^2, then $1500 \text{ mL} \times 0.5 \text{ m}^2 = 750 \text{ mL}/24 \text{ hours}$.

279

Weight Method

The **weight method** uses the child's weight in kilograms to estimate the fluid needs. This method uses 100 to 150 mL/kg for estimating maintenance fluid requirements and is most useful in children weighing less than 10 kg. Use of the square meter method is recommended in children weighing more than 10 kg.

ADVANTAGE
Simple to use

DISADVANTAGE
Inaccurate in a child who weighs more than 10 kg

Example

In a child weighing 10 kg, 100 × 10 kg = 1000 mL in 24 hours.

Caloric Method

The **caloric method** calculates the usual metabolic expenditure of fluid. It is based on the following metabolic expenditure:

Child weighing 0 to 10 kg expends approximately 100 calories/kg per day.

Child weighing 10 to 20 kg expends approximately 1000 calories, plus 50 calories/kg for each kg over 10 kg.

Child weighing 20 kg or more expends approximately 1500 calories, plus 20 calories/kg for each kg over 20 kg.

ADVANTAGE
Simple to calculate

DISADVANTAGE
Not totally accurate unless actual calorie requirements and energy intake are continuously assessed

The formula for calculating fluid requirement is 100 to 150 mL/100 calories metabolized.

Example

If weight of child is 30 kg and child expends 1700 calories/day, fluid requirement is 1700 to 2550 mL/24 hours.

Factors Affecting Fluid Needs in the Pediatric Patient

The most common cause of increased fluid and calorie needs in children is temperature elevation. An increase in temperature of 1° C, increases a child's calorie needs by 12 percent. Fluid requirements in a child who is hypothermic decrease by 12 percent (Teitell, cited in Plumer & Cosentino, 1987). In children, losses of gastrointestinal fluids, ongoing diarrhea, and small intestinal drainages can seriously affect fluid balance.

✎ **Note:** To ensure accuracy of fluid needs, most pediatric patients should be on strict intake and output monitoring, including diaper weighing.

Diaper Weighing

The weight difference in a dry and a wet piece of linen represents the amount of liquid that it has absorbed. The weight of the fluid measured in grams is the same as the volume measured in milliliters (Marlow & Redding, 1988, p 266).

Intravenous Equipment

The nurse must be aware of the special needs of the pediatric patient in selection of appropriate equipment. Intravenous Nursing Society (INS) (1990) standards of practice recommend:

1. An electronic infusion device for administration of therapy
2. Volume of solution container used, based on the age, height, and weight of the patient, to contain no more than 500 mL of fluid (preferably 250 mL)
3. Special pediatric equipment, such as volume chamber, for delivery of therapy
4. Monitoring at least every 2 hours and sometimes more frequently, depending on patient's age and size or type of therapy
5. Cannula site to be visible (S67)

Needle Selection

The choice of needle depends on the site selected. Refer to Figure 9–1 for scalp vein sites. A 23- or 25-gauge scalp vein (butterfly) needle is easy to insert but

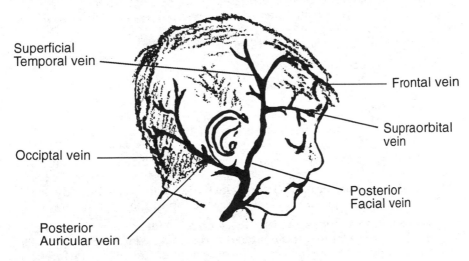

Figure 9–1 □ Scalp vein sites. (Drawing by Timothy D. Mitas.)

has the risk of infiltrating easily. The over-the-needle catheter (ONC), gauges 22 to 24, can be used in infants from birth to 1 year old. These catheters usually last longer than scalp vein needles but are more difficult to insert. The ONCs are also easier to stabilize.

Site Selection

The following sites are most frequently used in pediatric patients.

Dorsum of the Hand

Because veins over the metacarpal area are mobile and not well supported by surrounding subcutaneous tissue, the limb must be immobilized with a splint and tape prior to cannulation. It is difficult to insert the needle into this site owing to the limited space for tape restraint and difficulty maintaining the proper angle of the needle as it enters the vessel. The antecubital fossa should not be routinely used because of the use of the antecubital area for blood drawing and the mobility problems resulting from use of this site.

Dorsum of the Foot

The infant's foot has a great deal of subcutaneous adipose tissue and the veins are small, making visualization difficult. Because the neonate has very little subcutaneous adipose tissue, the veins are easily identified and cannulated just beneath the skin. Splinting of this site is awkward.

Scalp Veins

The major superficial veins of the scalp can be used. There are six scalp veins accessible to the practitioner. A scalp vein needle or an ONC can be used in a scalp vein, depending on the size of the vein.
Major veins in the scalp include:

Frontal, which is the best access
Superficial temporal
Posterior auricular
Supraorbital
Occipital
Posterior facial

The I.V. needle must be placed in the direction of blood flow to ensure that the I.V. fluid will flow in the same direction as the blood returning to the heart. When using a vein in the hand or foot, aim the needle toward the body. In the scalp, venous blood generally flows from the top of the head down.

✎ **Note:** A rubberband can be used as a tourniquet for location of scalp veins. Fold a piece of tape over the rubberband to make a tab that you can hold on to when removing the band. Place the rubberband low on the forehead like a headband. It is also recommended that the rubberband be cut to decrease the chances of dislodging the I.V. after cannulation (Arthur, 1984). Shaving is not recommended; if necessary, clip the hair on the infant (Fabian, 1991).

✎ **Note:** When choosing site on infant take into consideration cultural and family preferences (Wheeler, 1992).

PROCEDURE
1. The venipuncture should be performed in a room separate from the child's room.
2. Always use a saline-filled syringe with the scalp vein infusion device.
3. Use mummy and clove-hitch restraints as needed. The infant should be covered with a blanket to minimize cold stress. If the dorsum of the hand is used, place the extremity on an armboard before venipuncture.
4. Omit tourniquet use if possible. Use rubberband to dilate scalp veins.
5. Warm hands, wash in hot water before gloving.
6. Use a pacifier for neonates and infants.
7. Use direct entry approach with a 30-degree angle.
8. Flush the needle immediately with saline upon flashback of blood.
9. Stabilize the catheter with a tongue blade. Use only hypoallergenic or paper tape.

✎ **Note:** The preferred site for an infant I.V. is on the dorsal hand veins, because placement there allows for the greatest degree of mobility (Oelerich & Dombrowski, 1981; Wheeler, 1992).

When securing the child's extremity to an armboard, use clear tape to allow visualization of the I.V. site and digits or skin immediately adjacent to the site (Delaney & Lauer, 1988; Tietjen, 1990; Blatz & Paes, 1990).

✎ **Note:** The use of a paper cup is not recommended to cover the infusion site on the scalp (Jarmen, 1985). A clear medicine cup can offer protection when positioned over the site.

For children, illness and hospitalization constitute a major life crisis. Children are vulnerable to the crises of illness and hospitalization because stress represents a change from the usual state of health and environmental routine and children have a limited number of coping mechanisms to resolve the stressful events.

Children's reactions to these crisis are influenced by

Developmental age
Previous experiences with illness
Separation or hospitalization
Available support system
Seriousness of the illness

Children's understanding of, reaction to, and method of coping with illness or hospitalization are influenced by the significance of individual stressors during each developmental phase. The major stressors are separation, loss of control, and bodily injury. Table 9–3 summarizes the principle behavioral responses to each stressor as related to the function of I.V. therapy.

Table 9–3 □ **NURSING INTERVENTIONS FOR THE CHILD REQUIRING INTRAVENOUS THERAPY AS RELATED TO PHYSICAL AND PSYCHOLOGIC DEVELOPMENT**

Age	Development/Stressor	Behavior	Intervention
Infant	Trust versus mistrust *Stressor:* Pain	Cries, screams, clings in protest; neonate easily distracted—total body reaction Infants: localized reaction; often uncooperative	Consistency in assigning caregivers. Encourage parents to assist with care Explain I.V. to parents Have assistance starting I.V.
Toddler	Autonomy versus shame and doubt *Stressor:* Loss of control Physical restriction Loss of routine and rituals Bodily injury and pain	Protests verbally Cries for parents Kicks, bites, tries to escape to find parents Resistance Verbally uncooperative	Allow to express feeling Encourage parental help Allow as much mobility as possible in securing I.V. Encourage presence of favorite toy or blanket during invasive procedure Use comfort after procedure

Preschool	Initiative versus guilt *Stressor:* Loss of control Sense of own power Bodily injury—intrusive procedures, mutilation	Protests less directly Anxiety, guilt, shame, physiologic responses Immature behavior	Allow child to express protest Provide play and diversional activity Encourage to play out feelings and fears Allow as much mobility as possible; limit invasive procedures; explain procedure in simple terms to child; start pretend I.V. on doll
School-age	Industry versus inferiority *Stressor:* Loss of control Enforced dependency Altered family roles Bodily injury and pain Fear of illness, death, intrusive procedures in genital area	Loneliness, boredom, isolation, hostility, and frustration Depression and displaced anger Seeks information Passively accepts Communicates about pain	Allow to express feelings, both verbally and nonverbally Involve child in starting I.V. by tearing tape or holding tubing Encourage peer contacts Use diversional activities
Adolescent	Identity vs role diffusion *Stressor:* Loss of control Loss of identity, enforced dependency. Bodily injury and mutilation	Rejection Uncooperativeness Self-assertion Overconfidence Boredom	Explore feelings regarding hospitalization Help to adjust to authority Explain all procedures Allow choices in sites Provide privacy

Source: From *Essentials of Pediatric Nursing*, second edition (p. 501) by L.F. Whaley and D.L. Wong, 1985, St. Louis: C.V. Mosby Company, Copyright 1985 by C.V. Mosby Company. Reprinted by permission.

Intraosseous Infusions

The intraosseous route is a safe alternative for fluid and drug administration in an emergency situation for the infant or child. Between 1940 and 1950 the use of intraosseous infusion for both adults and children was widely used. By the late 1950s the use of the intraosseous route was replaced by the development of plastic catheters and newer infusion techniques (Peck & Altieri, 1988).

The revised standards and guidelines outlined in the *Textbook of Pediatric Advanced Life Support* by the American Heart Association recognize **intraosseous infusion** as an effective route for the administration of emergency medications or fluids or both to children under 6. These guidelines further emphasize the importance of establishing and maintaining an infusion route during the resuscitation of critically ill children (Chameides, 1988).

Intraosseous infusion uses the rich vascular network of the long bones to transport fluids and medications from the medullary cavity to the circulation. The medullary cavity is composed of a spongy network of venous sinusoids that drain into a central venous canal. Blood exits the venous canal by the nutrient and emissary veins into the circulation. Fluids infused into the medullary space diffuse a short space then are absorbed into the venous circulation, and the distribution is similar to I.V. injection (Spivey, 1987) (Fig. 9–2).

USES
1. Provides a quick access in emergency cases when life-sustaining medication must be administered
2. In difficult-to-access patients, provides an accessible entry for delivery of volume resuscitation

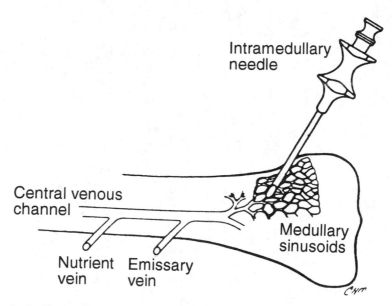

Figure 9–2 □ Intramedullary venous system. (From "Intraosseous Infusions" by W.H. Spivey, 1987, *The Journal of Pediatrics, 111*, p. 644. Copyright 1987 by C.V. Mosby Company. Reprinted by permission.)

3. Useful in cardiac arrest, shock, trauma, or any situation in which the potential benefit of rapid venous access outweighs the low incidence of complications

DISADVANTAGES
1. Potential for osteomyelitis (low incidence reported)
2. Potential for cellulitis; however, studies report only a 0.6 percent incidence (Rossetti, Thompson, & Miller, 1985)
3. Potential damage to the epiphyseal plate
4. Although not reported in the literature, potential embolus caused by fat dislodged from marrow cavity

Intraosseous Insertion Technique

The potential sites for intraosseous infusion are the sternum, iliac crest, femur, and distal and proximal tibia (Fig. 9–3).

1. Assemble equipment.

   Povidone iodine solution (Betadine)
   Jamshidi-Kormed bone marrow biopsy needle, 18-gauge spinal needle with stylet, or commercially prepared disposable intraosseous infusion needle by Cook Critical Care (Bloomington, IN)
   One 10-mL syringe filled with saline

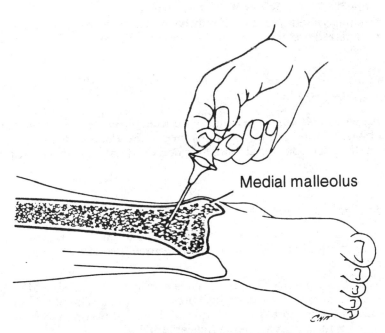

Medial malleolus

Figure 9–3 ☐ Position of intraosseous needle in the distal tibial intraosseous site. (From "Intraosseous Infusions" by W.H. Spivey, 1987, *The Journal of Pediatrics, 111*, pp. 639–643. Copyright 1987 by C.V. Mosby Company. Reprinted by permission.)

Fluid and medications to be administered with administration set
Tape or Elastoplast

2. Prepare the child's skin using povidone iodine solution
3. Wear gloves, mask, gown, and goggles.
4. Select site. Most common sites are the proximal tibia and distal tibia. Use of sternum in children is discouraged because it is too thin and poorly developed to guarantee safe placement.
5. Use local anesthesia of 1% lidocaine hydrochloride if patient is awake and alert.
6. Insert the needle at a 30-degree angle with the point directed away from the epiphyseal plate. Use a twisting or boring motion until needle penetrates the cortex.
7. Remove the stylet.
8. Infuse saline by syringe to clear the needle of marrow, as well as to check for placement.
9. Start infusion of fluid or medications under gravity pressure.
10. Apply sterile dressing.
11. Regulate infusion.
12. Chart the site, needle type and size, type of fluid and medication, as well as the patient response to the treatment (Peck & Altieri, 1988; INS, 1990, S74).

✎ **Note:** INS standards of practice for intraosseous access (INS, 1990, S74) recommend:

- Intraosseous access should only be used for 24 hours; then a conventional I.V. access should be established.
- Intraosseous access should only be used in patients aged 6 and younger.
- Preferred sites for intraosseous access are distal tibia, proximal tibia, and distal femur.

Contraindications

Patients who have areas of cellulitis or infected burns, as well as recently fractured bones, should not undergo this procedure. Patients with osteogenesis imperfecta or osteoporosis also are not good candidates for this route (Hodge, 1985).

Nursing Management

The nursing staff is responsible for managing the site and assessment, administration of the fluid or medication or both, proper use of I.V. equipment, and documentation.

✎ **Note:** Once the needle is removed, a sterile gauze pad should be placed over the puncture site and direct pressure applied. The site should be inspected daily and redressed. After 48 hours, if no drainage is seen, the dressing may be removed (Wheeler, 1989).

SPECIAL CONSIDERATIONS OF THE GERIATRIC PATIENT

By the year 2000 geriatric patients will represent 13 percent of the population, and it is expected that this percentage will increase to 21 percent by 2030 (AARP, 1985). Among the elderly the proportions of the "old-old" (ages 75 to 79) will increase faster than those of the "young-old" (ages 65 to 74). The "frail-old" (age 80+) will constitute 12 percent of the elderly population (Burnside, 1981). Health care practitioners will need a heightened awareness and understanding of the special needs of the elderly (Mellema & Poniatowski, 1989).

Physiologic Changes

Aging occurs on all levels of bodily function: cellular, organic, and systemic. "Loss of cells and loss of physiologic reserve make up the dominant processes of aging" (Smeltzer & Bare, 1992, p 170). The major systems changes the nurse must be aware of related to infusion therapy are homeostatic changes, cardiovascular changes, and skin and connective tissue changes.

Homeostasis is the body's ability to maintain a stable internal environment. The homeostatic mechanisms in the aging become less efficient, and reserve power is lost. When external stressors such as trauma or infection occur, there is minimal reserve capacity. This creates a situation in which the person is more vulnerable to disease.

Cardiovascular changes related to arteriosclerosis become clinically recognizable. Arteries show progressive chemical and anatomic changes, with an increase in cholesterol, other lipids, and calcium. The elastic fibers progressively straighten, fray, split, and fragment. There is an increase in density and amount of collagen fibers in the vessel walls, along with the decreasing elasticity of the wall.

The skin is one of the first systems to show signs of the aging process. As a person ages, there is loss of subcutaneous supporting tissue and resultant thinning of the skin. Folds, lines, wrinkles, and slackness appear as the skin ages. **Purpura** and **ecchymoses** may appear owing to greater fragility of the dermal and subcutaneous vessels and loss of support for the skin capillaries. Minor trauma can easily cause bruising. The dermis becomes relatively dehydrated and looses strength and elasticity (Smeltzer & Bare, 1992, p 170).

Fluid Balance in the Aging

Fluid balance in the elderly is affected by the physiologic changes associated with aging. The older person does not possess the fluid reserves or the ability to adapt readily to rapid changes. Alterations in fluid and electrolyte balance frequently accompany illness.

Renal structural changes associated with the aging process result in decreased glomerular filtration rate. When fluid is restricted for any reason, the

Table 9–4 □ ASSESSMENT OF FLUID VOLUME DISTURBANCES IN THE ELDERLY

Skin turgor of forehead or sternum
Temperature (normal body temperature often below 98.6°F)
Rate and filling of veins in hand or foot
Daily weight possibly a more accurate measure of patient's fluid balance (Pflaum, 1979)
Intake and output
Tongue—center should be moist, with observable pool of saliva beneath the tongue (even though aged have decreased saliva, this method useful in evaluating hydration) (Robinson & Demuth, 1985)
Orthostatic (postural) blood pressure changes
Swallowing ability
Functional assessment of patient's ability to obtain fluids

nurse must be aware that there will be a slower conservation of fluids in response to the fluid restriction.

The total body water is reduced by 6 percent, which creates a potential for fluid volume deficit. Gastrointestinal changes such as decreased volume of saliva, gastric juice, and calcium absorption cause the mouth to be drier in the aged, along with the potential for sodium and potassium deficit during episodes of vomiting and gastric suction and calcium deficit.

Cardiovascular changes and respiratory changes combine to contribute to a slower response to the stress of blood loss, fluid depletion, shock, and acid-base imbalances (Metheny, 1987, p 348). Table 9–4 provides assessment guidelines for fluid volume disturbances in the elderly.

Sites

The flexion areas should be avoided in the elderly. Avoid areas with bruising because the **oncotic** pressure is increased in these areas and may cause collapse of vessels. Avoid rolling or fragile veins if possible.

TECHNIQUES
✓ If the patient is hypertensive, do not use a tourniquet.
✓ If you use a tourniquet, apply it lightly to avoid overdistension of fragile veins.
✓ Use an assistant and have the extra person apply digital pressure with their hand above the site of venipuncture and release once the vein has been entered.
✓ Use a small-gauge needle (22 or 23).
✓ Enter the vein directly and gently.
✓ Use warm compresses to distend the vein.
✓ Use hypoallergenic or paper tape for fragile skin.

VENIPUNCTURE TECHNIQUES FOR THE DIFFICULT PATIENT

Special Problems

Before initiating therapy on a patient the I.V. nurse must know the diagnosis and allergies. The diagnosis affects the technique the therapist will use for a successful venipuncture (Table 9–5).

Alterations in Skin Surfaces

The I.V. nurse must take precautions in patients with damaged skin due to lesions, burns, or disease process. The two major problems the nurse must be aware of in a patient with altered skin integrity is that the patient often is photosensitive and that the already damaged tissue must be protected. It is recommended that **tangential lighting** be used. This indirect light does not flatten veins or cause damage to the skin. Use a light directed to the side of the patient's extremity, which will illuminate the blue veins and provide a guide for venipuncture.

✎ **Note:** This technique can also be used on dark-skinned patients.

Hard Sclerosed Vessels

If the peripheral vessels are hard and sclerosed because of a disease process, personal misuse, or frequent drug therapy, access presents a unique problem. The practitioner should assess for collateral circulation because venipuncture through hard sclerosed veins is difficult. In order to find collateral veins the nurse can use the multiple-tourniquet technique. By gradually increasing the oncotic pressure inside the tissue, blood is forced into the small vessels of the periphery.

PROCEDURE
Place one tourniquet high on the arm for 2 minutes and leave in place. Place a second tourniquet at midarm below the elbow for 2 minutes.

Table 9–5 □ **SPECIAL PROBLEMS**

Alterations in skin surfaces
Systemic lupus erythematosus
Dermatitis
Skin lesions
Burns
Hard sclerosed veins
Renal failure
Intravenous drug abuse
Sickle cell disease
Obese patient
Edematous patient

If soft collateral veins do not appear in the forearm, place a third tourniquet at the wrist.

Usually veins will appear in the hand with this approach (Fabian, 1991).

✎ **Note:** Only leave the tourniquets on 6 to 8 minutes.

Using this method to discover new vessels in patients with sclerosed vessels, the nurse will begin to discover, through palpation, the differences between the collateral veins and the sclerosed vessels.

Obese Patients

In patients with excessive adipose tissue the veins in the extremities react in one of two ways to the subcutaneous fat:

1. The vessels will be buried deep in the tissue; therefore, a 2-in catheter must be used to access the vein.
2. The vasculature will be forced to the surface because the veins have been displaced by the adipose tissue. A vessel can usually be located below the antecubital site, on the lateral dorsum of the forearm.

Multiple tourniquets can also be used to visualize veins. Place one tourniquet on the lower forearm and another tourniquet 2 minutes later at the wrist, to visualize hand veins.

✎ **Note:** The use of a blood pressure cuff is not recommended on obese patients because increased pressure from the cuff can cause backflash of blood.

Edematous Patients

In locating accessible vasculature in the edematous patient, the nurse must displace the tissue fluid with digital pressure. Often this will allow for visualization of an accessible vein. Care must be taken not to contaminate the site once the area is prepared. Venipuncture must be done quickly after the area is prepped to prevent the edematous fluid from obscuring the site.

✎ **Note:** Edematous fluid causes an increase in oncotic pressure. Therefore, if the fluid is not infusing once the catheter is in place, suspect that the vein may have collapsed as a result of the oncotic pressure in the tissue (Fabian, 1991).

SUMMARY OF CHAPTER 9

INTRAVENOUS THERAPY: SPECIAL PROBLEMS

Special Considerations of the Pediatric Patient

PHYSIOLOGIC CHARACTERISTIC OF THE NEONATE
Total body weight 90 percent water; high ratio of extracellular water to intracellular water

Metabolic demand influenced by increased muscular activity, thermal stress, congenital abnormalities, and respiratory distress syndrome
Heat production increased by 7 percent per degree of temperature elevation
Immature renal system
Integumentary system important in regulation of fluid and electrolyte needs

RISK FACTORS
Prematurity
Catabolic disease states
Hypothermia and hyperthermia
Metabolic and respiratory acid-base imbalance

COMPONENTS OF PHYSICAL EXAMINATION
Head circumference measurement up to 1 year
Height or length measurement
Vital signs assessment
Skin turgor assessment
Check for presence of tears
Assessment of moistness and color of mucous membranes
Urinary output monitoring
Checking characteristics of fontanelles
Assessment of level of child's activity

METHODS OF EVALUATION OF FLUID NEEDS
Weight method
Caloric method
Meter square method

INTRAVENOUS TECHNIQUES
Needle choice: 23- to 25-gauge scalp vein catheter or 22- to 24-gauge ONC
Site selection:
Dorsum of hand
Dorsum of foot
Scalp

- Frontal
- Superficial temporal
- Posterior auricular
- Supraorbital
- Occipital
- Posterior facial

INTRAOSSEOUS INFUSIONS
Good route in emergency for delivery of fluids and medications
Limited site for 24 hours
Sites: Proximal tibia, distal tibia, and femur
Used only in children less than 6 years old

CONTRAINDICATIONS FOR INTRAOSSEOUS INFUSION
Cellulitis or infected burn
Fractured limb
Osteoporosis
Osteogenesis imperfecta

Special Considerations of the Geriatric Patient

PHYSIOLOGIC CHARACTERISTICS
Homeostatic mechanisms less efficient
Cardiovascular: Arteries chemically and anatomically changed, elastic fibers frayed and split, increased collagen fibers, and decreased elasticity of wall
Skin: Loss of subcutaneous supporting tissue, thinning of the skin
Renal structures: Decreased glomerular filtration rate
Total body weight water decreased by 6 percent (which leads to potential fluid volume deficit)

ASSESSMENT OF ELDERLY
Skin turgor
Temperature
Rate and filling of veins in hand or foot
Daily weight
Intake and output
Center of tongue should be moist
Postural blood pressure
Swallowing ability
Functional assessment of patient's ability to obtain fluids

TECHNIQUES FOR VENIPUNCTURE
- If patient is hypertensive, do not use a tourniquet.
- Apply tourniquet lightly.
- Use an assistant if necessary to apply digital pressure.
- Use small-gauge needles.
- Enter vein directly.

Venipuncture Techniques for the Difficult Patient

ALTERATIONS IN SKIN SURFACES
Use of tangential lighting
Consideration of patient's photosensitivity and potential for skin damage

HARD SCLEROSED VESSELS
Multiple tourniquet technique
Palpitation of hard piano wire veins versus softer collateral circulation

OBESE PATIENT
Use of multiple-tourniquet technique
Use of 2-in catheters
Use of lateral veins displaced by adipose tissue

EDEMATOUS PATIENT
Edema displaced with digital pressure

Activity Journal

1. You are working on a pediatric ward and are assigned a 6-month-old baby with meningitis. The baby has the I.V. catheter placed in the scalp. You assess the baby and find the site covered with a white paper cup and lots of tape, and the baby's eye beneath the cup is swollen. What is the problem? How do you remedy this situation?

2. You have to start an I.V. infusion on a 70-year-old obese patient with systemic lupus erythematosus. What do you need to consider prior to venipuncture and what techniques should you use to be successful?

3. You must start an I.V. infusion on a 10-year-old who has never been hospitalized before. His diagnosis is osteomyelitis. How would you approach this patient?

4. You are working in an emergency room and a 2-year-old near-drowning victim is brought in and is in respiratory distress. Would you consider intraosseous infusion?

Quality Assessment Model

Instructions: Use this quality assessment model to conduct retrospective audits of charts, establish quality control standards, or develop outcome criteria for quality assurance. Refer to Chapter 2 for details on quality assessment.

STRUCTURE

(Resource that affects outcome)
Human Resource: I.V. Therapist
↓

PROCESS

(Actual giving and receiving of care)
Therapist activities related to care of the patient with special needs are:

1. Assessment of I.V. site every 2 hours or more frequently as needed with pediatric patients.
2. Fluid container on a pediatric patient will be according to weight and age but not to exceed 500 mL.
3. A volume-control chamber within the administration set should be in use on all pediatric patients.
4. Electronic volume control device will be used on all children.
5. Geriatric infusions will be monitored frequently and kept within 10 percent of the prescribed rate.
↓

OUTCOME STANDARDS

(Effects of care)
Documentation will reflect standards of practice for delivery of safe, practical care of the patient with special needs:

1. Evidence of documented site checks every 2 hours on pediatric catheter sites.
2. Evidence of documented use of volume control chamber and amount of fluid hanging.
3. Evidence of documented site checks every 4 hours and appearance of skin on patients age 65 years and older.
4. Evidence of site change within 24 hours when an intraosseous infusion has been started.

Post-test, Chapter 9

Fill in the missing terms in the sentences.

1. _____ infusion is the delivery of fluids and electrolytes into the medullary cavity in the bone.

2. The _____ method calculates the metabolic expenditure of energy in figuring fluid replacement.

3. The period of extrauterine life up to the first 28 days of life is called the _____ period.

4. The breakdown of chemical compounds into more elementary principles by the body is referred to as _____.

5. The _____ _____ _____ is determined through use of a nomogram.

6. List three of the six common reasons for I.V. therapy in an infant.

   A. _____

   B. _____

   C. _____

7. The preferred choice for I.V. site in the young infant under age 9 months is the:
   A. Frontal vein in the scalp
   B. Dorsum of the foot
   C. Dorsum of the hand
   D. Occipital vein on the head

8. The weight method of estimating fluid requirements in a child is:
   A. Weighing diapers and estimating output to replace sensible losses
   B. Formula based on weight in kilograms to estimate fluid needs
   C. Calculation of metabolic expenditure of energy based on weight
   D. Determined by use of a nomogram

9. In a dark-skinned person the best method for locating an accessible vein is:
   A. Multiple tourniquets
   B. Tangential lighting
   C. Direct overhead lighting
   D. Light application of tourniquet

10. What is the most appropriate needle for use on a 2-month-old infant?
    A. 18-gauge ONC
    B. 21-gauge scalp vein needle
    C. 16-gauge scalp vein needle
    D. 23- to 25-gauge scalp vein needle

11. Intraosseous infusion is contraindicated in patients with:
    A. Fractures in the extremities
    B. Infected burns

C. Osteoporosis
D. All of the above

12. When performing an I.V. on a toddler, methods that can be used to assist the therapist in this invasive procedure, based on developmental age, would include:
    A. Letting the child express feelings and scream
    B. Encouraging the child to hold a favorite toy or blanket
    C. Performing the procedure quickly with assistance from parents or other staff
    D. All of the above

13. When performing an I.V. infusion on a school-age child, it is important to:
    A. Explain procedure to patient in simple terms
    B. Limit explanations and perform procedure quickly
    C. Demonstrate procedure using doll or stuffed animal
    D. Have extra help in holding the child during the venipuncture

14. List six of the nine key points in assessment of fluid status in the elderly.

    A. _____

    B. _____

    C. _____

    D. _____

    E. _____

    F. _____

15. Discuss some of the postoperative complications for the elderly related to fluid and electrolyte needs.

Answers to Post-test, Chapter 9

1. Intraosseous
2. Caloric
3. Neonatal
4. Catabolism
5. Body surface area
6. Fluid volume deficit, electrolyte imbalance, nutritional support, antibiotic therapy, and chemotherapy
7. C
8. B
9. B
10. B
11. D
12. D
13. A
14. Skin turgor, temperature, rate and filling of veins in hand or foot, intake and output, daily weight, center of tongue for moisture, positional changes for blood pressure, swallowing ability, functional assessment of patient's ability to obtain fluids
15. Potential for fluid volume deficit, renal insufficiency, respiratory acidosis due to diminished respiratory function, tendency toward metabolic acidosis due to slower renal response to pH changes, hypotension, potential for sodium deficit, preoperative malnutrition (which would contribute to postoperative complications), decreased mobility (which leads to negative nitrogen balance), osteoporosis, muscle weakness, pneumonia, phlebitis, skin breakdown, bladder and bowel dysfunction, and respiratory function decrease

References

American Association of Retired Persons (AARP) (1985). *A profile of older Americans.* Washington, DC: US Department of Health and Human Services.

Arthur, G.M. (1984). When your littlest patients need IVs. *RN, 7,* 30–34.

Blatz, S., & Paes, B.A. (1990). Intravenous infusion by superficial vein in the neonate. *Journal of Intravenous Nursing, 13*(2), 122–128.

Burnside, I.M. (1981). *Nursing and the aged* (2nd ed.). New York: McGraw-Hill.

Chameides, L. (1988). *Textbook of pediatric advanced life support.* Dallas: American Heart Association.

Delaney, C.W., & Lauer, M.L. (1988). *Intravenous therapy: A guide to quality care.* Philadelphia: J.B. Lippincott.

Fabian, B. (1991). *I.V. therapy across the generations.* Paper presented at the Intravenous Nurses Society Annual Conference, Miami Beach, Florida.

Intravenous Nursing Society. (1990). *Standards of practice.* Philadelphia: J.B. Lippincott.

Hodge, D. (1985). Intraosseous infusions: A review. *Pediatric Emergency Care, 1,* 215–218.

Jarmen, C. (1985). Vein trauma—its complications and prevention. *Intravenous Therapy News, 7,*4.

Marlow, D.R., & Redding, B.A. (1988). *Textbook of pediatric nursing* (6th ed.). Philadelphia: W.B. Saunders.

Maxwell, M., & Kleeman, C. (1980). *Clinical disorders of fluid and electrolyte metabolism* (3rd ed.). New York: McGraw-Hill.

Mellema, S.J., Poniatowski, B.C. (1989). Geriatric I.V. therapy. *Journal of Intravenous Therapy, 11*(1), 56–62.

Metheny, N.M. (1987). *Fluid and electrolyte balance nursing considerations.* Philadelphia: J.B. Lippincott.

Oelerich, W.J., & Dombrowski, J.M. (1981). Mini IV patients: Maximum precautions. *RN*, *12*, 43–47.

Peck, K.R., & Altieri, M. (1988). Intraosseous infusions: An old technique with modern applications. *Pediatric Nursing*, *14*(4), 296–298.

Plumer, A.L., & Cosentino, F. (1987). *Principles and practices of intravenous therapy* (4th ed.). Boston: Little, Brown.

Robinson, S., & Demuth, P. (1985). Diagnostic studies for the aged: What are the dangers. *Journal of Gerontological Nursing*, *85*(6), 11.

Rossetti, V.A., Thompson, B.M., & Miller, J. (1985). Intraosseous infusion: An alternative route of pediatric intravascular access. *Annals of Emergency Medicine*, *14*, 885–888.

Smeltzer, S.C. & Bare, B.G. (1992). *Brunner and Suddaith's textbook of medical-surgical nursing (7th ed.)*. Philadelphia: J.B. Lippincott.

Spivey, W.H. (1987). Intraosseous infusions. *Journal of Pediatrics*, *111*(5), 639–643.

Teitell, B.C. (1984). Considerations for neonatal I.V. therapy. *National Intravenous Therapy Association*, *7*(6), 521–524.

Tietjen, S.D. (1990). Starting an infant's I.V. *American Journal of Nursing*, *5*, 44–46.

Weinstein, S.M. (1990). Math calculations for intravenous nurses. *Journal of Intravenous Nursing*, *13*(4), 231–236.

Whaley, L.F., & Wong, D.L. (1985). *Essentials of pediatric nursing*. St. Louis: C.V. Mosby.

Wheeler, C.A. (1989). Pediatric intraosseous infusion: An old technique in modern health care technology. *Journal of Intravenous Nursing*, *12*(6), 371–376.

Wheeler, C.A. (1992). *Pediatric I.V. Therapy*. Intravenous Nurses Society Annual Conference, Dallas, Texas.

Bibliography

Pflaum, S. (1979). Investigation of intake-output as a means of assessing body fluid balance. *Heart Lung*, *8*, 495.

UNIT THREE

ADVANCED PRACTICE

CHAPTER 10

Transfusion Therapy

LESLIE BARANOWSKI and LYNN DIANNE PHILLIPS

PART I

BASIC IMMUNOHEMATOLOGY AND BLOOD COMPONENT THERAPY

Glossary

ABO system: Human blood groups that are inherited; groups determined according to which antigens are present on the surfaces of red blood cells and which antibodies are present in the plasma

Agglutinin: An antibody that causes particulate antigens, such as other cells, to adhere to one another, forming clumps (antibody)

Agglutinogen: An antigenic substance that stimulates the formation of a particular antibody (antigen)

Alloimmunization: Development of an immune response to alloantigens; occurs during pregnancy, blood transfusions, and organ transplantation

Antibody: Protein produced by the immune system that destroys or inactivates a particular antigen

Antigen: Any substance eliciting an immunologic response, such as the production of antibody specific for that substance

Autologous donation: Blood donated before it was needed, to be used only by donor

CPD: Citrate-phosphate-dextrose; a preservative for collected blood

CPDA-1: Citrate-phosphate-dextrose-adenine; a preservative that extends the shelf life of stored blood to 35 days

Designated donation: Transfer of blood directly from one donor to specified recipient

Hemolysis: Rupture of red blood cells, with the release of hemoglobin

HLA: Human leukocyte antigen, used for tissue typing and relevant for transplant histocompatibility

Homologous donation: Donation of blood in similar structure, from a volunteer donor

Immunohematology: Study of blood and blood reactions

IgG: Gamma immunoglobulin

IgM: Immunoglobulin mu

Rh system: Second most important system; Rh antigens are inherited and found on surface of red blood cells; classified as positive or negative based on whether D antigen is present

LEARNING OBJECTIVES

Upon completion of this part of the chapter, the reader will be able to:
- [ ] State the antigens of the ABO system
- [ ] Define the terms related to basic immunohematology
- [ ] State the definition of human leukocyte antigen

☐ Identify the universal blood donor type
☐ State the antibodies in the ABO system
☐ Describe the Rh antigen
☐ Identify the preservatives used in donor blood storage
☐ Summarize the tests used to screen donor blood
☐ Distinguish among homologous, autologous, and designated blood donations

Pre-test, Chapter 10, Part I

Instructions: The pre-test is to review prior knowledge of the theory related to basic immunohematology. Each question in the pre-test is based on the learning objectives of the chapter.

Match the definition in column 2 to the correct term in column 1.

Column 1

1. _____ Agglutinin
2. _____ Antigen
3. _____ Alloimmunization
4. _____ Agglutinogen
5. _____ Designated donor
6. _____ Autologous donor
7. _____ HLA
8. _____ Immunohematology
9. _____ ABO
10. _____ Rh

Column 2

A. Found on the surface of red blood cells, positive or negative

B. Antigenic substance that stimulates the formation of an antibody

C. Substance eliciting an immunologic response

D. Study of blood and blood reactions

E. Antigens present on the surface of red blood cells

F. Human leukocyte antigen

G. Development of immune response to alloantigens

H. Antibody that causes particulate antigens to adhere to one another

I. Concept of donating one's own blood prior to transfusion

J. Donation of blood from selected friends or relatives of the patient

11. The preservative CPDA-1 extends the life of collected cells to:
    A. 25 days
    B. 30 days
    C. 35 days
    D. 42 days

12. The universal plasma donor type is:
    A. A
    B. O

C. AB
D. B

13. Transfusions are screened for all of the following *except*:
    A. Syphilis
    B. Human immunodeficiency virus (HIV)
    C. Surface hepatitis B
    D. Mononucleosis
    E. Hepatitis C

14. The antigens in the blood system would include all of the following *except*:
    A. ABO
    B. Rh
    C. HLA
    D. IgM

ANSWERS TO PRE-TEST, CHAPTER 10, PART I

1. H 2. B 3. G 4. C 5. J 6. I 7. F 8. D 9. E
10. A 11. C 12. C 13. D 14. D

Because the knowledge necessary for the nurse to deliver safe transfusion therapy depends on an understanding of the blood system, this chapter is divided into two parts. The first part establishes an understanding of basic immunohematology, and the second discusses the theory and practical management of blood component therapy. These sections may be used independently, but knowledge of basic immunohematology is crucial to delivery of safe transfusions.

Part I of this chapter introduces the reader to fundamental concepts of immunohematology, blood grouping, and the criteria for donor blood, including autologous, designated, and homologous donation. Fundamental concepts of blood component therapy, administration equipment, administration techniques for each blood component, and management of transfusion reactions are also presented here.

BASIC IMMUNOHEMATOLOGY

Immunohematology is the science that deals with antigens of the blood and their antibodies. The antigens and antibodies are genetically inherited and determine the blood group. An **antigen** is a substance capable of stimulating the production of an **antibody** and then reacting with that antibody in a specific way. It is also referred to as an **agglutinogen**. Antigens are any substance that elicit an immunologic response. The three antigens on the red cells that can cause problems and are routinely tested for are A, B, and Rh D. The human leukocyte antigen **(HLA)** is located on most cells in the body except mature erythrocytes. Antibodies are found in the plasma or serum.

Antigens (Agglutinogens)

ABO, Rh, HLA

ABO System

The most important antigens in the blood are the surface antigens A and B, which are located on the red cell membranes in the **ABO system** (see Table 10–1). Individuals who have A antigen on the red cell membrane are classified as group A; B antigens, group B; A and B antigens, group AB; and neither A nor B antigens, group O. This ABO system was discovered in 1901 by Dr. Karl Landsteiner.

Rh System

The second most important antigen system is the **Rh system**, discovered in 1940 by Drs. Landsteiner and Wiener, and so called because of its relationship to the substance in the red cells of the Rhesus monkey. The antigens in the Rh system are C, D, E, c, and e. A person who has D antigen is classified as Rh positive, one lacking D is Rh negative. Classification in 85 percent of the population is D-Rh positive (Widmann, 1981). D antibodies build up easily; therefore, typing is done to ensure that D-negative recipients receive D-negative blood. Rh-negative recipients should receive Rh-negative whole blood and red blood cell components.

HLA System

The HLA antigen was originally identified on the leukocytes but it has been established that HLA is present on most cells in the body. It is located on the surface of white blood cells, platelets, and most tissue cells. HLA typing, or tissue typing, is important in patients with transplants or multiple transfusions and for paternity testing. The HLA system is very complex and is involved in immune regulation and cellular differentiation.

The HLA system is important in transfusion therapy because of **alloimmunization** of the donor unit HLA antigens that occur in the recipient. This

Table 10–1 □ **BLOOD GROUPING CHART***†

Blood Groupings	Recipient Antigens on RBC's	Antibodies Present in Plasma	Compatible Donor Type
A	A	Anti-B	A, O
B	B	Anti-A	B, O
AB	A and B	None	A, B, AB, and O
O	None	Anti-A and Anti-B	O

*Universal plasma donor is AB; AB has no anti-A or anti-B antibodies in the plasma. Universal blood donor is O negative.
†When giving O negative to an uncrossmatched patient, administer packed cells so that the anti-A and anti-B antibodies within the serum are removed. Uncrossmatched whole blood must not be given.

alloimmunization is important in transplantation and has been found to be a major factor in the onset of refractoriness to random donor platelet support. HLA incompatibility is a possible cause of hemolytic transfusion reactions, and HLA antibodies as well as granulocyte- and platelet-specific antibodies have been implicated in the development of nonhemolytic transfusion reactions.

Methods used to decrease HLA alloimmunization include HLA matching and leukocyte depletion of the donor unit (American Association of Blood Banks [AABB], 1990).

✎ **Note:** Leukocyte antibodies have been shown to be the clinical cause of febrile transfusion reactions (Widmann, 1981). Patients receiving multiple transfusions are at particular risk for developing complications due to HLA alloimmunization.

Antibodies (Agglutinin)

Antibodies within the blood system are proteins that react with a specific antigen. Antigens are **agglutinins** in that particulate antigens, such as other cells, adhere to one another in response to a specific antigen. The antibodies anti-A and anti-B are produced spontaneously in the plasma. Each antibody has the same name as the antigen with which it reacts. For example, anti-A reacts to antigen A.

Naturally occurring antibodies, like those in the ABO system, are blood group antibodies that agglutinate erythrocytes containing corresponding antigens in a saline solution and are called saline antibodies. The naturally occurring antibody in the blood, which occurs within the inherited blood group, is called immunoglobulin mu **(IgM)**. Complete antibodies is the term for naturally occurring antibodies. Intravascular **hemolysis** may occur in vivo with naturally occurring antibodies (IgM).

Immune antibodies that do not agglutinate corresponding antigens in saline solutions are called incomplete antibodies or immunoglobulin **(IgG)**. These antibodies are produced by the immune system in response to previous exposure to the antigen via prior transfusion or pregnancy; they are not genetically inherited. When these antibodies meet with their corresponding antigen, the cells are affected but not destroyed in the intravascular system. The sensitized cells are removed intact by the reticuloendothelial system, primarily the spleen and liver. Albumin can sometimes bridge the molecules together; hence the term albumin agglutinins (Pauley, 1984).

Blood Group System

More than 300 blood group systems are identified, and references may vary on the most important ones; however, nine main blood systems have been defined on the basis of reaction to cells with antibodies. The following lists the most common groups identified:

ABO	Lewis
Rh	MNS
Kell	P
Duffy	Lutheran
Kidd	

Corresponding antibodies to all but ABO and Rh systems are found so infrequently that they do not usually cause common problems in transfusion therapy.

Testing of Donor Blood

At the time of donation, every unit of blood intended for **homologous donation** transfusion must undergo the following tests by the blood bank; Table 10–2 summarizes testing of donor blood.

1. The ABO group must be determined by testing the red blood cells with anti-A and anti-B serums and by testing the serum or plasma with A and B cells.
2. The Rh type must be determined with anti-D serum. *Units that are D positive must be labeled Rh positive.*
3. Most blood blanks test all donor blood for unexpected antibodies. If all donors are not tested, then at least blood from donors with a history of prior transfusion or pregnancy should be tested for unexpected antibodies before the crossmatch. If antibodies are found, then the blood should be processed into component parts that contain only minimal amounts of plasma.
4. All donor blood must be tested to detect transmissible disease. The blood component must not be used for transfusion unless the tests are nonreactive, negative, or within the normal range. Current required tests include:

    Surface hepatitis B (HBsAg)
    Acquired immune deficiency syndrome virus (anti-HIV-1)
    Human T-cell lymphotropic virus (anti-HTLV-1)
    Anticore hepatitis B (anti-HBc)
    Alanine aminotransaminase (ALT) liver test
    Serologic test for syphilis
    Hepatitis C (HCV)
    Cytomegalovirus (CMV) (on units identified for use in pediatric or transplant patients.)

5. Each unit must be appropriately labeled. The label must include the

Table 10–2 □ **SUMMARY OF TESTING OF DONOR BLOOD**

ABO group
Rh type
Testing for unexpected antibodies (escpecially from donors with history of pregnancy or prior transfusion)
Test for transmissible disease:
Syphilis
Anticore and surface hepatitis B
Acquired immune deficiency syndrome virus
Alanine transaminase liver test
Hepatitis C
Appropriate labeling
Compatibility testing on attached segment to blood bag

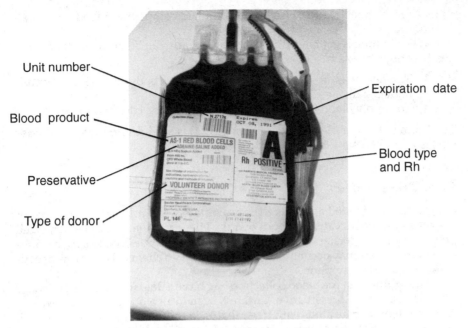

Figure 10–1 □ Correct labeling of blood unit.

following information: name of component, type and amount of anti-coagulant, volume of unit, required storage temperature, name and address of collecting facility, a reference to the circular of information, type of donor (volunteer, autologous, or paid), expiration date, and donor number. See Figure 10–1 for picture of correct labeling of blood unit.

✎ **Note:** The label should also include statements indicating that "this product may transmit infectious agents, and properly identify intended recipient."

6. The facility performing the compatibility testing must do ABO group and Rh type confirmation tests on a sample obtained from the originally attached segment of all units of whole or red cells (AABB, 1990).

Compatibility Testing

Recipients of transfusions must be tested for ABO and Rh grouping. In addition, antibody screening and a compatibility test must be performed. Previous exposure to an antigen by pregnancy or transfusion may have caused the patient to develop an antibody against an antigen.

Compatibility testing is performed between the recipient's plasma and the donor's red cells to ensure that the specific unit intended for transfusion to the recipient is not incompatible. Blood from the donor and recipient are mixed and incubated under a variety of conditions and suspending media. If the cells do not agglutinate, the donor's blood indicates compatibility. Blood bank per-

311

sonnel are responsible for providing serologic compatible blood for transfusion.

When testing is complete, transfusion therapy can begin. The blood bank has two objectives:

1. To prevent antigen-antibody reactions in the body and to identify antibodies that the recipient may have
2. To supply blood from a donation that lacks the corresponding antigen

The testing of donor blood and recipient blood is intended to prevent adverse effects of transfusion therapy.

Blood Preservatives

One donation of blood amounts to approximately 450 mL, and the volume of anticoagulant preservative is about 65 mL. There are several available red cell preservatives. Understanding of the red cell preservative is necessary because adverse reactions may occur in some patients due to chemicals in the anticoagulant-preservative solution.

The solutions in the blood collection bag have a dual function: as anticoagulant and as red cell preservative. Citrate is used in all blood preservatives as an anticoagulant. Citrate binds with free calcium in the donor's plasma. Blood will not clot in the absence of free or ionized calcium. Citrate prevents coagulation by inhibiting the calcium-dependent steps of the coagulation cascade. Preservatives provide proper nutrients to maintain red cell viability, function, and metabolism. Additionally, refrigeration at 1° to 6°C preserves red blood cells and minimizes proliferation of bacteria (Widmann, 1981).

The first preservative, acid-citrate-dextrose (ACD), was introduced in 1944 and used until replaced in 1971 by citrate-phosphate-dextrose **(CPD)**. The purpose of each of these chemicals is explained here.

Acid is used to prevent caramelization of the glucose if autoclaved in an alkaline environment and thus maintains the level of glucose to provide adequate viability to the red cell for 21 days. Dextrose is used as a nutrient to the red cell and supports continuing adenosine triphosphate (ATP) generation necessary for red cell viability. The expiration of red cells preserved in ACD is 21 days.

In 1971, CPD became a common preservative for blood. Compared with ACD, it offers a higher pH to prevent acid buildup in stored red blood cells. Phosphate is added to buffer the decrease in pH. The compound in the red blood cell that facilitates the transport of oxygen is 2,3-diphosphoglycerate (2,3-DPG). When the pH of the blood drops there is a decrease in 2,3-DPG and therefore a lowering of the oxygen-carrying capacity of the blood. The 2,3-DPG levels remain higher in blood stored in CPD versus ACD preservative. The expiration of red blood cells preserved in CPD is 21 days stored at 1° to 6° F.

CPD-adenine **(CPDA-1)** was licensed in 1978. This preservative contains adenine, which helps the red blood cells synthesize ATP during storage. Cells have improved viability in this anticoagulant-preservative because ATP is better preserved than in ACD or plain CPD. This preservative lengthens the shelf life of the blood to 35 days. CPDA-1 is beneficial for blood bank inventory, but its disadvantage is that it can cause adenine toxicity.

The newest anticoagulant-preservative is CPD-AS. Manufactured by Fenwal Laboratories and known as AS-1 or ADSOL, this solution is added to packed red blood cells and extends their expiration to 42 days after the day of collection. This preservative was licensed in 1983 by the Food and Drug Administration (FDA), and a similar preservative manufactured by Cutter Laboratories, known as AS-2 or Nutrice, has an expiration date of 35 days. Both solutions have a 100-mL volume and contain dextrose, adenine, and saline, with AS-1 additionally containing mannitol. These additives are added to packed red blood cells only after removal from the plasma.

✎ **Note:** Red cells prepared with ADSOL have better flow rates and do not require dilution with saline.

✎ **Note:** Hypocalcemia is an adverse reaction that can occur when large amounts of citrated blood are infused in an individual with impaired liver function.

BLOOD DONOR COLLECTION METHODS

Homologous

The term **homologous donation** describes transfusion of any blood component that was donated by someone other than the intended recipient. Most transfusions depend on homologous sources and are provided by volunteer donors.

Guidelines for Homologous Donor

Donor selection for homologous collection is based on a limited physical examination and a medical history to determine the safety of the donated unit. Strict criteria have been established for selection of prospective donors:

1. Brief health history, including illnesses, surgeries, drugs and medications, along with immunization information
2. Screening for diseases
3. Stable vital signs
4. Age
5. Weight (smaller volume should be drawn from donors weighing less than 110 lb)
6. No evidence of skin lesions at site of venipuncture
7. Adequate venous access for venipuncture
8. No donation of blood or plasma within last 8 weeks or hemapheresis within last 48 hours
9. Hemoglobin and hematocrit of at least 12.5 g/dL and 38 percent (male) or 12.0 g/dL and 36 percent (female).

Autologous

Autologous transfusion refers to the collection, storage, and delivery of a patient's own blood. This option is considered for patients who are likely to re-

313

ceive a transfusion during elective surgery. Patients may be able to donate their own blood before the operation.

The use of autologous blood avoids the possibility of alloimmunization because it does not contain foreign red blood cells, platelets, and leukocyte antigens. The risk of exposure and disease transmission is also eliminated. Because of this the use of autologous blood is regarded as safer than homologous transfusion. However, risks associated with labeling and documentation are still present. The same precautions used for preparing and administering a homologous blood component must be observed (Popovsky, 1986).

Guidelines for Autologous Donor

Autologous transfusion can be accomplished through preoperative collection or from intraoperative or postoperative blood salvage. For preoperative collection, blood is collected into an anticoagulant-preservative solution and stored. The 42-day shelf life of red cells needs to be considered. If necessary, red cells can be stored frozen. Frozen storage is not routinely recommended owing to considerable expense and the limitation of some blood banks.

The criteria for patient selection for autologous donation is not as restrictive as with homologous donations. Typically, autologous blood is not drawn more often than once a week. The last donation should be at least 72 hours and preferably 1 week before an operation to avoid hypovolemia during surgery. It is best to collect blood as far in advance of the intended date of surgery as is feasible. Except in special circumstances, the hemoglobin should be 11 g/dL and the hematocrit 33 percent or greater prior to each donation.

Oral iron supplementation should be considered to replenish bone marrow iron reserves for autologous donors (AABB, 1990).

Designated (Directed)

Designated donation, also called directed donation, refers to the donation of blood from selected friends or relatives of the patient. Most blood centers and hospitals provide this service. Designated donations have been requested more frequently owing to the concern over the risk of transfusion-transmitted diseases. However, there is no evidence that designated donations are safer than blood provided by transfusion service (AABB, 1990). Relatives or friends who may be members of a risk group may feel forced into donating and hesitate to identify themselves as a risk group member.

Figure 10–2 is of a designated donor unit.

Guidelines for Designated Donor

The selection and screening of designated donors is the same as for other homologous donors, except the units collected are labeled for a specific recipient. The designated donor must pass all the history and screening tests required and the unit must be compatible with the intended recipient (AABB, 1990).

314

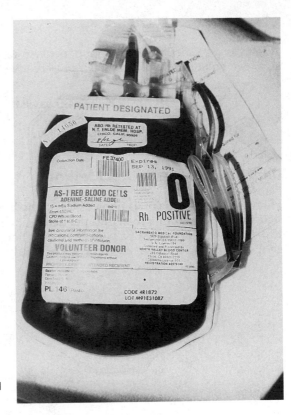

Figure 10-2 □ Designated donor unit.

SUMMARY OF CHAPTER 10, PART I

BASIC IMMUNOHEMATOLOGY

Immunohematology is the science that deals with antigens of the blood and their antibodies. Human blood can be typed on the basis of presence or absence of certain antigens and antibodies. Blood types are differentiated by their antigen and antibody content. Antigens are found in the red cell; antibodies, in the plasma or serum. Several different blood grouping systems are used to type blood. The most important antigen systems are the ABO and Rh systems.

Compatibility Testing

The testing of donor and recipient blood is done to prevent adverse and possibly fatal effects of transfusion therapy. Recipients of transfusions must be tested for ABO and Rh grouping. Crossmatching of the donor's blood is done with a sample of the recipient's blood. Antibody screening and a compatibility test must be performed. *Universal red cell donor type is O negative.*

315

Blood Preservatives

Additives are added to red cell components to act as an anticoagulant and preservative solution. Several red cell preservative solutions are available:

CPD

CPDA-1: extends life of cells to 35 days; the preservative used most frequently today

CPD-AS: extends life of cells to 49 days

Blood Donor Collection Methods

Homologous transfusion is transfusion of any blood component that was donated by someone other than the intended recipient. Autologous transfusion is the storage and delivery of a patient's own blood. Designated transfusion describes the blood from selected friends or relatives of the patient or recipient.

1. The universal blood donor is:
   A. O positive
   B. O negative
   C. AB positive
   D. AB negative

Match the definition in column 2 to the correct term in column 1.

Column 1

2. _____ HLA

3. _____ Antibody

4. _____ CPD

5. _____ Antigen

6. _____ ABO system

7. _____ Homologous transfusion

8. _____ Designated transfusion

9. _____ Autologous transfusion

10. _____ Rh system

Column 2

A. A preservative used for collected blood

B. Antigen used for tissue typing and relevant for transplant

C. Substance eliciting immunologic response

D. Protein produced by the immune system that destroys or inactivates an antigen

E. The most important antigen system in the blood

F. Concept of donating one's own blood prior to transfusion

G. Antigens found on the surface of red blood cells, positive or negative

H. Transfer of blood directly from one donor to a specified recipient

I. Donation of blood in similar structure, from volunteer donor

11. All of the following statements related to the HLA system are true *except*:
    A. HLA is located on the surface of white blood cells.
    B. Alloimmunization to HLA antigens is a factor in refractoriness to platelets.
    C. The use of type and crossmatch reduces the alloimmunization to the HLA antigen.
    D. The use of leukocyte-depleted blood can reduce the sensitization to HLA antigens.

12. Antibodies are found in the:
    A. Red cells
    B. White cells
    C. Plasma
    D. Antigens

13. Previous exposure to an antigen by pregnancy or previous transfusion may cause:
    A. The patient to develop an antibody to the antigen
    B. The patient to develop more antigens
    C. The patient to develop alloimmunization to the antibody
    D. The patient to develop a tolerance to the transfusion

14. A chemical added to donor units to preserve the blood is:
    A. Sodium heparin
    B. Sodium citrate
    C. Sodium phosphate
    D. Dextrose aluminum

15. Blood bank testing for donor blood includes tests for the following diseases *except*:
    A. HBsAg
    B. Anti-HIV-1
    C. Anti-HTLV-1
    D. Epstein-Barr virus (EBV)

Answers to Post-test, Chapter 10, Part I

1. B
2. B
3. D
4. A
5. C
6. E
7. I
8. H

9. F
10. G
11. C
12. C
13. A
14. B
15. D

PART II

BLOOD COMPONENT THERAPY

PART II CONTENTS

320

Glossary

Allergic reaction: Exposure to an antigen to which the person has become sensitized

Blood component: Product made from a unit of whole blood such as platelets, concentrate, red blood cells, fresh frozen plasma, cryoprecipitate

Delayed transfusion reaction: Adverse effect occurring after 48 hours and up to 180 days after transfusion

Febrile reaction: Nonhemolytic reaction to antibodies formed against leukocytes

Hemoglobin: Respiratory pigment of red blood cells having the reversible property of taking up oxygen or of releasing oxygen

Hemolysis: Rupture of red cells, with the release of hemoglobin

Hemolytic transfusion reaction: Blood transfusion reaction in which an antigen-antibody reaction in the recipient is due to incompatibility between red cell antigens and antibodies

Hypothermia: Abnormally low body temperature

Immediate reaction: Adverse effect occurring immediately or up to 48 hours after infusion

Microaggregate: Microscopic collection of particles such as platelets, leukocytes, and fibrin, which occurs in stored blood

Pheresis: Derived from the Greek word "aphairesis," which means "to take away;" used to denote the removal of blood, the separation into component parts, the retention of only the parts needed, and the return of the rest to donor (e.g., removal of plasma is plasmapheresis)

Plasma: The fluid portion of blood, composed of a mixture of proteins in solution

Refractory: Not responsive or readily yielding to treatment

Serum: The cells and fibrinogen-free amber fluid after blood or plasma clots

Thrombocytopenia: Abnormally small number of platelets in the blood

LEARNING OBJECTIVES

Upon completion of this part of the chapter, the reader will be able to:

☐ Define the terminology related to transfusion therapy
☐ Describe each of the blood components
☐ List the indications for use of each blood component
☐ State the key points in the administration of red cells, platelets, granulocytes, fresh frozen plasma, and cryoprecipitate.
☐ Describe the procedure for administration of blood components
☐ List the symptoms of hemolytic transfusion reaction, both acute and delayed

☐ State the signs and symptoms of febrile transfusion reaction and allergic transfusion reaction
☐ Differentiate between febrile and allergic transfusion reactions
☐ Identify the nursing interventions to deliver safe transfusion therapy
☐ Determine nursing diagnoses appropriate for the patient experiencing transfusion therapy

Pre-test, Chapter 10, Part II

Instructions: The pre-test is to review prior knowledge of the theory related to blood component therapy. Each question in the pre-test is based on the learning objectives of the chapter.
   Match the definition in column 2 to the correct term in column 1.

Column 1	Column 2
1. _____ Blood component	A. Respiratory pigment of red blood cell
2. _____ Microaggregate	B. Fluid portion of blood
3. _____ Plasma	C. Removal of blood, separation into component parts, and retention of part
4. _____ Delayed reaction	
5. _____ Hemolytic transfusion reaction	D. Adverse effect occurring immediately or up to 48 hours after transfusion
6. _____ Pheresis	E. Not responsive nor readily yielding to treatment
7. _____ Immediate reaction	
8. _____ Hemoglobin	F. Adverse effect occurring 48 hours up to 180 days after transfusion
9. _____ Refractory	G. Rupture of red cells
10. _____ Hemolysis	H. Product made from a unit of whole blood
	I. Microscopic collection of particles, which occurs in stored blood
	J. Red cells destroyed in the recipient during a transfusion

11. Cryoprecipitate is the component used to treat:
    A. Bleeding disorders related to factor VIII deficiency
    B. Acute massive blood loss
    C. Chronic anemia
    D. Bleeding disorders related to factor IX deficiency

12. Platelets are used to provide:
    A. Protein
    B. Clotting factors
    C. Red blood cells
    D. Granulocytes

13. Whole blood is used to treat:
    A. Chronic anemia
    B. Deficiency in factor VIII
    C. Massive blood loss
    D. White blood cell deficiency

14. The recommended rate of infusion for 1 U of packed red blood cells is no longer than
    A. 1 hour
    B. 2 hours
    C. 4 hours
    D. 6 hours

15. The nurse must check which of the following with another nurse before initiating the transfusion?
    A. ABO and Rh
    B. Patient name
    C. Unit number
    D. Expiration date
    E. All of the above

ANSWERS TO PRE-TEST, Chapter 10, Part II

1. H   2. I   3. B   4. F   5. J   6. C   7. D   8. A   9. E

10. G   11. A   12. B   13. C   14. C   15. E

BLOOD

The fluid tissue that circulates through the heart, arteries, capillaries, and veins, supplies oxygen and food to the other tissues of the body, and removes from them carbon dioxide, as well as waste products of metabolism, is called blood. Blood is a "liquid organ" with functions as extraordinary and unique as those of any other body organ. Fifty-five percent of blood is **plasma** (fluid); the remaining cellular portion (45 percent) is composed of solids — red cells, white cells, and platelets. Table 10–3 summarizes actions, uses, infusion guides, and special considerations of blood components.

> **BLOOD COMPONENT THERAPY**
> Whole blood
> Packed red blood cells
> Washed red blood cells
> Deglycerolized red blood cells
> Granulocytes
> Platelets
> Fresh frozen plasma
> Cryoprecipitate
> Albumin and plasma protein fraction
> Immune serum globulin

Table 10-3 □ **SUMMARY OF BLOOD COMPONENTS**

Blood Component	Volume	Action and Uses	Infusion Guide	Special Considerations
Whole blood	200 mL RBCs 300 mL plasma Total = 500 mL	Massive blood loss Restore blood volume Raise hemoglobin and hematocrit	0.9% sodium chloride primer Transfuse over 2–4 h Y blood set necessary Shelf life: 35 d (1,2) CPDA-1 ADSOL 49 d Filter	Always ABO and Rh Identical 1 unit whole blood raises the hemoglobin 1 g and hematocrit 3–4%
Red cells PRBCs	250 mL (same amount of hemoglobin and hematocrit as whole blood)	Acute anemia with hypoxia Chronic symptomatic anemia Aplastic anemia Bone marrow failure due to malignancy or chemotherapy	Same as whole blood Transfuse over 1-1/2–2 h	May add 50 mL normal saline to RBCs to decrease viscosity ABO and Rh identical 1 U PRBCs raises the hemoglobin 1 g and hematocrit 3–4%
Washed red cells	200–250 mL	Provides leukocyte-poor RBCs for patient with recurrent allergic or febrile transfusion reactions	Same as whole blood 24 h expiration date	Lab needs advanced notice to prepare cells This procedure is an open system: once ordered and the process of washing started, it must be used

(continued)

Table 10–3 □ **SUMMARY OF BLOOD COMPONENTS—Continued**

Blood Component	Volume	Action and Uses	Infusion Guide	Special Considerations
Deglycerolized red cells (frozen)	200–250 mL	Prolonged storage of blood, especially rare blood types Minimizes febrile or allergic reactions	Same as whole blood Infuse over 1-1/2–2 h Expires in 24 h	Blood bank will not deglycerolize until requested, and takes about 1 h
Granulocytes Leukopheresis	300–400 mL Note: Suspended in 200–200 mL of plasma	Patients with neutropenia, fever, or significant infection unresponsive to antibiotics	Usually administered for 4 consecutive days Standard blood filter Administer slowly over 2–4 hours Administer as soon as collected or at least within 24 h	ABO/Rh compatible Reactions are common Check vitals every 15 min Note: Febrile reactions occur in about two thirds of patients. Chills, fever, and allergic reactions common Requires premedication to control reactions
Platelets Random	60–70 mL/U minimum Usual dose: 6–10 U	Control bleeding in platelet deficiencies Thrombocytopenia Bone marrow	Administer as rapidly as patient can tolerate; 1–2 mL/min	Requires 20 min pooling time by laboratory ABO/Rh preferred

				but not necessary
		hypoplasia due to chemotherapy	Recommended 150–200 mL/h, platelet administration set (syringe push or Y type) Use a Y filter with saline as primer	
Fresh frozen plasma (FFP)	200–250 mL	Replacement of coagulation factors Increases clotting factors Factor deficiencies (e.g., factor V or XI) Thrombotic thrombocytopenia purpura	Storage is at 18°C for 1 y Standard blood filter	Does not provide platelets 1 mL of FFP raises the level of clotting factor 2–3%
Cryoprecipitate (concentrated fibrinogen)	Each unit contains 150 mg fibrinogen/15 mL plasma (5–10 mL U) with 10 mL saline added. Usual order is for 6–10 U	Used to control bleeding associated with deficiency in coagulation factors Treatment of hemophilia A, von Willebrand's disease, hypofibrinogenemia, factor VIII deficiency, DIC associated with obstetric complications	Administer with filter provided with product Give as fast as patient tolerates Monitor pulse while infusing	ABO compatible with patient's red cells If blood group unknown, use AB blood Rh match not required Must be used within 3 h after reconstituted

(continued)

Table 10–3 □ **SUMMARY OF BLOOD COMPONENTS—Continued**

Blood Component	Volume	Action and Uses	Infusion Guide	Special Considerations
Albumin 5% = 12.5 g/250 mL 25% = 12.5 g/50 mL	5% solution is in concentration of 250 mL or 500 mL; 25% solution is in 50–100 mL concentration	Plasma volume expander Hypovolemic shock Support blood pressure during hypotensive episodes Induce diuresis in fluid overload	May be administered as rapidly as tolerated if for reduced blood volume Normal rates: 2–4 mL/min for 5% solution; 1 mL/min for 25% solution Supplied in glass bottles with tubing for administration	25% albumin is hypertonic and is five times more concentrated than 5% solutions. Give with extreme caution; can cause circulatory overload No type or cross-match is necessary Store at room temperature
Plasma protein fraction (PPF)	Glass bottle with tubing, 250 mL	Same as albumin	Equivalent to 5% albumin Do not need saline primer	Has fewer purification steps than albumin No type and cross-match necessary Has a high sodium content
Intravenous serum globulin (IVIgG)	Lyophilized powder reconstituted with sterile water for injection following manufacturer directions	Primary immunodeficiency disorders Idiopathic thrombocytopenic purpura (ITP) Chronic B-cell lymphocytic leukemia Restores, strengthens, or modifies immunity	Standard administration set with vented airway Some manufacturers supply administration set Dose range: 200–400 mg/kg Rates of infusion are specific Rates are increased gradually	Severe reactions are rare No type and cross-match necessary Anaphylactic reaction can occur and is the greatest risk

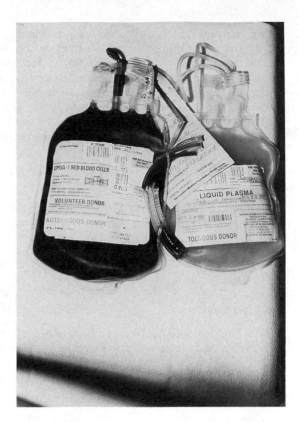

Figure 10–3 □ Whole blood components: Red blood cells and liquid plasma.

Whole Blood

Whole blood is composed of red blood cells (RBCs), plasma, white blood cells, and platelets (Fig. 10–3). The volume of each unit is approximately 500 mL and consists of 200 mL RBCs and 300 mL of plasma. Advances in the use of blood components have made the administration of whole blood rarely necessary.

Uses

Most whole blood units are now used to prepare valuable separate red cell and plasma components to meet specific clinical needs. A whole blood unit can be centrifuged and separated into three components: red blood cells, plasma, and platelet concentrates. By transfusing the patient with the specific component needed rather than with whole blood, the patient is not exposed to unnecessary portions of the blood product, and valuable blood resources are conserved.

Few conditions require transfusion of whole blood. A unit of whole blood increases red cell mass, which provides oxygen-carrying capacity and provides plasma for blood volume expansion. The primary indication for use is for patients experiencing acute massive blood loss of greater than 25 percent of their

329

blood volume. This type of patient requires both increased oxygen-carrying capacity and restoration of blood volume, or hemorrhagic shock could develop.

When whole blood has been stored for over 24 hours, degeneration of some of the components of whole blood occurs, resulting in nonviable platelets and granulocytes. In addition, levels of factor V and factor VIII decrease with storage. Therefore, a whole blood transfusion would not provide a therapeutic platelet transfusion or replace several clotting factors. Stable coagulation factors II, VII, IX, and X, and fibrinogen are well maintained throughout the storage period for whole blood units.

✎ **Note:** In an adult, 1 U of whole blood increases the **hemoglobin** by about 1 g/dL or the hematocrit by about 3 to 4 percent (AABB, 1989).

✎ **Note:** Unless a patient who receives whole blood needs volume replacement, in addition to oxygen-carrying capacity, fluid overload may occur. Plasma contained in whole blood provides an unnecessary volume load to patients who do not require or cannot tolerate excessive volume expansion.

Administration

Whole blood should not be given to patients with chronic anemia who are normovolemic and require only an increase in red cell mass. The administration of whole blood is indicated for neonatal exchange transfusion.

Whole Blood Administration Summary

Amount: 500 mL
Catheter choice: 20- to 18-gauge preferred
Usual rate: 2 to 4 hours
Administration set: Straight or Y type with filter or microaggregate recipient set

Compatibility

✎ **Note:** Whole blood requires type and crossmatching and must be ABO *identical*.

Packed Red Blood Cells

Packed red blood cell (PRBC) units are prepared by removing 200 to 250 mL of plasma from a whole blood unit by centrifugation. The remaining PRBC concentrate has a volume of approximately 300 mL, depending on the type of additive. Each unit contains the same red cell mass as whole blood, as well as 20 to 30 percent of the original plasma, leukocytes, and some platelets. The advantages to PRBCs over whole blood are decreased plasma volume in a red cell unit and decreased risk of circulatory overload. Another advantage is that because most of the plasma has been removed, less citrate, potassium, ammonia, and other metabolic byproducts are transfused.

✎ **Note:** In a normal adult patient, 1 U of PRBCs should raise the hemoglobin level approximately 1 g/dL or the hematocrit 3 percent (AABB, 1986b).

Uses

PRBCs are the component of choice for patients with chronic symptomatic anemia, liver, cardiac, or kidney disease, and patients who do not require restoration of blood volume. With each of these conditions the administration of PRBCs should be considered only if improvement of the red cell count cannot be achieved by nutrition, drug therapy, or treatment of the underlying disease. A definitive level has not been established for when transfusion of PRBCs is indicated or above which transfusion would be inappropriate. The traditional approach has been to transfuse patients when their hemoglobin drops below 10 g/dL or their hematocrit falls to 30 percent. Nevertheless, the decision to transfuse a patient with PRBCs should be based on the patient's clinical status rather than exclusively on the hemoglobin or hematocrit level (AABB, 1990). Patients with chronic anemia should be transfused only if they are symptomatic owing to a decrease in oxygen-carrying capacity because they usually adjust to the lower hemoglobin level and may not require a costly transfusion. Even if large volumes of blood are lost, other components such as platelets and plasma coagulation factors can be provided, rather than using whole blood (Baranowski, 1992).

Administration

PRBC administration is used for an operative blood loss of more than 1200 mL of blood. An operative blood loss of less than 1000 to 1200 mL of blood can be replaced by crystalloid or colloid solutions rather than with PRBCs. When the blood loss is greater than 1500 mL, PRBCs have a greater benefit than the use of whole blood (AABB, 1990).

TRANSFUSE RED BLOOD CELLS
To increase oxygen-carrying capacity in anemic patients

DO NOT TRANSFUSE RED BLOOD CELLS
For volume expansion
In place of a hematinic
To enhance wound healing
To improve general "well being"

(NIH, 1989)

Packed Cells Administration Summary

Amount: 250 mL
Catheter choice: 20- to 18-gauge preferred, as use of a 22-gauge does not always allow free flow and may require an infusion pump
Usual rate: 1-1/2 to 2 hours
Administration set: Straight or Y type with 170-micron microaggregate or leukocyte-depleting filters.

Compatibility

PRBCs require type and crossmatching before being transfused into a patient.

✎ **Note:** If the plasma has been removed, the unit of PRBC does not have to be ABO identical but it must be ABO compatible.

Washed Red Blood Cells

PRBCs can be "washed" with sterile saline using machines specially designed for this purpose. Saline washing removes most of the plasma, reduces the concentration of leukocytes, and removes platelets, along with cellular debris. Some red cell loss also occurs in the washing process, resulting in a reduced hematocrit. Washing may be performed at any time during the shelf life of a unit of blood.

✎ **Note:** The washing procedure is an open system process; therefore, once a unit of blood has been washed it must be used within 24 hours following preparation because of the risk of bacterial contamination (AABB, 1989).

Uses

Washed cells are used to provide leukocyte-poor RBCs for patients who have had recurrent or severe allergic or febrile transfusion reactions. The amount of leukocyte removal provided by washing does not meet the required depletion for prevention of HLA alloimmunization but may reduce **febrile reactions**. Because washing removes plasma proteins, the use of washed cells is indicated for patients with a history of severe **allergic reactions** (AABB, 1986b).

✎ **Note:** Washed cells are currently used with less frequency owing to the recent development of leukocyte-depleting filters, which are more efficient at removing leukocytes and more cost effective than the washing process.

Compatibility

Type and crossmatch are required, and the unit must be ABO compatible.

Deglycerolized Red Blood Cells

Deglycerolized red blood cells are prepared to allow for freezing of cells for long-term storage to preserve rare units of red blood cells and autologous donor units. The red cells are frozen after removal of the plasma by adding glycerol, a cryoprotective agent. Glycerol enters the cell and protects the cell from damage due to cell dehydration and mechanical injury from ice formation. Before transfusion, glycerol is removed by washing to prevent osmotic **hemolysis**. This washing process has the advantage of removing leukocytes, platelets, and plasma.

Uses

Deglycerolized red cells are suitable for transfusing patients who are sensitized to gamma A immunoglobulin (IgA) protein or to leukocyte or platelet antigens. Because of the extensive preparation and cost associated with this procedure, its use is not practical for prophylactic prevention of febrile transfusion reactions. As with washed cells, this process results in a decreased red cell mass.

✎ **Note:** Deglycerolization of red blood cells extends storage to 3 years or more; a thawed unit is stored at 4°C and must be used within 24 hours.

Granulocytes

Granulocyte concentrations are prepared by leukopheresis from a single donor. Each unit contains granulocytes, as well as variable amounts of lymphocytes, platelets, and red cells, suspended in 200 to 300 mL of plasma.

Uses

Prophylactic use of granulocyte transfusion is of questionable therapeutic value, and it is given infrequently. The use of granulocytes is indicated for patients with neutropenia who have been febrile for 24 to 48 hours and have evidence of significant infection that is unresponsive to appropriate antibiotic therapy or other modes of therapy. The patient should have a reasonable chance of recovering from the episode of neutropenia with an expected eventual chance for recovery of bone marrow function. Granulocyte transfusion has not been proved effective in patients with localized infections or infections with agents other than bacteria. Septicemia should be documented by cultures to identify the infecting organism and sensitivities.

Administration

It is expected that the patient will experience chills, fever, and allergic reactions to the transfusion. These side effects can be managed with diphenhydramine or meperidine or both, steroids and nonaspirin antipyretics, and slowing of the transfusion rate. The transfusion should not be discontinued unless severe respiratory distress occurs. The concentrate must be infused within 24 hours after collection, and to achieve maximal clinical effect it should be delivered as soon as possible (AABB, 1990).

Granulocyte Administration Summary

Amount: 300 to 400 mL suspended in 200 to 300 mL of plasma
Catheter choice: 20- to 18-gauge preferred
Usual rate: 1 to 2 hours; slower if reaction occurs
Administration set: Straight or Y type with filter; microaggregate filter contraindicated

Compatibility

Donor blood must be ABO and Rh compatible because a unit of granulocytes is usually heavily contaminated with red cells. There is no set standard regarding the amount or duration of granulocyte therapy but generally transfusion therapy is delivered for at least four consecutive days.

Platelets

Platelets can be supplied as either random-donor or single-donor concentrates. Platelet concentrates (random donor) are prepared from individual units of whole blood by centrifugation. The platelets are stored at room temperature (20 to 24°C) with constant, gentle agitation to maintain viability of the platelets. Platelets can be stored for up to 5 days, depending on the plastic formation of the storage bag. Single-donor platelet **pheresis** products are collected from a single donor, and all unneeded portions of the donor's blood are returned back to the donor. A single pheresis unit is equivalent to 6 to 8 U of random-donor platelets. The use of a single-donor unit has the obvious advantage of exposing the recipient to fewer donors and is ideal for treating patients who have developed HLA antibodies from previous transfusion and have become refractory or unresponsive to random-donor platelets. HLA typing may be indicated when patients become refractory to platelets after multiple transfusion. Platelet crossmatch procedures are also being evaluated for their usefulness with **refractory** patients.

✎ **Note:** One platelet concentrate should raise the recipient's platelet count 5000 to 10,000. The usual dose is 6 to 10 U of concentrate (AABB, 1990).

Uses

Platelets are administered to control or prevent bleeding from platelet deficiencies resulting in **thrombocytopenia** or for the presence of functionally abnormal platelets. Indications for platelet transfusion include:

- Hemorrhage with platelet count less than 50,000
- Surgery with platelet count less than 100,000
- Nonbleeding patients with rapidly dropping counts, less than 15,000 to 20,000

Platelet transfusions at higher platelet counts may be required for patients with systemic bleeding and for patients at high risk of bleeding because of additional coagulation defects, sepsis, or platelet dysfunctions related to medication or disease. Significant spontaneous bleeding with platelet counts of more than 20,000 are rare. Platelet transfusions are usually not effective in patients with conditions in which rapid platelet destruction occurs, such as idiopathic thrombocytopenic purpura (ITP) and untreated disseminated intravascular coagulation (DIC). With these conditions platelet transfusions should be used only in the presence of active bleeding (Rutman & Miller, 1981, p 45).

TRANSFUSE PLATELETS
To control or prevent bleeding associated with deficiencies in platelet number or function

DO NOT TRANSFUSE PLATELETS

To patients with ITP (unless there is life-threatening bleeding)
Prophylactically with massive blood transfusions
Prophylactically following cardiopulmonary bypass

(National Institute of Health, Publication No 89-2974a, 1989)

Administration

The half-life of platelets is 3 to 4 days; transfusions may be repeated every 1 to 3 days. The platelets may be infused as rapidly as the patient tolerates, with infusion rates ranging from 1 to 2 mL/minute up to 5 minutes/bag. Platelets should be delivered to infants using a syringe-type device and can be transfused at a rate of 1 mL/minute.

The effectiveness of platelet transfusions may be altered if fever, infection, or active bleeding is present. To determine the effectiveness of a transfusion, platelet counts may be checked at 1 hour and 18 to 24 hours after transfusion. Patients who repeatedly have poor clinical response or poor 1-hour platelet count increment responses are likely to be alloimmunized and are considered refractory to platelet transfusions.

Platelet Administration Summary

Amount: 30 to 50 mL/U; usual dose 6 to 8 U
Catheter choice: 20- to 22-gauge
Usual rate: 1 U in 5 to 10 minutes as tolerated
Administration set: Component syringe or Y drip set; tubing should be rubber free to prevent platelets from sticking; use saline as primer

Platelet concentrates may be pooled before administration or infused individually. If pooled, platelets should be transfused within 6 hours.

Compatibility

Preferably, platelets should be ABO compatible; but when ABO compatibility is unavailable, mismatched platelets may be given. Crossmatching is not required. Rh matching is also preferred. Standard pretransfusion compatibility testing is not done for platelets.

Fresh Frozen Plasma

Fresh frozen plasma (FFP) is prepared from whole blood by separating and freezing the plasma within 6 hours of collection. FFP may be stored for up to 1 year at $-18\,^{\circ}$C or lower. The volume of a typical unit is 200 to 250 mL. FFP does not provide platelets, and loss of factors V and VIII, the labile clotting factors, is minimal.

Uses

FFP is primarily used to provide replacement coagulation factors. FFP is indicated for patients with multiple coagulation factor deficiencies secondary to

335

liver disease, DIC, and the dilutional coagulopathy resulting from massive volume load or volume replacement. FFP is indicated for patients with demonstrated factor deficiencies for which no coagulation concentrate is available, such as deficiencies of factor V or XI (AABB, 1989a). FFP may be used also for coumarin drug reversal when time does not permit reversal by stopping the drug or administering vitamin K. Patients with other rare deficiencies such as antithrombin III deficiency and thrombotic thrombocytopenic purpura may also benefit from FFP.

✎ **Note:** FFP contains optimal levels of all plasma clotting factors with approximately 200 U factor activity per bag and 200 to 400 mg fibrinogen per bag (AABB, 1986b).

TRANSFUSE FRESH FROZEN PLASMA
To increase the level of clotting factors in patients with a demonstrated
deficiency

DO NOT TRANSFUSE FRESH FROZEN PLASMA
For volume expansion
As a nutritional supplement
Prophylactically with massive blood transfusion

(National Institutes of Health, Publication No. 89-2974a, 1989)

Administration

Before being transfused, FFP must be thawed in a 30 to 37°C waterbath with gentle agitation or kneading. The thawing process takes approximately 30 minutes and the FFP should be transfused as soon as possible after thawing or within 6 hours. FFP must be delivered through a standard blood filter. It can be infused as fast as the patient tolerates or condition indicates. Rates of 4 to 10 mL/minute have been suggested, and most units are generally completed within 1 to 2 hours.

Fresh Frozen Plasma Administration Summary

Amount: 200 to 300 mL
Catheter choice: 20- to 22-gauge
Usual rate: 1 to 2 hours
Administration set: Straight or Y type with filter

Compatibility

Compatibility testing is not required, but the patient's ABO group must be known before product selection to make sure A or B antibodies present in the plasma are compatible with the patient's red cells. The small amount of antibodies possibly present in plasma are not considered clinically important. If the patient's blood type is not known, group AB can be safely given. Rh match is not required.

336

Cryoprecipitate

Cryoprecipitate is the insoluble portion of plasma that remains as a white precipitate after FFP is thawed at 4°C under special conditions. Cryoprecipitate is separated from plasma and refrozen. Cryoprecipitate has a shelf life of 1 year and contains concentrated factor VIII, vWF (von Willebrand factor), fibrinogen, and factor XIII. It is the only concentrated source of fibrinogen.

Uses

Cryoprecipitate is primarily used to control bleeding associated with a deficiency or defect in one of the coagulation factors. Its use is indicated for the treatment of hemophilia A, von Willebrand's disease, hypofibrinogenemia, factor VIII deficiency, obstetric complications, or other situations associated with consumption of fibrinogen (e.g., DIC).

Administration

Cryoprecipitate is thawed before transfusion and must be used within 6 hours. The inside of the bag should be rinsed with a small amount of saline to maximize recovery. Cryoprecipitate should be administered through a standard blood filter, and, as with platelet administration sets, small priming volumes are recommended to decrease loss of the product in the set. The cryoprecipitate units are usually pooled to simplify administration. Cryoprecipitate should be transfused as rapidly as the patient can tolerate.

Cryoprecipitate Administration Summary

Amount: 10 to 15 mL of diluent added to precipitate unit; usual dose 6 to 10 U
Catheter choice: 20- to 22-gauge
Usual rate: As rapidly as possible; approximately 10 mL/minute
Administration set: Component syringe or Y drip set

Compatibility

Compatibility testing is not done, but the cryoprecipitate should be ABO compatible with the patient's red cells because a very small volume of plasma is present. If the patient's blood group is not known, group AB is preferred, but any group can be given in an emergency because the plasma volume is small. Rh matching is not required.

COLLOID VOLUME EXPANDERS

Products are available that do not require screening techniques. These products are colloid volume expanders. These include albumin, plasma protein fraction (PPF), dextran, and hetastarch (HES).

Normal human serum albumin is the most widely used colloid solution. It is heat treated for viral inactivation and free from hepatitis risk. PPF is also a

337

hepatitis free plasma derivative and is less expensive than albumin. Dextran is a branched polysaccharide available in low molecular weights: 40,000 (dextran 40) and 70,000 (dextran 70). It is dissolved in either normal saline or dextrose. Dextran's use as a volume expander is limited by two factors. It can interfere with coagulation and platelet adhesion and it has been associated with rare anaphylactic reactions.

HES is an amylopectin derivative marketed in a 6% saline solution. Because of its structural similarity to glycogen, anaphylaxis is less likely than with dextran (Gridley, 1986).

Albumin and Plasma Protein Fraction

Albumin is a plasma protein that supplies 80 percent of plasma's osmotic activity and is the principal product of fractionation. Administered as PPF and as more purified albumin, albumin and PPF are derived from donor plasma and prepared by the cold alcohol fractionation process and then subsequently heated. Both products do not transmit viral diseases because of the extended heating process. Normal serum albumin is composed of 96 percent albumin and 4 percent globulin and other proteins. It is available as a 5% or 25% solution. PPF is a similar product except that it is subjected to fewer purification steps in the fractionation process and contains about 83 percent albumin and 17 percent globulins. PPF is available in only a 5% solution.

Uses

PPF and 5% albumin are isotonic solutions and, therefore, are osmotically equivalent to an equal volume of plasma. They cause a plasma volume increase and are used interchangeably and share the same clinical uses. They both are used primarily to increase plasma volume resulting from sudden loss of intravascular volume as seen in hypovolemic shock from trauma or surgery. Their use may also be indicated in individual cases to support blood pressure during hypotensive episodes or to induce diuresis in fluid overload to assist in mobilization of fluid. The plasma derivatives lack clotting factors and other plasma proteins and therefore should not be considered plasma substitutes. Neither component will correct nutritional deficits or chronic hypoalbuminemia. The 25% albumin is hypertonic and is five times more concentrated than 5% albumin. The 25% albumin is used to draw fluids out of tissues and body cavities into intravascular spaces. *This solution must be given with caution.* Principal uses for 25% albumin include plasma volume expansion, hypovolemic shock, burns, and prevention and treatment of cerebral edema.

✎ **Note:** Albumin 25% must not be used in dehydrated patients without supplemental fluids or in patients at risk of circulatory overload.

Administration

Albumin and PPF are supplied in glass bottles. Albumin 5% is available in 250 mL and 500 mL of saline, and albumin 25% is supplied in units of 50 mL and 100 mL of saline. Manufacturers recommend the solution be used within 4 hours of opening. Depending on the manufacturer, the solutions are sometimes supplied with an infusion set. Blood transfusion sets and filters are not required for infusion of albumin.

Albumin, 5% and 25%, may be given as rapidly as the patient tolerates for reduced blood volumes. When the blood volume is normal or only slightly reduced, rates of 2 to 4 mL/minute have been suggested for 5% albumin and 1 mL/minute for 25% albumin. More caution is used when infusing PPF because hypotension may occur with a rate greater than 10 mL/minute (AABB, 1986b).

Albumin and Plasma Protein Fraction Administration Summary

Amount: 5% solution 250 mL, 25% solution 50 to 100 mL
Catheter choice: 20- to 22-gauge
Usual rate: 5% solution 2 to 4 mL/minute; 25% solution 1 mL/minute
Administration set: Comes with administration set in package

Compatibility

ABO or Rh matching and compatibility testing are not necessary for these components because antigens and antibodies are not present in these products.

Immune Serum Globulin

In 1981, intravenous gamma globulin (IVIgG) became widely used in the United States to achieve higher serum levels of immunoglobulin (Frey, 1991). Recognition of immune dysfunction has increased and new therapies are being tested. An agent that restores, strengthens, and modifies immunity is gamma immunoglobulin (IgG). Since 1952, standard gamma globulin (SGG) has been administered by the intramuscular (IM) route for reducing frequency of immunodeficiencies. It has been difficult to achieve high **serum** levels of immunoglobulin by the IM route.

The FDA currently approves the following six IVIgG products:

Gammagard (Baxter-Hyland Therapeutics, Glendale, CA)
Sandoglobulin (Swiss Red Cross, distributed by Sandoz Pharmaceuticals, East Hanover, NJ)
Gamimune N (Cutter Biological, Berkeley, CA)
Venoglobulin-I (Alpha Therapeutic Corp., Los Angeles, CA)
Iveegam (Immuno-US, Rochester, MI)
Gammar-IV (Armour Pharmaceuticals, Blue Bell, PA)

IVIgG is derived from pools of at least 1000 screened blood donors (Frey, 1991).

Uses

The IVIgG products are approved by the FDA for I.V. usage in the treatment of primary immunodeficiency disorders and ITP; Gammagard is also approved

339

for treating patients with chronic B-cell lymphocytic leukemia. Infusions of gamma globulin do not cure the underlying disease, however.

✎ **Note:** A dose of 100 mg/kg results in a rise of IgG level by 200 mg/dL (Frey, 1991).

Administration

IVIgG can be administered via peripheral or central venous access devices. The patient with acquired immunodeficiency syndrome (AIDS) and other immune disorders receives infusions of IVIgG via a peripheral 24- or 22-gauge I.V. catheter. A universal administration set can be used to infuse IVIgG therapy. Gammagard and IVeegam provide a filtered administration set with their product; however, IVIgG can be administered by a vented administration set. The recommended filter size is from 5 to 15 microns.

IVIgG can be administered in a controlled setting such as a hospital or physician's office, as well as at home. Rates of administration vary with each manufacturer and are increased gradually while the patient's response is observed closely.

✎ **Note:** A gradual advancement of rate is recommended to minimize the side effects. Severe reactions are rare, however chills, fever, flushing, wheezing, and hypotension can occur (Miller, 1987).

As with other blood products, careful monitoring of the patient is required. Vital signs and weight are checked before administration and then every 15 minutes or before each rate change during the first half hour, followed by every 30 to 60 minutes during the remainder of the infusion. Blood tests may be ordered before and after infusion. These may include measuring IgG, IgA, and IgM levels.

Immune Serum Globulin Administration Summary

Amount: Single-dose vials, reconstituted per manufacturer recommendations 10 mL to 250 mL

Catheter choice: 22- to 24-gauge

Usual rates: Rates vary per manufacturer but range from 10 to 20 drops/minute, increasing to 40 to 50 drops/minute or 1 mL/minute up to 2 mL/minute

Administration set: Vented standard administration set with 5- to 15-micron filter.

Compatibility

IVIgG should not be mixed with any other fluids or medications. Refer to manufacturer recommendations before diluting with 5% dextrose or saline solutions.

ALTERNATIVE PHARMACOLOGIC THERAPIES

Alternatives for homologous blood continues. In recent years, this issue has been addressed by alternative therapies to blood components. Examples of alternative therapies include hematopoietic growth factor erythropoietin and Desmopressin Acetate (DDAVP). Erythropoietin is used for management of chronic anemia in dialysis patients. DDAVP is a synthetic analogue of L-arginine vasopressin and is used for increasing factor VIII and von Willebrand's factor (vWF) and management of patients with hemorrhagic disorders related to thrombocytopenia. These drugs decrease blood loss and the risk of bleeding, resulting in a reduced need for blood components (Baranowski, 1992).

BLOOD SUBSTITUTES

Efforts continue in the search to develop a practical red cell substitute. However, it may be several years before one is available for commercial use. Several products continue to be evaluated for their ability to serve as oxygen carriers as a substitute for red cells. One is a synthetic material, a perfluorocarbon emulsion, which was found to not carry enough oxygen under practical conditions (Baranowski, 1992). Other preparations being developed include intramolecular crosslinked or polymerized hemoglobin and products containing hemoglobin encapsulated in phospholipide liposomes (Pisiotto, 1989).

TECHNIQUES IN ADMINISTRATION OF BLOOD COMPONENTS

General Considerations

The procedure for obtaining a blood component from the hospital blood bank varies from institution to institution. Regardless of the specific institutional procedure, certain essential guidelines must be adhered to (Table 10–4).

Table 10–4 □ **SUMMARY OF STEPS IN ADMINISTRATION OF BLOOD COMPONENT**

Steps of Initiation of a Transfusion
Step 1: Physician's order
Step 2: Equipment setup
Step 3: Patient preparation
Step 4: Obtaining blood product from blood bank
Step 5: Preparation for administration of blood component
Step 6: Initiation of transfusion
Step 7: Monitoring of transfusion
Step 8: Discontinuation of transfusion

Step 1: Physician's Order

A physician's order for the blood component is required.

Step 2: Equipment Setup

Catheter

An I.V. line should be started, per institution protocol, using the gauge size recommended for the component to be administered. Usually an 18- or 20-gauge catheter is used to prevent cell damage. Free flow through a 22-gauge catheter is sometimes difficult with red cell units and requires the use of a pump. A 22-gauge catheter is appropriate for delivery of plasma products.

Solution

No solution other than 0.9% sodium chloride shall be added to blood or blood components (Intravenous Nursing Society [INS], 1990, S66). The use of dextrose and water can cause red cell hemolysis, and the use of lactated Ringer's solution is not recommended because it contains enough ionized calcium to overcome the anticoagulant effect of CPDA-1 and allows small clots to develop.

Administration Sets

Blood administration sets are available as a two-lead Y-type tubing or as single-lead tubing. Y-type administration sets allow for infusion of 0.9% saline before and after each blood component. A Y-type set also allows for dilution of PRBCs that are too viscous to be transfused at an appropriate rate. Platelets and cryoprecipitate should be infused through a filter similar to the standard blood filter but with a smaller drip chamber and shorter tubing so that less priming volume is needed. A syringe device designed specifically for platelets and cryoprecipitate may also be used to administer these products.

Blood administration sets come with an inline filter. Most routine blood filters have a pore size of 170 microns designed to remove the debris that accumulates in stored blood. It is necessary to fill the filter chamber completely to use all the surface area. One filter can usually be used for 2 to 4 U, depending on the manufacturer, the type of filter, the type of blood product, and the age of the cells. As debris in the filter accumulates, the rate of flow through the filter is slowed. Additionally, because of the hazards of hemolysis and bacterial contamination, the filter should not be left hanging in place for extended periods and then reused.

✎ **Note:** The maximum time for use of a blood filter is 4 to 6 hours.

Special Filters

Microaggregate filters and leukocyte-depleting filters are also available for use. These filters are designed to be added to a standard administration set or come already incorporated into the tubing. Microaggregate filters are designed to remove 20- to 40-micron particles, filtering out the microaggregates that develop in stored blood. Microaggregates consist primarily of degenerated platelets, leukocytes, and strands of fibrin. Leukocyte-depleting filters for use at the bedside are also available for delivery of PRBCs and platelets. These filters are capable of removing greater than 99 percent of the leukocytes present in the unit. These new-generation filters were developed in response to data supporting clinical benefits associated with the administration of leukocyte-poor blood products. These benefits include prevention of nonhemolytic transfusion reactions, HLA alloimmunization, and leukocyte-mediated viral transmission. These filters are more expensive than the standard blood filter, and therefore are generally used only per physician order. If using microaggregate or leukocyte-removal filters, follow manufacturer recommendations regarding the number of units that can be filtered through one filter (Baranowski, 1991).

Blood Warmers

Specific equipment is also available for use to warm blood if needed. Most transfusions do not require the use of a blood warmer. Warming of blood toward body temperature is indicated for rapid or massive transfusions, in neonatal exchange transfusions, or for patients with potent cold agglutinins. A blood warmer is a device that heats blood as it passes through sterile, disposable plastic coils. Electric blood warming machines are available that have heated plates that warm blood as it passes through a flat plastic bag placed between the plates.

✎ **Note:** Only temperture devices specifically designed to warm blood should be used. **Blood components** should not be placed in microwave ovens because damage to red cells occurs.

Electronic Monitoring Devices

Some transfusions may require an electronic monitoring device to control the flow. Only pumps designed for the infusion of whole blood and PRBCs may be used because other types of infusion pumps may cause hemolysis. Pumps require the use of special tubing and filters. Little if any increased hemolysis occurs secondary to the use of most infusion pumps. A specific manufacturer should be consulted for detailed information on the suitability of any particular infusion pump for transfusing blood components.

A pressure bag is a commonly used device for increasing flow rates during transfusion, usually in an emergency or during surgery. This device has a sleeve into which the blood bag is inserted and the sleeve is inflated by filling it with air from a pressure manometer. As the unit of blood empties, the pressure of the sleeve decreases; therefore, it should be observed frequently and reinflated when necessary.

Step 3: Patient Preparation

Patient preparation begins when transfusion of a blood component is anticipated. Urgency factors related to the transfusion may affect the amount of time available to prepare the patient for the transfusion. The steps of the nursing process are activated, including assessment and the establishment of new goals and interventions related to the transfusion.

The patient's and patient's family's understanding of the need for blood, procedure, and related concerns need to be assessed. Concerns are typically expressed regarding the risks of disease transmission, and these need to be addressed. The patient should be instructed regarding the length of time for the procedure and the need for monitoring of physical condition and vital signs. Signs and symptoms that may be associated with a complication of the component to be given should be explained to the patient or family or both. It is not necessary to offer graphic explanations regarding symptoms; rather, the patient should be asked to report any different sensations after the transfusion has been started along with a brief description of possible symptoms. Because transfusions typically take several hours, preparation also includes making the patient physically comfortable.

The final step of patient preparation includes a thorough assessment of the patient. Baseline vital signs should be taken. Consult with the physician before initiating the transfusion if the vital signs are abnormal. Premedication with diuretics or antipyretics may be necessary to help keep the vital signs at an acceptable level. Patients should also be questioned regarding any current symptoms they may be experiencing that could be confused with a transfusion reaction.

✎ **Note:** The patient teaching and assessment should be documented in the chart.

Step 4: Obtaining Blood Product from Blood Bank

As a rule, except in emergency situations, no more than one blood component per patient should be picked up at one time. The blood component should not be obtained until the patient is ready to receive the component. The transfusion must be initiated within 30 minutes from the time the component is released from the blood bank. If the transfusion is delayed more than 30 minutes, the component should be returned to the blood bank for proper storage. Whole blood and PRBCs must be refrigerated at a temperature between 1 and 6°C. Special refrigerators are available in the blood bank to maintain these temperatures and are equipped with an alarm that sounds if the temperature is outside the appropriate range.

✎ **Note:** *Refrigerators on the units may not be used to store blood products.*

Proper identification of the blood component and the recipient are essential. Several items must always be verified before the transfusion is initiated.

1. The physician's order should always be verified before picking up the component.
2. When the blood is issued, verification should include *name and identification number* of the recipient, which must be recorded on the blood request form.

✎ **Note:** The transfusion form becomes part of the patient's permanent record.

- *The notation of ABO group and Rh type* must be the same on the primary blood bag label and on the transfusion form. This information is to be recorded on the attached compatibility tag or label.
- *The donor number* must be identically recorded on the label of the blood bag, the transfusion form, and the attached compatibility tag.

344

- The color, appearance, and *expiration date* of the component must be checked.
- *The name of the person issuing the blood, the name of the person to whom the blood is issued, and the date and time of issue must be recorded.* Often this is in a book in the laboratory.

Step 5: Preparation for Administration of Blood Component

Before obtaining the blood component (step 4) the correct tubing, normal saline, and appropriate catheter should be in place. It is vitally important that the site be checked to ensure that the I.V. line is patent.

Baseline vital signs should be obtained, including temperature, blood pressure, pulse, and respirations. For example of transfusion record, refer to Figure 10–4.

TRANSFUSION PROCEDURE CHECKLIST

INITIAL

- Record Donor Number(s) and Component
- Information verified at bedside
- Normal Saline used with transfusion
- Record time started
- Record amount given
- Record time stopped
- Record reactions (if any)
- Vital Signs at 0, 15, 30, and every 30 minutes thereafter
- Infusion completed within 4 hours
- Copy of completed form and empty bag to laboratory - DO NOT REMOVE LABEL FROM BLOOD BAG

VITAL SIGNS

TIME	BLOOD PRESSURE	PULSE	RESPIRATION	TEMP
0				
15				
30				
60				
90				
120				
150				
180				
210				
240				

AT THE TIME OF TRANSFUSION PLEASE VERIFY:

I have verified the name, medical record number, transfusion armband number, blood group and type for the donor and recipient as recorded on labels and forms for the following units (one unit of WB, PC, FFP or maximum of 10 units platelet concentrate, or cryoprecipitate per transfusion procedure and report form). I have further verified the identification of the recipient.

DONOR NUMBER   COMPONENT

_____ _____

_____ _____

_____ _____

_____ _____

_____ _____

Signature of person initiating transfusion   Signature of verifier

TRANSFUSION RECORD:

Date and Time Started: _____

Date and Time Stopped: _____

Record Amount Given if Less Than Full Unit(s): _____

Record Initials if Blood Warmer Used: _____

Transfusion Armband Number: _____

REPORT OF SUSPECTED TRANSFUSION REACTION:

- ☐ Increased Pulse Rate
- ☐ Chills
- ☐ Elevation of temperature >2° F
- ☐ Headaches
- ☐ Nausea or Vomiting
- ☐ Flushing of skin
- ☐ Backpain/Muscle aching
- ☐ Darkening of urine (hemoglobinuria)
- ☐ Petechiae
- ☐ Hypotension
- ☐ Dyspnea
- ☐ Chest pain

If any of the above signs or symptoms are observed during or following the transfusion:

initial

- ☐ Stop the transfusion immediately, keep the IV open with normal saline
- ☐ Notify physician immediately _____ physician contacted
- ☐ Notify Transfusion Service immediately (x1187)

Technologist Notified

- ☐ Recheck the patient identification, crossmatch tag, and blood bag to determine if the patient received the correct unit.
- ☐ Send unit with administration set to the Transfusion Service.

Signature of Person Reporting Suspected Transfusion Reaction

Comments: _____

_____

_____

Figure 10–4 ☐ Transfusion record and report of suspected transfusion reactions. (Courtesy of Roseville Community Hospital, Roseville, California.)

345

- At the time of infusion, verification should include checking the component against the physician's order. The blood component should be verified with another registered nurse or a state certified licensed practical/vocational nurse or physician.
- *Compare donor numbers and the ABO group and Rh type* on the transfusion record with the information on the blood component. The information should be identical on the label and compatibility tag.

✎ **Note:** It is helpful if one nurse reads the information for verification to the other nurse; errors can be made if both nurses look at the tags together.

- *Check the expiration date* and time.

✎ **Note:** Unless the exact time is given, the component expires at midnight on the expiration date.

- At the bedside, *compare the full name and hospital identification number on the patient's identification wristband with the name and number that is on the form attached to the blood component.*

✎ **Note:** Watch for any discrepancies during any part of the identification process; the transfusion should not be initiated until the blood bank is notified and any discrepancies are resolved.

Step 6: Initiation of Transfusion

To administer whole blood or packed cells, spike the blood container with the Y set and hang. Turn off the 0.9% normal saline and turn on the blood component. It is recommended that transfusions be started at 2 mL/minute or no greater than 50 mL over the first 5 to 15 minutes of the transfusion. If the patient shows signs or has symptoms of an adverse reaction, the transfusion can be stopped immediately and only a small amount of blood product will have been infused. Once the first 15 minutes is safely over, the rate of flow can be increased to complete the transfusion within the amount of time indicated by the physician or by policy. The rate of infusion should be based on the patient's blood volume, hemodynamic condition, and cardiac status.

✎ **Note:** Blood should be infused within a 4-hour period. When a longer transfusion time is clinically indicated, the unit may be divided (split) by the blood bank before administration, and the portion not being transfused can be properly refrigerated.

Step 7: Monitoring of Transfusion

The patient's vital signs should be monitored at the end of the first 15 minutes and then periodically throughout the transfusion. It is recommended that vital signs be checked every 15 minutes for the first half hour and then periodically during the transfusion (every half hour is often recommended until the transfusion is complete). Careful observation of the patient during and after a blood transfusion is necessary to provide a more reliable assessment.

✎ **Note:** The patient should be observed for at least 5 minutes after initiation of a blood component (INS, 1990, S66).

✎ **Note:** Patient teaching is required for conscious patients. They should be instructed to call if any unusual symptoms or sensations occur during a transfusion. Be sure to inform the patient that a nurse will be checking the transfusion and vital signs at least every 30 minutes.

Step 8: Discontinuation of Transfusion

When the unit is complete, flush the tubing with approximately 50 mL of 0.9% normal saline. Because of the sodium and chloride content of 0.9% normal saline, a minimal amount should be used to complete the transfusion. At this point, another unit may be infused, the unit and line discontinued, the line can be capped with prn adaptor, or a new infusion line and solution container may be administered.

✎ **Note:** Do not save previous solutions and tubing, which were interrupted to give the blood component; they are considered contaminated. Restart with a fresh set and solution (AABB, 1986b).

When the unit of blood has infused, the time, volume given, and patient's condition should be documented. Some transfusion service departments require that a copy of the completed transfusion form be returned to them. Returning the blood component after an uncomplicated transfusion is not required in all facilities. If disposal is on the unit, use hospital standards in disposing of the blood bag in contaminated trash.

A Note on Medications

Drugs should never be mixed with the blood component to be administered. There are several reasons for this. One is the indeterminate effect the medication may have on the blood component. Also, if a reaction occurs, it would be difficult to ascertain whether the drug or the blood component was responsible for the adverse effect. Another reason is that if the transfusion needs to be interrupted, it would be impossible to calculate the amount of drug the patient received. If a patient required I.V. medications during the course of the transfusion, a separate I.V. site should be started for the blood.

✎ **Note:** Absolutely no medications or solutions other than 0.9% sodium chloride shall be added to blood or blood components (INS, 1990, S66; AABB, 1990).

Summary Worksheet

STEPS IN INITIATING A TRANSFUSION

Step 1:

Step 2: *Catheter:*
Solution:
Administration set:

Step 3:

Step 4: *Criteria:*

Step 5: *Prior:*
Criteria:

Step 6:

Step 7: *Guidelines:*

Step 8:

HOME TRANSFUSION THERAPY

Transfusion services can be delivered safely and efficiently in the home setting. With patients taking a more active role in the management of their health care, and third-party payers willing to reimburse for home care, the frequency of home transfusions should increase in the future.

Home transfusion therapy can be a safe and viable service. Guidelines and standards need to be set with the patient's best interest in mind. The AABB is currently creating standards for the home transfusion procedure, and the INS standards should also be considered in the formulation of home transfusion therapy (Monks, 1988).

Transfusions in the home setting include:

1. PRBCs
2. Leukocyte-poor red blood cells
3. Platelets
4. Cryoprecipitate
5. Plasma

6. Immune serum globulin
7. Factor VIII concentrate

✎ **Note:** Whole blood is not an alternative in the home setting (Monks, 1988).

The same guidelines for administration of blood components used in the hospital setting should be instituted in the home setting to ensure patient safety.

GUIDELINES FOR HOME TRANSFUSION THERAPY

1. Written physician's order is required.
2. Transportation of blood component to the home setting must use blood bank standards.
3. Blood and patient must be properly identified.
4. Baseline assessments must use INS standards for monitoring the infusion.
5. Use an appropriate blood filter.
6. Electromechanical devices may be used, but the product information should be checked to ensure the pump is indicated for transfusion delivery and will not cause hemolysis of the red blood cells.
7. Use only 0.9% sodium chloride solutions to prime the administration set.
8. The registered nurse administering the transfusion must remain in the home setting throughout the transfusion and for an appropriate time afterward to check for complications.
9. Blood warming should not be considered for home transfusion because no more than 2 U of blood should be administered at one time in the home setting.
10. A biohazard bag should be brought to the home and all contaminated equipment disposed of according to state regulations.
11. Review written transfusion instructions that include but are not limited to:
    - Emergency telephone numbers
    - Information regarding signs and symptoms of delayed reactions

    Schedule the post-transfusion assessment visit with the patient before leaving.
12. Notify physician of the transfusion completion and patient's response to therapy.
13. Charting must include but is not limited to:
    - Type of I.V. solution and time started
    - Type of blood product
    - Vital signs, skin condition, and appearance
    - Any patient symptoms and/or complaints
    - Time blood product discontinued
    - Volume infused
    - Reason for discontinuing the transfusion if done before completion of the infusion
    - Patient reactions to the procedure

349

TRANSFUSION REACTIONS

INS standards of practice (1990) dictate that a transfusion reaction requires immediate intervention.

Interventions include but are not limited to:

- Terminating the transfusion
- Maintaining patency of the cannula with 0.9% sodium chloride
- Notifying the physician and hospital blood bank or transfusion services
- Implementing other interventions as indicated

Transfusions can cause **immediate reactions**, which occur immediately or up to 48 hours after the transfusion; or **delayed reactions**, which occur after 48 hours up to 180 days after the transfusion.

Hemolytic Transfusion Reaction (Acute and Delayed)

Acute Transfusion Reaction

The most serious and potentially life-threatening reaction is acute **hemolytic transfusion reaction**. This type of reaction occurs after infusion of incompatible red blood cells. There are two types of red cell destruction. First, intravascular hemolysis, in which the red cells are destroyed with hemolysis directly in the bloodstream, is usually seen with ABO-incompatible red blood cells. Second, extravascular hemolysis, in which the cells are coated with the antibody and subsequently removed by the reticuloendothelial system, is seen in Rh incompatibility. These incompatibilities may lead to an activation of the coagulation system and release of vasoactive enzymes, which can result in vasomotor instability, cardiorespiratory collapse, or DIC. Intravascular hemolysis is the most serious and is usually fatal (National Blood Resource Group, 1991).

Incompatibilities involving other red cell antigens and IgG antibodies can result in fever, anemia, hyperbilirubinemia, and development of a positive direct antibody test. The severity of the reaction can be dose related, but reactions can occur with less than 30 mL of blood administered. Most hemolytic reactions are a result of *clerical errors*, such as incorrect labeling of the blood specimen or errors in identifying the patient.

Common transfusion reactions are listed in Table 10–5.

Table 10–5 □ **COMMON TRANSFUSION REACTIONS**

Hemolytic, acute and delayed
Febrile reactions
Allergic reactions
Circulatory overload

Signs and Symptoms

The first symptoms are burning sensation along the vein in which the blood is being infused:

Lumbar pain
Flank pain
Flushing of face
Chest pain

If infusion is allowed to continue:

Fever
Chills
Hemoglobinemia
Oozing of blood at the injection site
Shock
DIC

Interventions

Stop the transfusion. However, disconnect the tubing from the I.V. catheter and infuse fresh saline not contaminated by the blood.

✎ **Note:** In acute hemolytic transfusion reaction you *must not* give the patient another drop of donor blood.

Notify the physician and blood bank or transfusion service *immediately*. Monitor vital signs and maintain intravascular volume with fluids to prevent renal constriction. Additionally, diuretics, mannitol, and dopamine can support the renal and vascular systems. This is an emergency situation. The patient's respiratory status may have to be supported.

Prevention

Extreme care during the entire identification process is the first step in prevention. The transfusion must be started slowly, and the nurse must remain with the patient during the first 5 to 15 minutes of the transfusion.

Delayed Transfusion Reaction

Delayed reaction is a result of red blood cell antigen incompatibility other than the ABO group. Rapid production of red blood cell antibody occurs shortly after transfusion of the corresponding antigen, as a result of sensitization during previous transfusions or pregnancies. Destruction of the transfused red cells gradually occurs over 2 or more days, or up to several weeks, after the transfusion. Most reactions of this type go unnoticed and are common.

Signs and Symptoms

Decrease in hemoglobin and hematocrit levels
Persistent low-grade fever

351

Malaise
Indirect hyperbilirubinemia

Interventions

No acute treatment is usually required. Monitor hematocrit, renal function, and coagulation profile routinely for all patients receiving transfusions. Notify physician and transfusion services if delayed reaction suspected.

Prevention

Avoid clerical errors.

Nonhemolytic Febrile Reactions

Nonhemolytic febrile transfusion reactions usually are a reaction to antibodies formed directed against leukocytes or platelets. A febrile reaction is the most common acute transfusion reaction. It can occur immediately or within 1 to 2 hours after transfusion is completed. Fever is the symptom most closely associated with this type of transfusion reaction.

Signs and Symptoms

Fever
Chills
Headache
Nausea and vomiting
Hypotension
Chest pain
Dyspnea and nonproductive cough
Malaise

Interventions

Stop transfusion.
Keep vein open with normal saline.
Notify physician.
Monitor vital signs.
Physician might order antipyretics.

✎ **Note:** In this type of reaction you may turn off the blood and turn on the normal saline primer and infuse slowly. Do not take the blood bag down until notified by physician. Leave the blood bag hanging, but clamp the Y connector to the blood unit

Prevention

This type of reaction can be prevented or reduced by the use of leukocyte-poor blood components. HLA-compatible products may also be indicated (National Blood Resource Group, 1991).

Allergic Reactions

In its mild form, this is the second most common type of reaction and is probably caused by antibodies against plasma proteins. The patient may experience mild localized urticaria or a full systemic anaphylactic reaction. This can occur immediately or within 1 hour after infusion. Most reactions are mild and respond to antihistamines.

Signs and Symptoms

Itching
Hives (local erythema)
Rash
Urticaria
Runny eyes
Anxiety
Dyspnea
Wheezing
Decreased blood pressure
Shock
Gastrointestinal distress
Cardiac arrest and death

Treatment

Stop transfusion. Keep vein open with normal saline. Notify the physician. Monitor the vital signs. For a mild reaction, administer antihistamines per physician's order, and continue transfusion if symptoms subside. For severe anaphylactic reactions, administer epinephrine, steroids, and dopamine, and maintain intravascular volume with fluids as ordered by the physician.

✎ **Note:** A report of suspected transfusion reaction should be completed (Fig. 10–4).

Prevention

For mild reactions, the patient may receive antihistamines, such as Benadryl, before the transfusion. Transfuse patients with a history of anaphylaxis with IgA-deficient blood products, washed red blood cells, or deglycerolized red cells.

With a mild reaction, the transfusion may be continued after antihistamines are administered and the symptoms have subsided. Severe reactions may require discontinuation of the transfusion and drug therapy to support vascular system.

Circulatory Overload

This complication can occur when rapid or excessive blood is infused over a short period of time. Be aware of the amount of sodium chloride that is being administered to the patient in conjunction with the transfusion.

Signs and Symptoms

Onset of dyspnea
Enlarged neck veins
Congestive heart failure
Pulmonary edema

Treatment

Stop the transfusion.
Elevate the patient's head.
Notify the physician.
Phlebotomize, if necessary.
Administer diuretics, if necessary.

Prevention

Minimize the risk of overload by using PRBCs instead of whole blood, infusing at a reduced rate for the high-risk patient. Also, use a diuretic when beginning the transfusion in high-risk patients to decrease the risk of circulatory overload.

COMPLICATIONS ASSOCIATED WITH TRANSFUSIONS

Potassium Intoxication

Potassium toxicity is a rare complication. As the blood ages during storage, potassium is released from the cell into the plasma during red cell lysis. This increases the amount of potassium the patient receives and depends on the number of units the patient receives along with the age of the blood when administered. Patients at risk for this complication are those with renal failure and those who receive massive transfusions of aged blood.

Signs and Symptoms

Immediate onset of hyperkalemia
Slow, irregular heartbeat
Nausea and muscle weakness
Electrocardiographic (ECG)

Hypothermia

When large volumes of blood are administered, **hypothermia** can occur owing to the consistently cool temperature of the blood. This risk brings about decreased temperature and chills. Treatment is to warm the patient with blankets. The use of a blood warmer during transfusions can be helpful to minimize this risk.

Hypocalcemia

A reaction to toxic proportions of citrate, which is used as a preservative in blood, can cause hypocalcemia. The citrate ion can combine with calcium, causing a calcium deficiency, or normal citrate metabolism is hindered by the presence of liver disease.

Signs and Symptoms

Tingling sensation in fingers
Muscle cramps
Hypotension
Tetany

Calcium levels should be carefully monitored in patients with liver disease. The use of washed red cells helps to prevent this risk.

Risks of Transfusion Therapy

Despite dynamic advances in blood banking and transfusion medicine, there are still risks to blood component therapy. The patient should be told of alternatives to transfusion, including those risks to the patient if the patient does not undergo transfusion. Further, patients need to know about the blood centers' autologous transfusion and patient designated donor programs, without implication that there is added safety to the latter.

There are a number of potential risks surrounding transfusions. The most significant risks are identified in Table 10–6. Fevers, chills, and urticaria are among the most common adverse effects of transfusion but are usually not a major concern. A hemolytic transfusion reaction may occur with 1 of every 6000 transfusions and result in a fatality in 1 of every 100,000 transfusion recipients.

Viral hepatitis is still a serious and not infrequent risk of transfusion. With the current screening procedures, a patient's chance is 1 in 1000 that a pint of blood may result in a non-A or non-B viral hepatitis. This is an appreciable risk and may have long-term consequences for the recipient.

Currently, the risk of a transfusion-associated HIV infection is remote, no more than 1 in 150,000. However, because AIDS may follow HIV infection,

Table 10–6 ☐ **RISKS OF TRANSFUSION**

Risks of Transfusion	Chance of Occurrence/U
Fever, chill, urticaria	1:100
Hemolytic transfusion reaction	1:6000
Fatal hemolytic transfusion reaction	1:100,000
Viral hepatitis	1:1000
HIV infection (and thus AIDS)	1:150,000

Source: Courtesy of P. Holland, 1991, Sacramento Medical Foundation Blood Center, Sacramento, California, with permission.

patients should be warned of the potential risk of this dreadful and usually fatal disease (Sacramento Medical Foundation Blood Center, 1991).

PHYSICAL ASSESSMENT (BLOOD COMPONENTS)

The nurse must use a systems approach to assess for both local and systemic complications associated with the infusion of blood components. The nursing assessment should include infusion rate, intake and output, and an awareness of agency policy and procedures to prevent complications associated with transfusions. The following body systems should be assessed at the beginning of each transfusion and every 15 minutes thereafter. Symptoms listed with each system may indicate local problems or life-threatening complications. All laboratory findings should be monitored.

NEUROMUSCULAR
Anxiety
Change in level of consciousness
Confusion
Malaise
Fatigue
Headache
Complaints of pain
Impending sense of doom
Tremors
Tetany
Paresthesia of the extremities
Muscle weakness
Muscle cramps
Seizures

CARDIOVASCULAR
Increased or decreased blood pressure
Increased heart rate
Irregular heart rate
Extra cardiac sounds
Distended neck veins
Bleeding from the site
Degeneralized bleeding (DK)

RESPIRATORY
Shortness of breath
Hypoxia
Dyspnea
Cyanosis
Rales
Respiratory distress
Wheezing
Nonproductive cough

GASTROINTESTINAL
Nausea
Vomiting
Diarrhea (may be bloody)
Abdominal cramping

RENAL
Flank pain, lumbar pain
Decreased urinary output
Variance between intake and output
Changes in urine color—red, brown, amber

INTEGUMENTARY
Fever
Tender, cordlike vein

Profuse sweating
Itching
Urticaria, hives rash
Flushing of the face
Change in skin color
Edema at or near insertion site
Sensation of heat at or near insertion site

Bruising around or near the site of the insertion
Sluggish flow rate
Back flow absent
Coolness of the skin
Taut skin around venipuncture site

BODY WEIGHT
Rapid weight gain

SPECIAL SENSES
Runny eyes
Sneezing

NURSING DIAGNOSES RELATED TO TRANSFUSION THERAPY

1. Anxiety (mild, moderate, severe) related to threat to or change in health status; misconceptions regarding therapy
2. Decreased cardiac output related to sepsis, contamination
3. Fear related to homologous blood transfusion and the transmission of disease; fear of "needles."
4. Fluid volume excess related to fluid administration; excess sodium
5. Hyperthermia related to increased metabolic rate; illness; dehydration
6. Hypothermia related to exposure to cool or cold blood
7. Impaired physical mobility related to pain or discomfort resulting from placement and maintenance of I.V. catheter
8. Impaired skin integrity related to I.V. catheter; irritating I.V. solution; inflammation; infection; infiltration
9. Impaired tissue integrity related to altered circulation; fluid deficit or excess; irritating solution; inflammation; infection; infiltration
10. Impaired gas exchange related to ventilation perfusion imbalance; decreased oxygen-carrying capacity of the blood
11. Knowledge deficit related to purpose of blood component therapy; signs and symptoms of complications
12. Pain related to physical trauma (e.g., catheter insertion)
13. Risk for infection related to broken skin or traumatized tissue

---

SUMMARY OF CHAPTER 10, PART II

BLOOD COMPONENT THERAPY

The administration of blood components allows for no margin of error. Therefore, when involved in the administration of blood components, it is essential to have a knowledge and understanding of immunohematology, blood grouping, blood components, administration equipment, techniques of administration, and management of transfusion reactions.

357

Component Therapy

Component therapy refers to the delivery of components obtained from a unit of whole blood. Whole blood is composed of red blood cells, plasma, white blood cells, and platelets. Platelets and granulocytes can be obtained using pheresis procedures. Albumin and PPF products are prepared from plasma donors. The following components can be prepared to form a whole blood unit:

Component	Indications
Packed red cells	Symptomatic acute and chronic anemia
Washed red cells	Provides leukocyte-poor red blood cells for patients with recurrent allergic or febrile reactions
Deglycerolized red cells	Long-term storage of red cells to minimize febrile and allergic reactions
Platelets	Control of bleeding in platelet deficiencies
Fresh frozen plasma	Replacement of coagulation factors
Cryoprecipitate	Deficiency of factor VIII, von Willebrand's disease, Hemophilia A, fibrinogen replacement
Granulocytes	Febrile patients with neutropenia unresponsive to antibiotic therapy
Immune serum globulin	

Administration of Blood Products

According to the standards of I.V. nursing, responsibilities for the administration of blood components include:

- Blood product inspection
- Verification of product expiration date
- Confirmation of compatibility between recipient and donor
- Confirmation of informed patient consent
- Patient education
- Monitoring during and after administration
- Identification of immediate and delayed reactions
- Accountability for initiating appropriate intervention
- Written documentation
- Communication of pertinent data to physician and other health care providers
- Adherence to aseptic technique

The initiation and administration of blood products involves detailed and rigid procedures that must be followed exactly. Keep the following points in mind:

- A physician's order is required for administration of all blood components.
- Normal saline is the only solution that may be used with blood components.
- All blood components must be filtered. A standard 170-micron filter is

typically used. Special filters that remove microaggregates and leuko-
cytes are also available if indicated.
- Proper identification of the blood component and the recipient is essential.
- All blood products must be delivered within 4 hours.
- Medications may not be added to blood components.
- The patient's physical condition and vital signs must be monitored throughout the transfusion to assess for transfusion reactions.

COMPLICATIONS OF TRANSFUSION THERAPY

Possible reactions that may occur during transfusion include:

Acute and delayed hemolytic reactions
Febrile reactions
Allergic reactions
Potassium intoxication
Hypocalcemia

Post-test, Chapter 10, Part II

1. Whole blood is indicated for:
   A. Treatment of anemia
   B. Red cells and platelet replacement
   C. Acute massive blood loss

2. Washed red blood cells are used to:
   A. Provide leukocyte-poor red cells
   B. Prevent or delay febrile transfusion reactions
   C. Prevent or delay allergic reactions
   D. All of the above

3. Indications for platelet transfusion include:
   A. Hemorrhage with a platelet count less than 50,000
   B. Nonbleeding patients with a platelet count of 80,000
   C. Preoperative patients with a platelet count of 150,000

4. Which of the following is a symptom of a *febrile* transfusion reaction?
   A. Itching
   B. Hives
   C. Rash
   D. Chills and fever

5. The nursing interventions for an *acute hemolytic reaction* would be to:
   A. Slow the transfusion and call the physician
   B. Stop the transfusion and turn on the saline side of the administration set
   C. Stop the transfusion, disconnect the tubing from the I.V. catheter, and initiate new saline and tubing to keep the vein open

6. The component albumin 25% is hypertonic. Caution should be used by the nurse when infusing 25% albumin because this product can:
   A. Cause circulatory overload
   B. Cause clotting disorders
   C. Increase red cell hemoglobin
   D. Lower the blood pressure

7. The component FFP is used
   A. For patients with hemophilia A
   B. For patients who have developed HLA antibodies
   C. To expand the plasma volume
   D. All of the above

8. The nurse must check all of the following with another nurse before initiating the transfusion *except*.
   A. ABO and Rh
   B. Patient name
   C. Unit number
   D. Expiration date
   E. Preservative

True-False

9. **T F** Lactated Ringer's solution is an acceptable solution to use with blood components.

10. **T F** Platelets may be given through unfiltered tubing.

11. **T F** Pressure bag sleeves may be used to increase flow rates when transfusing PRBCs.

12. **T F** Blood warmers may be used as an adjunct to the transfusion when the patient is hypothermic.

13. List the eight steps in initiation of a transfusion.

Step 1

Step 2

Step 3

Step 4

Step 5

Step 6

Step 7

Step 8

Match the definition in column 2 to the correct term in column 1.

Column 1

14. _____ Thrombocytopenia

15. _____ Delayed reaction

16. _____ Febrile reaction

17. _____ Allergic reaction

18. _____ Hemolytic transfusion reaction

19. _____ Blood component

20. _____ Hemolysis

21. _____ Plasma

22. _____ Hypothermia

23. _____ Immediate reaction

Column 2

A. Adverse effect occurring immediately or up to 48 hours later

B. Adverse effect occurring after 48 hours later, and up to 180 days after transfusion

C. A product made from a unit of blood

D. Rupture of red cells, with release of hemoglobin

E. Fluid portion of blood

F. Abnormally low body temperature

G. Exposure to antigen to which the person has become sensitized

H. Abnormally small number of platelets in the blood

I. Destruction of red blood cells by antibodies present in the blood of either donor or recipient

J. Nonhemolytic reaction to antibodies formed against leukocytes

Answers to Post-test, Chapter 10, Part II

1. C
2. D
3. A
4. D
5. C
6. A
7. D
8. E
9. F
10. F
11. T
12. T
13. Step 1: Physician's order
    Step 2: Equipment setup
    Step 3: Patient preparation
    Step 4: Obtaining blood product
      from blood bank

Step 5: Preparation for
  administration of blood
  component
Step 6: Initiation of transfusion
Step 7: Monitoring of transfusion
Step 8: Discontinuation of
  transfusion
14. H
15. B
16. J
17. G
18. I
19. C
20. D
21. E
22. F
23. A

Activity Journal

1. A friend wants to know if she can donate blood directly to be designated for her father. What do you tell her?

2. While caring for a patient who is to receive a unit of packed cells, the patient expresses his fear of contracting AIDS from the transfusion. What do you tell him? Are there risks?

3. As a new graduate, what resources are available to you in providing patient teaching related to the donation of blood?

4. Review the policy and procedure for blood transfusion at the agency in which you work. Does the policy designate who should pick the blood up from the laboratory? Is the procedure clear on how to check blood out from the laboratory and how to administer the component safely?

5. If you were unclear on how to administer cryoprecipitate, what would you do?

6. Your patient develops an increase in temperature during a transfusion of packed cells. The pulse rate is 120 and the patient is slightly short of breath. Your discover baseline vital signs had not been taken, as you had directed a nurse's aide to do prior to administering the transfusion. What would you do? Also, who is at fault?

7. At the beginning of your shift, you check on a unit of blood that had been hung before your shift. The unit of packed cells is infusing slowly, with approximately 100 mL left. You agitate the bag slightly and discover a pinhole at the top of the bag. What do you do?

Quality Assessment Model

Instructions: Use this quality assessment model to conduct retrospective audits of charges, establish quality control standards, or develop outcome criteria for quality assurance. Refer to Chapter 2 for details on quality assessment.

STRUCTURE

(Resource that affects outcome)
Human Resource: Nurse or Transfusion Therapist

PROCESS

(Actual giving and receiving of care)
Therapist activities related to quality and safety of transfusion are:

1. Take baseline vital signs before transfusion.
2. Record vital signs every 15 minutes for first half hour and every half hour thereafter.
3. Check blood component with another nurse before administration for unit number, ABO and Rh compatibility, expiration date, and patient name.
4. Initiate only one transfusion at a time.
5. Assess patient during and after transfusion for signs and symptoms of transfusion reactions
6. Use only 0.9% sodium chloride with blood components.

OUTCOME STANDARDS

(Effects of care)
Documentation will reflect standards of practice for delivery of safe transfusions:

1. Documentation of baseline vital signs and interval vital signs on transfusion record.
2. Patient response to transfusion documented in nursing notes.
3. Documentation of blood component check with another nurse before transfusion.
4. Documentation on transfusion record of 0.9% sodium chloride as primer for blood component.

References

AABB. (1986a). The latest protocols for blood transfusions. *Nursing 86, 16*(10), 34–42.
AABB. (1986b). *Practical aspects of blood administration.* Philadelphia: J.B. Lippincott.

AABB. (1989). *Blood transfusion therapy—a physician's handbook* (3rd ed.). Philadelphia: J.B. Lippincott.

AABB. (1990). *Technical manual* (10th ed.). Philadelphia: J.B. Lippincott.

Baranowski, L. (1991). Filtering out the confusion about leukocyte-poor blood components. *Journal of Intravenous Nursing, 14*(5), 298–305.

Baranowski, L. (1992). Current trends in blood component therapy: The evolution of a softer, more effective product. *Journal of Intravenous Therapy, 15*(3), 136–149.

Frey, A.M. (1991). The immune system part II: I.V. administration of immune globulin. *Journal of Intravenous Nursing, 6*(14), 396–420.

Gridley, J.H. (1986). Blood component therapy. *Trauma Quarterly, 2*(3), 45–54.

Intravenous Nursing Society. (1990). *Standards of practice*. Philadelphia: J.B. Lippincott.

Miller, D. (1987). Intravenous immune globulin for treating primary immunodeficiency disease. *Maternal Child Nursing, 14*(4), 244–248.

Monks, M.L. (1988). Home transfusion therapy. *Journal of Intravenous Nursing, 11*(6), 389–396.

National Blood Resource Education Program's Nursing Education Working Group. (1991): *Transfusion nursing trends and practices for the 90's*. American Journal of Nursing, *91*(6), 42–56.

National Institutes of Health. (1989). NIH publication No. 89-2974a. Bethesda: National Blood Resource Education Program, US Department of Health and Human Services

Pauley, S.Y. (1984). Transfusion therapy for nurses, part I. *National Intravenous Therapy Association, 7*(6), 501–511.

Plumer, A.L., & Cosentino, F. (1987). *Principles and practice of intravenous therapy*. Boston: Little, Brown.

Popovsky, M.A. (1986). Autologous transfusion: Present practice and future trends. *National Intravenous Therapy Association, 9*(5), 292–294.

Popovsky, M.A., & Taswell, H.F. (1984). Role of I.V. and transfusion nurses in autologous transfusion. *National Intravenous Therapy Association, 7*(4), 385–386.

Widmann, F.K., (1981). *Technical manual* (8th ed.). Washington, DC: American Association of Blood Banks.

Rutman & Miller (1985). *Transfusion therapy principles and procedures*. Baltimore: Aspen Publications.

Bibliography

Birdsall, C. (1985). How do you avoid transfusion complications? *American Journal of Nursing, 85*(4), 312.

Madden, K., & Adams, L. (1983). Autotransfusions: Now it's saving lives. *RN, 46*(12), 50–53.

Masoorli, S.T., & Piercy, S. (1984). A lifesaving guide to blood products. *RN, 9*, 32–37.

Nicholson, E. (1988). Autologous blood transfusion. *Nursing Times, 84*(2), 33–36.

Pittiglio, D.H. (1984). *Modern blood banking and transfusion practices*. Philadelphia: F.A. Davis.

Richards, C.A. (1989). *Blood—a gift of life*. Sacramento: Sacramento Medical Foundation Blood Center.

Rutman, R.C., & Miller, W.V. (1982). *Transfusion therapy: Principles and procedures*. Baltimore: Aspen Publications.

Smith, L. (1984). Homologous blood transfusion reactions. *American Journal of Nursing, 84*(9), 1096–1101.

Administration of Intravenous Medications

CHAPTER CONTENTS

Glossary

Absorption: Process of movement of medication from drug administration sites to the vasculature

Adsorption: Attachment of one substance to the surface of another

Admixing: Combining two or more medications

Ambulatory drug pump: An electronic infusion device specifically designed in size to be worn on the body to promote patient mobility and independence

Antineoplastic: Medication for the treatment of cancer

Bolus: Concentrated medication or solution given rapidly over a short time; may be given by direct intravenous injection or by intravenous drip

Chemical incompatibility: Change that may or may not be visually observed in the molecular structure or pharmacologic properties of a substance

Clinical trial: Planned experiments that involve patients and are designed to evoke an appropriate treatment of future patients with a given medical condition

Compatibility: Capable of being mixed and administered without undergoing undesirable chemical and/or physical changes or loss of therapeutic action

Curative: Therapy that is either healing or corrective

Distribution: Process of delivering a drug to the various tissues of the body

Drug interactions: Interactions between two drugs; also, drug that causes an increase or decrease in another drug's pharmacologic effects

369

Epidural: Situated on or over the dura mater

Incompatibility: Chemical or physical reaction that occurs among two or more drugs or between drug and delivery device

Intermittent drug infusion: Intravenous therapy administered at prescribed intervals

Intraperitoneal (IP): Within the peritoneal cavity

Intraspinal: Spaces surrounding the spinal cord, including epidural and intrathecal

Intrathecal: Within a sheath, surrounded by the epidural space and separated from it by the dura mater; contains cerebral spinal fluid

Intravenous push: Manual administration of medication under pressure over 1 minute or as manufacturer of medication recommends

Multiple-dose vial: Medication bottle that is hermetically sealed with a rubber stopper and designed to be entered more than once

Nonvesicant: Intravenous medication that includes but is not limited to medications administered for cancer, which generally does not damage or cause sloughing of tissue

Palliative: Treatment that may be provided for comfort or temporary relief of symptoms

Physical incompatibility: An undesirable change that is visually observed

Single-dose vial: Medication bottle that is hermetically sealed with a rubber stopper and is intended for one-time use

Therapeutic incompatibility: Undesirable effect occurring within a patient as a result of two or more drugs being given concurrently

Vesicant: Intravenous medication that causes blisters and tissue injury when it escapes into surrounding tissue

---

LEARNING OBJECTIVES

Upon completion of this chapter, the reader will be able to:

☐ Define terminology related to administration of intravenous medications
☐ Identify the advantages of intravenous medications
☐ List the hazards associated with intravenous medications
☐ Identify the methods through which medications may be delivered by the intravenous route
☐ Identify three incompatibilities related to intravenous therapy
☐ Describe the proper technique in delivery of intravenous push medication
☐ Describe the treatment of adverse effects of intravenous medications
☐ State the precautions to be followed when medication is infused via the epidural route
☐ List the key steps in dressing management of an intraspinal catheter
☐ Describe the method of delivery and nursing consideration for intraperitoneal therapy
☐ Describe the special considerations when administering anti-infective therapy, chemotherapeutic agents, and narcotics via the intravenous route
☐ Identify the general side effects of chemotherapeutic agents
☐ List the phases of the cell cycle
☐ List the key points in delivering medications intravenously for pain control

☐ Describe the nurse's role in delivery of investigational drugs
☐ Determine the nursing diagnoses appropriate for patients receiving intravenous medications

Pre-test, Chapter 11

Instructions: The pre-test is to review prior knowledge of the theory related to administration of intravenous medications. Each question in the pre-test is based on the learning objectives of the chapter.

Match the definition in column 2 to the correct term in column 1.

Column 1

1. _____ Adsorption
2. _____ Absorption
3. _____ Palliative
4. _____ Curative
5. _____ Therapeutic incompatibility
6. _____ Chemical incompatibility
7. _____ Physical incompatibility
8. _____ Drug interaction
9. _____ Clinical trials
10. _____ Distribution

Column 2

A. Planned experiment designed to evoke an appropriate treatment for a given medical condition

B. A change in the molecular structure or properties of a substance

C. An undesirable effect when two or more drugs are given concurrently

D. An interaction between a drug and another drug that results in increase or decrease in pharmacologic effects

E. A process of delivering a drug to the various tissues

F. Process of movement of medication from drug administration sites to the musculature

G. An undesirable change that is visual

H. A remedy

I. Alleviating, temporary relief

J. Attachment of one substance to the surface of another

11. Which of the following are advantages of intravenous medications?
   A. Route for irritating substances, instant drug action, and better control over administration
   B. Allows for rapid onset of action and allows for absorption of drugs in gastric juices
   C. Prevents errors in compounding of medication, low risk of infiltration, and low risk of phlebitis
   D. Allows for uninterrupted control of rate, low risk of side effects, and low risk of adsorption

12. Incompatibilities of drugs fall into three classes, which include:
   A. Physical, incompatible, and chemical
   B. Physical, chemical, and therapeutic
   C. Therapeutic, absorption, and distribution

Match the description of the following catheters in column 1 to the correct term in column 2:

Column 1

13. _____ Epidural

14. _____ Intraperitoneal

15. _____ Intrathecal

16. _____ Subcutaneous infusion

Column 2

A. Catheter is placed over the dura mater

B. Needle is inserted into the tissue spaces

C. Catheter is within a sheath and contains spinal fluid

D. Catheter is placed in the peritoneal cavity

True-False

17. **T F** Intravenous push medication should be given slowly and according to manufacturer's recommendations.

18. **T F** Alcohol should not be used in epidural catheter dressing management because of the risk of migration of alcohol into the epidural space.

19. **T F** A hazard related to administration of intravenous medication is extravasation.

20. **T F** The intermittent infusion route can be piggyback or by intravenous push.

21. There are _____ phases of the cell cycle.
   A. Three
   B. Six
   C. Five
   D. Two

22. Side effects from antineoplastic agents most often affect which of the following general systems?
   A. Immune system, integumentary, and gastrointestinal
   B. Integumentary system, cardiovascular, and respiratory
   C. Gastrointestinal system, neurologic, and genitourinary

ANSWERS TO PRE-TEST, Chapter 11

1. J   2. F   3. I   4. H   5. C   6. B   7. G   8. D   9. A

10. E   11. A   12. B   13. A   14. D   15. C   16. B   17. T

18. T   19. T   20. T   21. C   22. A

Table 11–1 □ **ADVANTAGES OF INTRAVENOUS MEDICATION ADMINISTRATION**

1. Provides a direct access to the circulatory system
2. Provides a route for drugs that irritate the gastric mucosa
3. Provides a route for instant drug action
4. Provides a route to deliver high drug concentrations
5. Provides for instant drug termination if sensitivity or adverse reaction occurs
6. Provides for better control over rate of drug administration
7. Provides a route of administration in patients in whom use of the gastrointestinal tract is limited

ADVANTAGES OF INTRAVENOUS MEDICATION

The infusion of intravenous (I.V.) medication offers pronounced advantages over subcutaneous, intramuscular, or oral routes (Table 11–1). The advantages of I.V. medications include a direct access to the circulatory system, a route for administration of fluids and drugs to patients who cannot tolerate oral medications, a method of instant drug action, and a method of instant drug administration termination.

Drugs that cannot be absorbed by other routes because of large molecular size of the drug or destruction of the drug by gastric juices, can be administered directly to the site of **distribution**, the circulatory system, via I.V. infusion. Drugs with irritating properties that cause pain and trauma when given by the intramuscular or subcutaneous route can be given intravenously. When a drug is administered intravenously there is instant drug action, which is an advantage in emergency situations. The I.V. route also allows instant drug termination if sensitivity or adverse reactions occur. The I.V. route provides for control over the rate at which drugs are administered; prolonged action can be controlled by administering a dilute medication infusion intermittently over a prolonged time (Plumer & Cosentino, 1987).

HAZARDS OF INTRAVENOUS MEDICATION

The number of drug combinations, along with the ever-increasing production of drugs and parenteral fluids, has compounded the hazards associated with I.V. medications. Despite the many advantages of I.V. medication there are hazards to this venous route that are not found in other drug therapies. The hazards that are specific to the administration of I.V. drugs include drug interactions, drug loss via adsorption to I.V. containers and administration sets, errors in mixing techniques, the complications of speed shock, extravasation of vesicant drugs, and phlebitis (Todd, 1988) (Table 11–2).

The nurse responsible for delivery of I.V. medications must have the necessary skills of organization, technical knowledge of mechanism of drug delivery, and awareness of drug action and adverse effects to ensure safe delivery of the medication.

Table 11-2 □ **DISADVANTAGES OF INTRAVENOUS MEDICATION ADMINISTRATION**

1. Drug interaction due to incompatibilities
2. Absorption of the drug impaired due to leaching into I.V. container or administration set
3. Errors in compounding (mixing) of medication
4. Speed shock
5. Extravasation of a vesicant drug
6. Chemical phlebitis

Drug Interactions

Drug interactions are not always clear-cut. Many factors affect drug solubility and **compatibility**. The potential for **incompatibility** is unique to the injectable drugs. Mixing of two incompatible drugs in a solution can cause an adverse interaction.

Factors affecting drug solubility and compatibility include:

1. Drug concentration
2. Brand of I.V. fluid or drug
3. Type of administration set
4. Preparation technique; duration of drug-drug or drug-solution contact
5. pH value
6. Temperature of the room and light

Drugs can be compatible when mixed in certain solutions yet incompatible when mixed with others. Mixing two incompatible drugs in solution in a particular order may be enough to avoid a potentially adverse interaction (Gahart, 1991).

The pH of both solution and drug must be considered when compounding medication. Drugs that are widely dissimilar in their pH values are unlikely to be compatible in solution. For example, dextrose solutions are slightly acidic, with a pH of 4.5 to 5.5. There are several antibiotics on the market with an acidic pH that are stable in dextrose; however, alkaline antibiotics, such as carbenicillin, are unstable when mixed with dextrose.

✎ **Note:** Dextrose, with a pH of 4.5 to 5.5, should be used as a base for acidic drug dilution; normal saline, with a pH value of 6.8 to 8.5, should be used as a base for alkaline drug dilution.

✎ **Note:** When in doubt about I.V. drug incompatibilities, it is a good practice to flush the I.V. administration set with sodium chloride before and after medications are infused (Todd, 1988).

Adsorption

Adsorption refers to the attachment of one substance to the surface of another. Many drugs adsorb to glass or plastic. The hazard associated with adsorption is that the patient receives less drug than was actually intended. The amount of adsorption is difficult to predict; adsorption is affected by the concentration of

Table 11–3 □ **DRUGS THAT HAVE INCREASED ADSORPTION WHEN INFUSED IN PVC CONTAINERS**

Vitamin A acetate (but not the palmitate form)
Insulin
Phenothiazine tranquilizers (Thorazine, Compazine)
Hydralazine (Apresoline)
Warfarin (Coumadin)
Nitroglycerin

Source: Data from "Intravenous Hazards: Interaction, Absorption, Inadequate Mixing" by B. Todd, 1988, *Geriatric Nursing, 1,* 20–22. Copyright 1988.

the drug, the solution of the drug, the amount of surface contacted by the drug, and temperature changes (D'Arcy, 1983).

An example of adsorption would be the binding of insulin to plastic and glass containers. The insulin rapidly adsorbs to I.V. containers and tubing until all potential adsorption sites are saturated. During the initial part of an infusion, then, very little insulin may reach the patient; later, after adsorption sites are saturated, more of the insulin will be delivered to the patient. To prevent this occurrence, injecting the drug as close to the I.V. insertion site as possible will promote better therapeutic drug effects (Todd, 1988).

Polyvinylchloride (PVC) containers and plastic flexible I.V. bags promote drug adsorption. Several drugs undergo significant loss from adsorption during infusion in PVC plastic solution containers (Table 11–3).

When mixing medications into glass or plastic systems, refer to manufacturer's guidelines to prevent adsorption.

Errors in Mixing

Drug toxicity, subtherapeutic infusion, or erratic therapeutic effects can result from inadequate mixing of a drug into the infusion container. Inadequate mixing can contribute to a **bolus** of medication delivered to the patient, which may cause adverse effects (Gong & King, 1983).

✎ **Note:** Burning at the I.V. site from a presumably dilute drug is a warning that the concentration of the drug is too high and needs to be further diluted. (Refer to Chapter 8 for dilution guidelines.)

FACTORS THAT CONTRIBUTE TO INADEQUATE MIXING
1. Length of time required to mix drugs adequately in flexible bags
2. Addition of a drug to a hanging flexible bag
3. Insufficient needle length or incomplete needle insertion through the injection port (use at least a 1-in needle)
4. Additives injected at a slow rate into the primary bag (the turbulence of fast flow promotes mixing, especially in glass containers)
5. Inadequate movement of the additive from the injection port (e.g., the

375

long, narrow sleeve-type additive ports on some flexible bags, as op-
posed to the button type, hinder effective mixing)
6. Use of immiscible or very dense drugs
7. Nonexistent or improper mixing caused by human error (Gong & King, 1983)

Speed Shock

The nurse must be aware that speed shock can be caused by too rapid administration of a drug. Rapid onset of action is a double-edged sword: on one side, it
is to the patient's advantage to have rapid action in certain clinical situations;
on the other side, once infused, the rapid onset cannot be recalled. (Refer to
Chapter 8 for additional information on speed shock.)

Extravasation

The nurse must be aware of patency of the I.V. cannula before initiating an infusion to prevent extravasation of a **vesicant** drug. (Refer to Chapter 8 for additional information on extravasation.)

Chemical Phlebitis

Chemical phlebitis can occur from the pH of the medication; a pH greater than
11.0 or less than 4.3 is most irritating to the vein wall. Antibiotics, chemotherapeutic drugs, potassium chloride, and diazepam (Valium) are known to cause
irritation to the vein wall and promote phlebitis. (Refer to Chapter 8 for further
information on phlebitis.)

10 KEY RECOMMENDATIONS FOR ADEQUATE MIXING OF INTRAVENOUS MEDICATIONS

1. Gently invert the I.V. container several times to adequately mix the
   medication with the solution, taking care to avoid foaming the
   solution.
2. When inversion is impossible, gently swirl or rotate to mix, to prevent
   the drug from settling to the bottom of the container.
3. When agitating an intermittent infusion set, clamp off the air vent; if
   the vent becomes wet, the solution will not infuse properly after
   mixing.
4. Vacuum devices can facilitate mixing in plastic flexible bags by creating a vacuum and drawing any drug left in the port into the body of
   the bag.
5. When possible, use premixed solutions from the manufacturer; premixed heparin or potassium chloride solutions, for example, can save
   time and avoid dose errors as well as preclude mixing problems.
6. Add one drug at a time to the primary I.V. solution. Mix and examine
   thoroughly before adding the next drug.
7. Add the most concentrated or most soluble drug to the solution first

because some incompatibilities, such as precipitates, require a certain concentration or amount of time to develop. Mix it well, and then add the dilute drugs.

8. Add colored additives last to avoid masking possible precipitates or cloudiness.
9. Always remember to inspect containers visually after adding and mixing drugs; hold the container against a light or a white surface and check for particulate matter, obvious layering, or foaming.
10. If you do not have a clear understanding of the compatibility or stability of the admixtures you are using, check the manufacturer's recommendation, or consult a pharmacist (Todd, 1988).

✎ **Note:** Owing to the complexity of this subject, many hospitals allow only registered pharmacists to prepare admixtures.

DRUG COMPATIBILITY

According to the Intravenous Nursing Standards of Practice (1990, S49), compatibility is required for a therapeutic response to prescribed therapy. Chemical, physical, and therapeutic compatibilities must be identified before **admixing** and administering I.V. medications.

An incompatibility results when two or more substances react or interact so as to change the normal activity of one or more components. Incompatibility may be manifested by harmful or undesirable effects, and is likely to result in a loss of therapeutic effects.

Incompatibility may occur when:

1. Several drugs are added to a large volume of fluid to produce an admixture
2. Drugs in separate solutions are administered concurrently or in close succession via the same I.V. line
3. A single drug is reconstituted or diluted with the wrong solutions
4. One drug reacts with another drug's preservative

Specific incompatibilities fall into three categories:

Physical
Chemical
Therapeutic

Physical Incompatibility

A **physical incompatibility** is also called a pharmaceutic incompatibility. Pharmaceutic incompatibilities occur when one drug is mixed with other drugs or solutions to produce a product unsafe for administration.

Insolubility and **absorption** are the two types of physical incompatibility. Insolubility occurs when a drug is added to an inappropriate fluid solution, creating an incomplete solution or a precipitate. This risk occurs more frequently with multiple additives, which may interact to form an insoluble product.

Signs of insolubility include:

Visible precipitation
Haze
Gas bubbles
Cloudiness

Some precipitations may be microcrystalline, smaller than 50 microns, and not be apparent to the eye. The use of micropore filters is intended to prevent such particles from entering the vein. The use of a 0.22-micron inline filter reduces the amount of microcrystalline precipitates.

The presence of calcium in a drug or solution usually indicates that a precipitate might form if mixed with another drug. Ringer's solution preparations contain calcium, so check carefully for incompatibility before adding any drug to this solution.

Other physical incompatibilities caused by insolubility include the increased degradation of drugs added to sodium bicarbonate and the formation of an insoluble precipitate when sodium bicarbonate is combined with other medications in emergency situations.

✎ **Note:** Never administer a drug that forms a precipitate.

✎ **Note:** Drugs that are prepared in special diluents should not be mixed with other drugs.

✎ **Note:** When administering a series of medications, prepare each drug in a separate syringe. This will lessen the possibility of precipitation. Insolubility may also result from the use of an incorrect solution to reconstitute a drug.

✎ **Note:** Follow the manufacturer's directions for reconstituting drugs.

Chemical Incompatibility

A **chemical incompatibility** is defined as the reaction of a drug with other drugs or solutions, which results in alterations of the integrity and potency of the active ingredient. The most common cause of chemical incompatibilities is the reaction between acidic and alkaline drugs or solutions, resulting in a pH that is unstable for one of the drugs. A specific pH or a narrow range of pH values is required for the solubility of a drug and for the maintenance of its stability, once it has been mixed.

Therapeutic Incompatibility

A **therapeutic incompatibility** is an undesirable unexpected effect occurring within a patient as a result of two or more drugs being given concurrently. An increased or decreased therapeutic response may be produced.

This incompatibility often occurs when therapy dictates the use of two antibiotics. For example, in the use of chloramphenicol and penicillin, chloramphenicol has been reported to antagonize the bacterial activity of penicillin. If prescribed, penicillin should be administered at least 1 hour before the chloramphenicol to prevent therapeutic incompatibility.

Therapeutic incompatibility may go unnoticed until the patient fails to show the expected clinical response to the drug or until peak and trough levels of the drug show a lack of therapeutic levels. If an incompatibility is not suspected, the patient may be given increasingly higher doses of the drug to try to obtain the therapeutic effect (Lippincott Learning System, 1984).

A compatibility chart (Appendix B) identifies the physical and chemical incompatibilities of commonly prescribed drugs.

✎ **Note:** When more than one antibiotic is prescribed for intermittent infusion, stagger the time schedule so that each can be infused individually.

METHODS OF ADMINISTRATION OF INTRAVENOUS MEDICATIONS

Continuous infusions
Intermittent infusions
I.V. push
Subcutaneous infusions
Intraspinal infusions

  Epidural
  Intrathecal

Intraperitoneal
Other methods of medication administration

  Ventricular reservoir
  Arteriovenous fistulas

✎ General Points in Delivery of Intravenous Medications

NURSING RESPONSIBILITIES
1. To identify whether a prescribed method of drug administration (continuous, intermittent, or push) is appropriate
2. To use aseptic technique in the preparation of an admixture
3. To identify the expiration date on solutions and medications
4. To follow manufacturer's guidelines for preparation and storage of medication
5. To be knowledgeable of the pharmacologic implications relative to patient clinical status and diagnosis
6. To verify that all solution containers are free of cracks, leaks, and punctures
7. To monitor the patient for therapeutic response to medication

Continuous Infusions

Continuous infusion is defined as large-volume parenteral solutions of 250 to 1000 mL of infusate administered over 2 to 24 hours. Medication added to these large volume infusates are administered continuously. These infusions

379

should be regulated by an I.V. pump or controller to ensure an accurate flow rate.

KEY POINTS IN DELIVERY OF CONTINUOUS INFUSIONS

ADVANTAGES
1. Admixture and bag changes can be performed every 8 to 24 hours.
2. Constant serum levels of the drug are maintained.

DISADVANTAGES
1. Monitoring the drug rate can be erratic if not electronically controlled.
2. Higher risk of drug incompatibility problems.
3. Accidental bolus infusion if medication is not adequately mixed with I.V. solution.

PROCEDURE FOR ADMINISTRATION OF CONTINUOUS INFUSIONS
(Verify physician's order, educate patient regarding purpose of therapy, and document procedure.)
1. Spike the I.V. container with an I.V. administration set.
2. Regulate the flow rate.
3. Based on the type of drug being administered, monitor the patient at the recommended time intervals for therapeutic and nontherapeutic effects of the drug.
4. Place time-tape on bag, even when a pump or controller is used, to verify administration rate at a quick glance.

 Note: When adding medication to an infusion container, use **single-dose vials** instead of **multiple-dose vials** to decrease potential for infection, complications, and medication errors.

Intermittent Infusions

The administration of certain medications, often called "piggyback" or secondary infusions, for intermittent delivery of medication have become popular. This secondary administration container contains a single additive or multiple-dose admixture connected to a controlled-volume set.

TYPES OF INTERMITTENT INFUSIONS
1. Piggyback using a secondary set
2. prn infusion using heparin or saline locking device
3. Use of a volumetric chamber.

Piggyback

I.V. piggyback (Fig. 11–1) is a method of **intermittent drug infusion**. I.V. medication is diluted in 50 to 150 mL of 5% dextrose and water or sodium chlo-

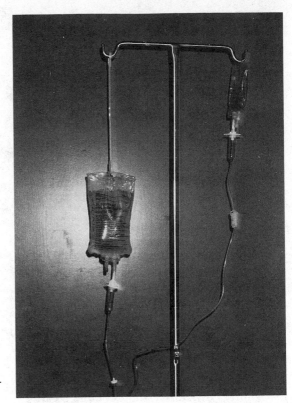

Figure 11–1 ☐ Delivery of secondary "piggyback" medication.

ride and administered over 30 to 60 minutes. The administration time varies according to the drug manufacturer's recommendations.

✎ KEY POINTS IN DELIVERY OF PIGGYBACK MEDICATIONS

ADVANTAGES
1. The risk of incompatibilities is reduced.
2. Larger drug doses can be administered at a lower concentration per milliliter than with the I.V. push method.

DISADVANTAGES
1. Administration rate may not be accurate unless electronically monitored.
2. I.V. set changes can result in wasting of a portion of the drug.
3. If the patient is not properly monitored, fluid overload or speed shock could result.
4. Drug incompatibility can occur if the administration set is not adequately flushed between medication administrations.

381

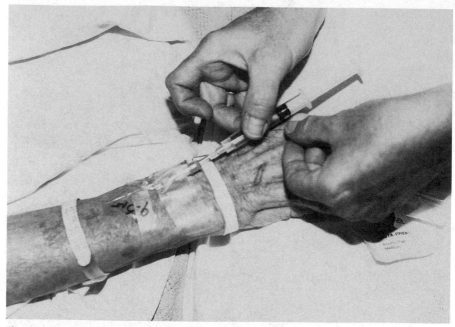

Figure 11–2 □ Delivery of intermittent medication via a locking device.

prn Administration Using Locking Device

Medication administered by this intermittent route (Fig. 11–2) is usually diluted in 1 to 50 mL of infusate and infused over a 1-minute to 15-minute period. An intermittent infusion is attached directly to an I.V. lock, and 0.9% sodium chloride or heparinized sodium chloride is used to maintain patency of the lock.

✎ **KEY POINTS IN DELIVERY OF INTERMITTENT DRUG THERAPY USING A LOCKING DEVICE**

ADVANTAGES
1. Incompatibilities are avoided.
2. A minimal amount of fluid is provided to the patient on restricted intake.
3. Minimal drug is wasted.

DISADVANTAGES
1. If the fluid container runs dry, blood backs into the cannula and tubing and could cause a clot (Plumer & Cosentino, 1987).
2. After each infusion of medication, the lock must be flushed with heparinized sodium chloride or 0.9% sodium chloride (depending on agency policy) to maintain patency.

✎ PROCEDURE FOR ADMINISTRATION OF MEDICATION THROUGH PRN DEVICE

(Verify physician's order, educate patient regarding purpose of therapy, and document procedure.)

1. Wash hands.
2. Flush lock with 1 to 2 mL of normal saline.
3. Infuse the drug at the prescribed rate.
4. After drug delivery, flush the lock with 0.9% sodium chloride or heparinized sodium chloride solution.

✎ **Note:** Exert a positive pressure on the syringe when withdrawing from the I.V. lock to prevent a backflow of blood into the I.V. catheter.

Volumetric Chamber

This method of intermittent delivery of medication (Fig. 11–3) is used most frequently with pediatric patients or when delivery of small amount of well-controlled drug needs to be administered to critical care patients. Medication is

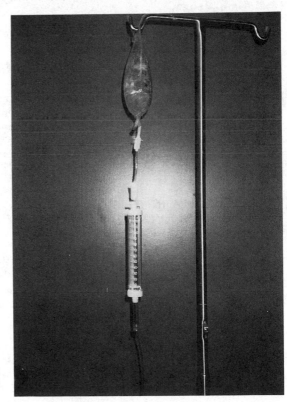

Figure 11–3 ☐ Administration of medication via volumetric chamber.

added to the volume control chamber and diluted with I.V. solution. The infusion is generally over 15 minutes to 1 hour. Volumes delivered vary from 25 to 150 mL per drug dose.

✎ KEY POINTS IN DELIVERY OF INTERMITTENT DRUG THERAPY VIA A VOLUMETRIC CHAMBER

ADVANTAGES
1. Runaway infusions are avoided without the use of electronic equipment.
2. Volume of fluid in which the drug is diluted can be adjusted.

DISADVANTAGES
1. Medication must travel the length of the tubing before it reaches the patient, so there is a significant time delay.
2. A portion of the medication can be left in the tubing after the chamber empties.
3. Incompatibilities may develop when the chamber, which is usually within the primary line, is used for multiple drug deliveries.
4. Labeling of the chamber must coincide with the drug being delivered. If multiple drugs are delivered this could present a problem (LaRocca & Otto, 1989).

Intravenous Push Administration of Medication

Intravenous push administration of a medication, referred to as "I.V. push," provides a method of administering high concentrations of medication. Administration via this route can be accomplished by direct penetration of a vein, by penetration of a vein using a syringe and needle scalp vein infusion set or over-the-needle infusion device, or by access of the low injection port of primary administration sets.

✎ KEY POINTS IN DELIVERY OF INTRAVENOUS PUSH MEDICATIONS

ADVANTAGES
1. Barriers of drug absorption are bypassed.
2. Drug response is rapid and usually predictable.
3. Patient is closely monitored during the full administration of the medication.

DISADVANTAGES
1. Adverse effects occur at the same time and rate as therapeutic effects.
2. The I.V. push method has the greatest risk of adverse effects and toxicity, because serum drug concentrations are sharply elevated.
3. Speed shock is possible from too rapid administration of medication.

Adverse effects that can occur during administration of a medication directly into a vein are changes in level of consciousness, vital functions, and reflex activity (Burman & Berkowitz, 1989).

✎ **Note:** If adverse effects occur, supportive care is the basis for treatment of most symptoms because specific antidotes are available for only certain drugs.

✎ **PROCEDURE FOR INTRAVENOUS PUSH DRUG ADMINISTRATION**

(Verify physician's order, educate patient regarding purpose of therapy, and document procedure.)

1. Check compatibility of drug with primary solution.
2. Dilute opioid narcotics and follow recommendation of manufacturer for administration.
3. Swab lowest Y port with alcohol or betadine.
4. Insert syringe with medication into Y site.
5. Pinch tubing to primary solution.
6. Inject one quarter of medication into patient over a 15- to 20-second period.
7. Unpinch tubing, allowing primary solution to flush. *Watch patient for any adverse effects.*
8. Repeat steps 5 through 7, delivering one quarter of drug each time for three more times.
9. When all the desired drug is delivered, remove syringe.

✎ **Note:** This process should take *at least* 1 minute; however, always follow recommendations of manufacturer for delivery of the drug. For example, drugs such as Dilantin and Valium must be delivered over a lengthy period of time; the manufacturer provides specific guidelines for administration.

Continuous Subcutaneous Infusion

Continuous subcutaneous infusion (CSQI) is a practical and simple approach to pain management. Pain affects approximately 65 to 85 percent of cancer patients (Murphy, 1990). Two factors that contribute to unsatisfactory pain management are inadequate dosage and titration of available pain medications and limited resources to educate and advise physicians and nurses properly on pain management. Patients who require parenteral narcotics are candidates for CSQI. This type of infusion therapy can be established for the following types of patients who require intermittent injection, usually longer than 48 hours (McLaughlin-Hagan, 1990):

- Patients unable to take medications by mouth
- Patients who require subcutaneous injections for more than 48 hours
- Patients who require parenteral narcotics but have poor venous access

✎ **KEY POINTS IN DELIVERY OF CONTINUOUS SUBCUTANEOUS INFUSION**

ADVANTAGES
1. Easy care for home management of pain
2. Decreased number of times tissue is traumatized by repeated injections

385

3. Better home management of pain, which decreases hospital time
4. Decrease in central nervous side effects associated with intermittent drug therapy, such as nausea, vomiting, and drowsiness
5. Decrease in pain breakthrough

DISADVANTAGES
1. Local irritation at infusion site
2. Rapidly escalating pain of dying patient requiring larger volumes of drug; this route is inappropriate for volumes larger than 1 mL/hour (Coyle, Mauskop, Maggard, & Foley, 1986)

✐ PROCEDURE FOR ADMINISTRATION OF CONTINUOUS SUBCUTANEOUS INFUSION (Fig. 11–4)
(Verify physician's order, educate patient regarding purpose of therapy, and document procedure.)

1. Establish baseline vital signs.
2. Have patients rate their pain on a scale of 1 to 10.
3. Establish subcutaneous access per hospital policy and use continuous infusion guidelines.
4. Use a 24-gauge catheter, with a 26-gauge insertion needle. The Soft-set (MiniMed Technologies) also has a 42-in microbore tubing attached to the infusion device, which can then be attached to a patient-controlled analgesia pump. This system has a Leur lock hub. The tubing is made of polyfin, which is compatible with most drug deliveries.
5. Prime tubing if needed.
6. Administer prescribed bolus dose and immediately begin the continuous infusion.
7. Obtain vital signs, neurologic signs, and pain level assessment every 30 minutes (number times four) and then as needed.

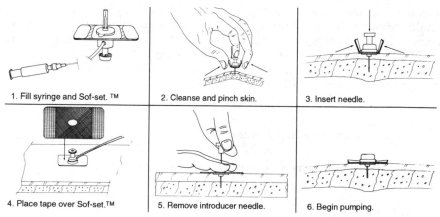

1. Fill syringe and Sof-set. ™
2. Cleanse and pinch skin.
3. Insert needle.
4. Place tape over Sof-set.™
5. Remove introducer needle.
6. Begin pumping.

Figure 11–4 □   Steps in subcutaneous infusion. (Courtesy of MiniMed Technologies, Sylmar, California.)

386

Intraspinal Medication Infusions

Spinal opiate receptor sites were discovered in 1973, and subsequently selective spinal opiate analgesia was developed—"selective" because only pain is alleviated (Bromage, 1980). The first controlled study describing the intrathecal administration of morphine in humans was reported in the late 1970s (Wang, Nauss, & Thomas, 1979). The rationale for this method of drug administration is that it allows for direct delivery of narcotic or dilute anesthetic to the receptors in the brain and spinal column. The spinal anatomy consists of two spaces, the epidural space and the intrathecal space. **Intraspinal** is the term used to encompass both the epidural and intrathecal spaces surrounding the spinal cord. **Intrathecal** space is surrounded by the epidural space and separated from it by the dura mater; the intrathecal space contains cerebral spinal fluid, which bathes the spinal cord. The epidural and intrathecal spaces share a common center, the spinal cord. **Epidural** space surrounds the spinal cord and intrathecal space and lies between the ligamentum flavum and the dura mater. This is a potential space, inasmuch as the ligamentum flavum and the dura mater are not separated until medication or air is injected between them. This potential space contains a network of veins that are large and thin-walled and has a strong leukocytic activity to reduce the risk of infection. Dividing epidural and intrathecal spaces is a tough, fatty membrane called the dura. The dura's permeability is important in determining how fast epidural drugs cross into the intrathecal space and how long they remain there to be active (St. Marie, 1989). The epidural space also contains fat in proportion to a person's body fat. Opiate receptor sites are cells contained in the dorsal horn of the spinal cord, at which point opioids combine with their respective receptor site to generate analgesia (Bonica, 1990).

Intraspinal analgesia can provide relief to patients suffering from intractable pain. Intraspinal analgesia does not cause the central nervous system side effects that systemic narcotic delivery can cause. Multiple studies show that in the surgical and postsurgical settings, epidural morphine is superior to a systemic narcotic for abdominal, pelvic, thoracic, spinal surgery, and obstetrics (Slater, Zeitlin, & Edwards, 1985; Zola & McLeod, 1983).

Local anesthetic agents are frequently used with intraspinal narcotics and are instrumental in controlling pain and reducing postoperative complications. When a patient experiences acute pain the sympathetic system, which is part of the autonomic nervous system, is activated, increasing the workload of the heart. When intraspinal local anesthetic agents are administered, a sympathetic block results, which produces a decrease in blood pressure, pulse, and respirations. The advantages of adding local anesthetic agents to an epidural narcotic are that it produces a sympathetic block, resulting in decreased workload on the heart and decreases incidence of thrombophlebitis and paralytic ileus. A disadvantage to local anesthetic agents is the nurse's lack of understanding of such agents. Nurses must be educated regarding the use of these agents (St. Marie, 1991). Refer to Table 11–4 for medications currently used for intraspinal administration.

Epidural Medication Administration

PATIENT SELECTION CRITERIA
1. Control of pain associated with cancer

Table 11–4 □ MEDICATIONS USED FOR INTRASPINAL ADMINISTRATION

Agonists	Antagonists	Anesthetics
Morphine (preservative-free)	Butorphanol tartrate (Stadol)	Bupivacaine (Marcaine)
Meperidine (Demerol)	Nalbuphine hydrochloride (nubain)	Lidocaine (Xylocaine)
Sublimaze (Fentanyl)	Pentazocine hydrochloride (Talwin)	Mepivacaine (Carbocaine)
Hydromorphone (Dilaudid)		Prilocaine (Citanest)
		Etidocaine (Duranest)
		Tetracaine (Pontocaine)
		Procaine (Novocaine)

2. Surgical patient about to have extensive surgery performed (e.g., thoracic or abdominal surgery)
3. Victims of trauma in the chest area or limbs who have no increased intracranial pressure and normal bleeding times

✎ **KEY POINTS IN DELIVERY OF EPIDURAL MEDICATIONS**

ADVANTAGES
1. Permits control or alleviation of severe pain without the sedative effects
2. Permits delivery of smaller doses of a narcotic to achieve desired level of analgesia
3. Prolongs the analgesia (average about 14 hours)
4. Allows for continuous infusion if needed
5. Allows terminal cancer patients treated with epidural narcotics to be more comfortable and mobile (Slater et al., 1985)
6. Can be used for short- or long-term therapy
7. Does not produce motor paralysis or hypotension

DISADVANTAGES
1. Only preservative-free narcotics can be used.
2. Complications such as paresthesia, urinary retention, and respiratory depression (greatest 6 to 10 hours after injection) can occur.
3. Catheter-related risks can occur (e.g., infection, dislodgment, and leaking.)
4. Pruritus can occur on face, head, and neck or be generalized.

✎ **Note:** Have naloxone (Narcan) 0.4 mg I.V. available to counteract respiratory depression.

Insertion and Maintenance of Epidural Catheters

1. The insertion of the epidural catheter is a sterile procedure and is a medical act performed by a physician or anesthesiologist.
2. Administration of medication by a nurse through an epidural catheter must be in accordance with each state's Nurse Practice Act.

3. The drug most frequently used is preservative-free morphine. Preservatives (mainly alcohol) have a destructive effect on neural tissue (Lieb & Hurtig, 1985). Examples of other preservatives are methylparaban, sodium bisulfite, sodium hydroxide, buffers, benzoalcohol, and phenol. Currently, preservative-free morphine is available in 0.5 mg/mL and 1 mg/mL concentrations.
4. The physician uses an 18-gauge needle inserted between L-2 and L-3, or L-3 and L-4.
5. Lidocaine is injected subcutaneously. The needle is inserted and the catheter is threaded through the needle so that the catheter tip is approximately at the dermatome level affected by the pain (Fig. 11-5).
6. After insertion, the exposed catheter length is then laid cephalad along the spine and over the shoulder. The entire length of the exposed catheter is taped in place to provide stability and protection. The end of the catheter and the filter is generally placed on the patient's chest wall and taped securely in a position that allows the patient or significant other to access the catheter for use.

✎ **Note:** The epidural catheter must be clearly labeled after placement to prevent accidental infusion of fluids or medications.

7. Epidural catheters can be connected in one of three ways: via an' implantable pump or implantable port or threaded subcutaneously so it exits out the side of the body.
8. Intravenous Nursing Standards of Practice (1990) recommend that

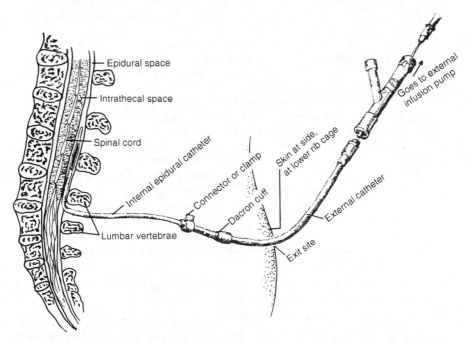

Figure 11-5 □ Epidural catheter for pain relief. (From "Administration of Intraspinal Analgesia in the Home Care Setting" by B. St. Marie, 1989, *National Intravenous Therapy Association, 12 (3)*, p. 166. Copyright 1989 by the National Intravenous Therapy Association. Reprinted by permission.)

medication infused via an epidural catheter should be administered via an electronic infusion device (S71).

✎ **Note:** Strict sterile technique must be used in caring for this catheter.

✎ **Note:** It is recommended that a 0.22-micron filter be used on the catheter to prevent introduction of particulate matter or bacteria into the epidural space (INS, 1990, S71).

NURSING RESPONSIBILITIES
1. Patient and family education
2. Site and dressing management
3. Medication administration
4. Evaluation of pain relief

✎ **Note:** Ineffective pain control should be reported to the physician or anesthesiologist managing care of the epidural catheter.

Administration of Medication via the Epidural Catheter

(Verify physician's order, educate patient regarding purpose of therapy, and document procedure.)

1. Assemble equipment; wash hands thoroughly.
2. Inspect insertion site for signs of infection or drainage.
3. Verify with another nurse that a preservative-free narcotic is mixed in normal saline solution.
4. Assess patient for baseline data and vital signs.
5. Use sterile gloves. Scrub the injection cap with povidone iodine and allow 2 minutes of contact time. Wipe with a sterile 2 × 2 gauze strip to remove any excess iodine.
6. Enter the injection cap using the 3-mL empty syringe and a 25-gauge 5/8-in needle. Gently aspirate to verify catheter tip is *not* in the subarachnoid space by observing that less than 1 mL of fluid returns. Discard any fluid withdrawn.
7. Rescrub injection cap with povidone iodine.
8. Begin infusion via pump connected to extension tubing and filter or inject intermittent dose at rate of approximately 5 mL/minute.
9. Check catheter cap for secureness. Tighten as needed.
10. Document.
11. Assess patient every 15 minutes twice, then every 4 hours for vital signs. Check level of consciousness every hour for 24 hours, then every 4 hours.

✎ **Note:** Have available naloxone (Narcan) 0.4 mg to treat respiratory depression or increased sedation.

✎ **Note:** Never use alcohol for site preparation or for accessing the catheter because of the potential for alcohol migration into the epidural space.

Nursing Dressing Management of Epidural Catheters

This is a sterile procedure.

1. Wash hands with antimicrobial soap and water for at least 1 minute.
2. Remove old dressing. Use cottonball soaked in sterile water to assist in lifting the edge of dressing.
3. Wet cotton-tipped applicator in povidone iodine solution and clean area starting at the catheter, working outward in a circular motion. Repeat this two more times, and allow area to dry. (Note if any crusted areas exist around the catheter and remove them by using a swab dipped in hydrogen peroxide before using the povidone iodine.)
4. Apply new transparent dressing.
5. Remove the tape holding the catheter end, clean skin under the tape, allow to dry, and retape for comfort and safety (Lonsway, 1988).

✎ **Note:** Do not use alcohol on skin or at dressing site due to the risk of migration of alcohol into the epidural space and possibility of neural damage.

Intrathecal Administration

The intrathecal injection of a narcotic requires approximately 10 times less medication than is needed in the epidural space. The intrathecal space, however, affords a greater risk for infection. When intrathecal catheters are used for long-term applications they are connected to an implantable pump to reduce the risk of infection.

✎ **KEY POINTS IN INTRATHECAL ADMINISTRATION**

ADVANTAGES
1. Useful for delivery of certain antineoplastic agents, antibiotics, analgesics, and anesthetic agents
2. Effective alternative to oral or parenteral therapy in abatement of pain associated with cancer because of direct delivery of narcotic to opiate receptors in the brain and spinal column
3. Allows for low doses of drug to produce the same degree of analgesia as high doses required systemically

DISADVANTAGES
1. Side effects that can be life threatening
2. Potential for spinal fluid leak
3. Potential infection (Akahoshi, Furuike-McLaughlin, & Enriquez, 1988)

✎ **PROCEDURE FOR ADMINISTRATION OF MEDICATION VIA THE INTRATHECAL CATHETER**
(Verify physician's order, educate patient regarding purpose of therapy, and document procedure.)

1. Use sterile gloves and mask.
2. Use noncoring needles to access ports and pumps.
3. Use preservative-free medication via an intrathecal catheter.
4. Alcohol is contraindicated for site preparation and for accessing the catheter because of the potential for alcohol migration into the intrathecal space.
5. A 0.22-micron filter without surfactant should be used for medication administration.
6. Assess for therapeutic response and complications.

✎ **Note:** When an intrathecal catheter is attached to an implanted pump, the manufacturer's guidelines regarding aspiration must be adhered to (INS, 1990, S72).

Side Effects of Intraspinal Medications

Side effects with intraspinal narcotic infusions include nausea, vomiting, urinary retention, pruritus, and respiratory depression. Nausea and vomiting can be controlled with antiemetics such as prochlorperazine (Compazine). An antagonist such as naloxone (Narcan) 0.2 mg I.V. or an agonist/antagonist such as nalbuphine (Nubain) 5 to 10 mg subcutaneously may reverse the narcotic enough to reverse side effects without reversing the analgesia (St. Marie, 1991).

Urinary retention is a common side effect and may occur 10 to 20 hours after the first injection of intraspinal narcotic. This may require either administration of bethanecol (Urecholine) or intermittent catheterization.

Pruritus is caused by the opiate's interacting with the dorsal horn and not by histamine release. This is best treated with an antagonist rather than with diphenhydramine (Benadryl). After an epidural injection, 8.5 percent of all patients experience pruritus; after an intrathecal injection, 46 percent experience pruritus.

Respiratory depression from epidural or intrathecal narcotic administration is a risk. Vital signs should be assessed and Narcan should be available to reverse depressant effects of a narcotic (Rosen, 1990).

Intraperitoneal Infusions

Intraperitoneal (IP) therapy is the administration of therapeutic agents directly into the peritoneal cavity. Many studies (Dedrick, 1985; McClay & Howell, 1990) have confirmed the advantages of this approach to chemotherapeutic management of cancer.

The purpose of IP therapy is to increase the **antineoplastic** agents' concentration at the tumor site (peritoneal cavity) in order to enhance its penetration and cell kill while limiting systemic effects. The peritoneal cavity acts as a reservoir for the drug. The goal is to decrease systemic toxic effects and increase the antitumor action of the antineoplastic agent (Zook-Enck, 1990). (Fig. 11–6).

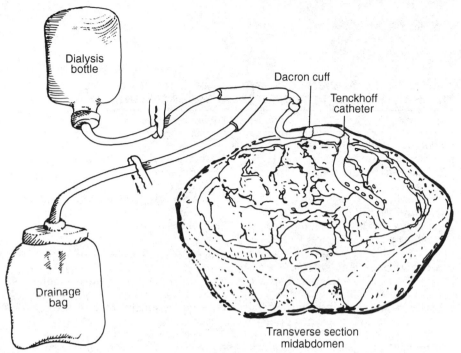

Figure 11–6 ☐ Transverse section midabdomen with Tenckhoff catheter for intraperitoneal therapy. (From "Intraperitoneal Chemotherapy I.V. Team Responsibility," by C. Vizcarra, 1988, *Journal of Intravenous Nursing, 11(3)*. Copyright 1988 by the Intravenous Nursing Society. Reprinted by permission.)

✎ KEY POINTS IN INTRAPERITONEAL THERAPY

1. The disease must be limited to the body region in which the antineoplastic agent is administered.
2. There are three types of IP access devices: temporary indwelling catheter, IP implantable port, and indwelling Tenckhoff catheter (Table 11–5).
3. Nursing staff must be well prepared to care for an IP catheter.
4. Nurse and family must be familiar with therapeutic effects of antineoplastic agent.

ADVANTAGES
1. When not in use, its presence is invisible, enhancing a positive body image
2. No catheter site care
3. Care free for patient
4. Cytotoxic drugs administered directly to tumor area (Malloy, 1991)

DISADVANTAGES
1. Device related—locating and accessing port
2. Catheter infections can occur
3. Build-up of fibrin sheath on distal catheter tip (Howell, 1990)

393

Table 11–5 □ **ADVANTAGES AND DISADVANTAGES OF THE THREE METHODS OF INTRAPERITONEAL MANAGEMENT**

Advantages	Disadvantages
Temporary Catheter	
1. May be inserted at the bedside	1. Increases risk of bowel or visceral perforation
2. Does not require surgical procedure for removal	2. Requires extra precautions to prevent displacement when patient is mobile
3. Is an inexpensive catheter	
4. Decreases risk of infection and fibrous sheath formation owing to its temporary presence	
Intraperitoneal Implantable Port	
1. Serves as a semipermanent access device	1. Requires the use of the operating room for insertion
2. Decreases risk of bowel or visceral perforation when inserted during laparotomy	2. Requires surgical procedure for removal
3. Implantable system, decreases risk of infection	3. Expensive access device
4. Provides a greater chance of patient acceptance owing to absence of external catheter	4. Does not allow for high-pressure, forced irrigation or manipulation to dislodge fibrin clot
	5. Requires a needlestick with each access
Indwelling Tenckhoff Catheter	
1. Serves as a semipermanent access device	1. Requires the use of the operating room for insertion
2. Decreases risk of bowel or visceral perforation	2. Increases the risk of infection with an external catheter component
3. Is an inexpensive catheter	3. Requires catheter home care by the patient
4. Allows for high-pressure, forced irrigation/manipulation to dislodge or loosen fibrin clots	4. May create body image changes with presence of long-term use
5. Permits rapid instillation of fluid	
6. Permits rapid drainage of peritoneal fluid	
7. Requires pulling to remove, no surgical incision	
8. May be preferred in an obese patient	

Source: From "Intraperitoneal Therapy via the Tenckhoff Catheter" by D. Zook-Enck, 1990, *Journal of Intravenous Nursing, 13,* pp. 375–382. Copyright 1990 by Intravenous Nursing Society. Reprinted by permission.

NURSING CONSIDERATIONS IN INTRAPERITONEAL THERAPY

1. Maintain strict sterile technique: use povidone iodine for washing hands before handling system.
2. Scrub all connectors with povidone iodine.
3. Use sterile gloves when separating a connection.
4. Minimize accessing the system when possible.
5. Be aware that a fibrin sheath may build up on the distal catheter tip resulting in a one-way flow problem. The injection of solution may be easily performed but withdrawal of solution difficult (Howell, 1990).
6. Irrigate catheter well before and after administering therapy or withdrawing or draining peritoneal fluid with 3 to 50 mL of normal saline (Piccart, Speyer, & Markman, 1985).
7. Ensure that administration and drainage tubing is free of kinks.
8. Maintain a sterile dressing in hospital environment. Teach home care to maintain clean and dry dressing.
9. Teach patient and family care of the dressing for home care.
10. If using Tenckhoff catheter, allow Dacron cuffs to heal for at least 1 to 2 weeks before initiating IP therapy.
11. Warm IP solution in a dry incubator prior to treatment (Swenson & Eriksson, 1986).
12. Observe catheter site for signs of infection (Zook-Enck, 1990).

Other Methods of Medication Delivery

Ventricular Reservoir

A ventricular reservoir allows for the administration of medications into the central nervous system. A physician must place the ventricular reservoir, and the nurse administering medications into the reservoir must follow the Nurse Practice Act.

✎ KEY POINTS IN DELIVERY OF MEDICATIONS VIA VENTRICULAR RESERVOIR

1. Patient should be taught the purpose of the reservoir.
2. When accessing the ventricular reservoir, sterile gloves and mask should be worn.
3. Use only preservative-free medications.
4. Aspirate to check placement before drug delivery. Spinal fluid should be present.
5. Withdrawal of spinal fluid for diagnostic purpose is a medical act.

Arteriovenous Fistulas

An arteriovenous (AV) fistula facilitates accessing of the vascular system. AV fistulas are used for administration of parenteral therapies.

✎ **KEY POINTS IN DELIVERY OF ARTERIOVENOUS PARENTERAL THERAPY**
1. Nurse must be knowledgeable regarding the type of fistula that is in place: synthetic, bovine graft, or anastomosis.
2. The integrity of the graft site must be determined before venipuncture by palpation and auscultation.
3. Use sterile technique; sterile gloves should be worn.
4. Arterial pressure within the AV fistula increases the potential for bleeding.
5. Potential complications include but are not limited to infection, occlusion, and thrombosis.

ANTI-INFECTIVE ADMINISTRATION CONSIDERATIONS

The nurse responsible for I.V. administration of antibiotic, antifungal, and antiviral agents should understand pharmacotherapeutics related to the administration of these drugs. Manufacturer recommendations for administration should be carefully followed. Anti-infectives are administered to achieve therapeutic coverage based on culture and sensitivity reports.

✎ **KEY QUESTIONS IN DELIVERY OF ANTIMICROBIAL AGENTS**
1. Has the infecting organism been identified (suspected or confirmed by culture)?
2. Is the organism resistant to any antimicrobial agents?
3. Is the site of infection identified?
4. What is the status of the host (patient) defenses?
5. Is the nurse familiar with the antimicrobial pharmacokinetics?
6. What is the status of the patient's renal and hepatic function?
7. Is monitoring the patient's blood levels necessary to avoid toxicity of dosage?
8. Does the patient have an allergy to the anti-infective agent? (Mathewson-Kuhn, 1991)

Antibiotics

Antibiotic action is either bacteriostatic, inhibiting bacterial cell wall synthesis and producing a defective cell wall, or bactericidal, altering intracellular function of the bacteria. A knowledge of each antibiotic administered is essential for safe delivery of the medication.

GENERAL NURSING CONSIDERATIONS
1. Be knowledgeable about the antibiotic ordered: its normal dosage, side effects, and compatibilities; and the purpose of the antibiotic in treating the patient's infection (Table 11–6).
2. Be sure the drug has not expired.
3. Be familiar with reconstitution, dilution, and storage information.

396

Table 11-6 □ **INTRAVENOUS ANTIBIOTICS ADMINISTRATION GUIDELINES**

Antibiotic	Key Points in Intravenous Administration
Penicillin	Can cause phlebitis. Never administer procaine penicillin by I.V. route. Interaction: Aspirin increases blood levels. Concomitant use of bacteriostatic agents decreases activity of penicillin.
Cephalosporin	Be aware of nephrotoxic effects. Do not administer if patient is penicillin sensitive. Rotate sites often; high risk for phlebitis. Monitor renal function with blood urea nitrogen and creatinine. Use cautiously in pregnant and lactating women.
Aminoglycosides	Assess for muscle weakness. Assess blood urea nitrogen and serum creatinine levels. Assess balance and hearing functions for any damage to the eighth cranial nerve.
Chloramphenicol	Only administer intravenously. Assess for bone marrow suppression.
Erythromycin	High risk of phlebitis. One of the safest antibiotics.
Tetracycline	Do not administer to patients with liver dysfunction. Do not administer to patients with renal failure. Assess for superinfections.

Source: Data from *Pharmacotherapeutics: A Nursing Process Approach*, 2nd edition (p. 1214–1227) by M. Mathewson-Kuhn, 1991, Philadelphia: F.A. Davis Company. Copyright 1991 by F.A. Davis Company; *Intravenous Therapy: A Guide to Quality Care* (p. 249) by C. W. Delaney and M. L. Lauer, 1988, Philadelphia: J.B. Lippincott Company. Copyright 1988 by J.B. Lippincott Company; and *Davis's Drug Guide for Nurses*, 3rd edition (p. 28) by J.H. Deglin and A.H. Vallerand, 1992, Philadelphia: F.A. Davis Company. Copyright 1992 by F.A. Davis Company.

4. Correctly label the admixture with drug name, concentration, diluent, date, time, and initials.
5. Be familiar with potential adverse effects of the drug.
6. Use strict aseptic technique throughout administration.
7. Be aware that the drug must be delivered at specified times to ensure maintenance of the proper drug levels and to identify therapeutic, subtherapeutic, and toxic drug levels.
8. Use assessment skills to monitor functions of organ(s) that metabolize(s) the antibiotic.
9. Evaluate the patient every shift for sensitivity to the drug.
10. Be prepared to respond to anaphylaxis (Delaney & Lauer, 1988, p 248).

Antibiotic Compatibility Issue

Nurse's Drug Alert (1985) addressed the issue of infusing morphine, hydromorphone, or meperidine via the same administration set used for infusing antibiotics. In this investigational study it was found that the following incompatibilities occurred:

397

1. Physical change in administration set (pale yellow to light green) when morphine, hydromorphone, or meperidine added to minocycline or tetracycline.
2. Physical incompatibility occurred immediately when meperidine was infused into a line with nafcillin, cefoperazone, or mezlocillin (Nieves-Cordero, 1985).

Home Antibiotic Therapy

I.V. therapy has moved to the home. Use of the computerized **ambulatory drug pump** has enabled safe and effective antimicrobial administration with minimal disruption of a patient's life. Considerations for home drug delivery of antimicrobials include

- Safety
- Effectiveness
- Acceptance
- Cost

Safety in the administration of drug therapy should be considered when choosing the computerized drug pump method of delivery. Self-care patients are most successful with ambulatory pumps and usually make the adjustment to ambulatory therapy quickly.

The effectiveness of therapy in the home is related to the patient's or patient's caregiver's ability to learn to participate in therapy. Patient education and the level of patient safety have made home therapy effective and safe. The patient, nurse, pharmacist, and physician must work as a team toward acceptance and management of this form of therapy for it to be successful in the home setting.

Cost is decreased in home therapy without sacrificing the level of care. Medicare and third-party payers have recognized financial savings (Brown, 1988).

Antifungal Agents

The antifungal agents' method of action is injury to the cell wall of the fungi. The drugs in this classification are specifically targeted for fungi. Three antifungal drugs can be given intravenously: amphotericin B, fluconazole, and miconazole (Table 11–7). The most frequently administered antifungal agent by intravenous route is amphotericin B.

✎ KEY POINTS IN DELIVERY OF ANTIFUNGAL AGENTS
1. Most are infused as a suspension.
2. These drugs should not be filtered.
3. These drugs should be administered slowly over 2 to 6 hours.

Antiviral Agents

Antiviral drugs are selectively toxic to viruses. A safe, broad-spectrum antiviral drug has yet to be discovered. Most chemicals administered by the I.V. route to

Table 11–7 □ **INTRAVENOUS ANTIFUNGAL ADMINISTRATION GUIDELINES**

Antifungal Agent	Key Points in Administration
Amphotericin B	Light-sensitive, but protection not necessary. Use on hospitalized patient only. Monitor vital signs, intake and output. During therapy, frequently test renal and liver function. To reduce nephrotoxic effects: Administer mannitol 12.5 g before and after each dose. *Incompatibility*: Not compatible with any solution with a pH below 4.2. Do not mix with any drug unless absolutely necessary; there are many incompatibilities.
Fluconazole	I.V. use only. Administered in a glass system. Inadequate treatment may lead to recurrent infection. Hepatotoxicity may occur. If any signs and symptoms of liver disease exist, laboratory analysis should be done and the drug discontinued. *Incompatibility*: Manufacturer states: "Do not add supplemental medication."
Miconazole (Monostat IV)	Hospitalize the patient for the first several days of initial treatment. Monitor blood counts, electrolytes, and lipids. Can be administered intrathecal and as bladder irrigant. Pruritis is common side effect. *Incompatibility*: Considered incompatible in syringe or solutions with any other drug

Source: Data from *Intravenous Medications*, 7th edition (pp. 24, 270, 420) by B.L. Gahart, 1991, Philadelphia: Mosby-Year Book, Inc. Copyright 1991 by Mosby-Year Book, Inc; *Davis's Drug Guide for Nurses*, 3rd edition (p. 21) by J.H. Deglin and A.H. Vallerand, 1992, Philadelphia: F.A. Davis Company. Copyright 1992 by F.A. Davis Company; and *Pharmacotherapeutics: A Nursing Process Approach*, 2nd edition (pp. 1263–1267) by M. Mathewson-Kuhn, 1991, Philadelphia: F.A. Davis Company.

combat virus growth are antimetabolites or are related to the antimetabolites used in treating malignant tumors. These drugs tend to be toxic, and usefulness is limited. These drugs are administered in selected situations. At present there are five antiviral agents infused by the I.V. route: acyclovir, ganciclovir, pentamide isethionate, vidarabine, and zidovudine (Table 11–8).

ANTINEOPLASTIC AGENT ADMINISTRATION CONSIDERATIONS

Over the past 15 years, nurses have actively participated in administration of chemotherapeutic agents. Any nurse who administers these agents must be technically skilled and knowledgeable regarding the pharmotherapeutic effects of these agents.

The majority of nurses administering chemotherapy agents in the past

399

Table 11–8 □ INTRAVENOUS ANTIVIRAL ADMINISTRATION GUIDELINES

Antiviral Agent	Key Points in Administration

Acylovir (Zovirax)
  Treats: Herpes simplex virus
  (HSV-1, HSV-2)
	Can cause renal tubular damage if too rapidly infused. Make sure patient is adequately hydrated.
	Incompatibility: Blood products, dobutamine, protein solutions, or dopamine.

Ganciclovir (Cytovene)
  Treats: Cytomegalovirus (CMV),
  varicella zoster (I.V. *only*)
	Follow guidelines for handling cytoxic drugs.
	Maintain hydration. Assess renal function.
	Do not use during pregnancy unless risk is justified.
	Incompatibility: Any other drug or solution because of alkaline pH.

Pentamidine isethionate (Pentam 300)
  Treats: *Pneumocystis carinii*
  Investigational use: Trypanosomiasis
  visceral
	Specific use only.
	Has numerous side effects: severe hypotension, hypoglycemia, cardiac dysrhythmias.
	Monitor blood glucose levels. Before and after therapy: blood urea nitrogen, complete blood count. Side effects 50%, may be life threatening.
	Incompatibility: All drugs.

Adenine arabinoside (Vidarabine)
  Treats: Herpes simplex encephalitis
  Investigational use:
    Immunocompromised patients
	I.V. infusion only.
	Confirm diagnosis of encephalitis with brain biopsy.
	Use caution in cerebral edema or potential fluid overload.
	Incompatibility: Blood products, protein solutions.

Zidovudine (AZT)
  Treats: Symptomatic AIDS, AIDS,
  and advanced ARC
	Specific use only; only a cure.
	Frequent blood counts.
	Anemia is a side effect.
	Toxicity may be increased by nephrotoxic or cytoxic drugs.
	Protect from light.
	Incompatibility: Blood products and protein solutions.

Source: Data from *Intravenous Medications,* 7th edition (pp. 2, 281, 461) by B.L. Gahart, 1991, Philadelphia: Mosby-Year Book, Inc. Copyright 1991 by Mosby-Year Book, Inc; *Davis's Drug Guide for Nurses,* 3rd edition (p. 44) by J.H. Deglin and A.H. Vallerand, 1992, Philadelphia: F.A. Davis Company. Copyright 1992 by F.A. Davis Company; and *Pharmacotherapeutics: A Nursing Process Approach,* 2nd edition (pp. 1270–1276) by M. Mathewson-Kuhn, 1991, Philadelphia: F.A. Davis Company. Copyright 1991 by F.A. Davis Company.

have received their training on the job. Today, because of the advancement of nursing's scope of practice, the Oncology Nurse Society offers credentialing in this specialty. Chemotherapy certification is generally established by policy and procedure at each facility. Refer to Table 11–9 for administration considerations.

Table 11–9 □ **INTRAVENOUS ANTINEOPLASTIC ADMINISTRATION (CONSIDERATIONS)**

Antineoplastic Agent	Key Points in Intravenous Administration
Alkalating Agents Mustargen Cytoxan TSPA	Cell-cycle nonspecific Keep patient well hydrated Monitor blood urea nitrogen, creatinine Monitor I.V. site
Antimetabolites 5-FU Mexate Cytosar-U	Works in S phase: cell-cycle specific Assess pain in chest, stomach, diarrhea, or black stools Monitor blood urea nitrogen, creatinine Leukovorin given with high doses to minimize side effects
Antitumor Antibiotics Doxorubicin (Adriamycin) Bleomycin (Blenoxane) Mitomycin-C (Mutamycin) Dactinomycin (Cosmegen) Mithramycin (Mithracin)	Cell-cycle nonspecific Administer antipyretics as ordered Assess stomach pain, black stools Ascultate lungs daily
Steroids Diethystilbesterol Betamethasone (Celestone)	Cell-cycle nonspecific Give emotional support for side effects
Plant Alkaloids Vinblastine (Velban) Vincristine (Oncovin)	Acts on M phase; cell-cycle specific Assess jaw pain, numbness, tingling, and loss of deep tendon reflexes Prevent constipation with high-fiber diet, activity, and stool softner
Nitrosureas Dacarbazine (DTIC-Dome) Cisplatin (Platinol) Carmustine (BiCNU)	Cell-cycle nonspecific Can cross blood-brain barrier

Source: Data from "Chemo: A Nurse's Guide to Action, Administration, and Side Effects" by P. Walters, 1990, *RN, 4*, pp. 52–57. Copyright 1990 by Medical Economics Co.; *Intravenous Therapy: A Guide to Quality Care* (p. 252) by C.W. Delaney and M.L. Lauer, 1988, Philadelphia: J.B. Lippincott Company. Copyright 1988 by J.B. Lippincott Company; and *Pharmacotherapeutics: A Nursing Process Approach*, 2nd edition (pp. 1342–1360) by M. Mathewson-Kuhn, 1991, Philadelphia: F.A. Davis Company. Copyright 1991 by F.A. Davis Company.

✎ KEY POINTS IN ADMINISTRATION OF ANTINEOPLASTIC AGENTS

NURSING RESPONSIBILITIES
1. Knowledge of the cell cycle and malignant cell growth
2. Knowledge regarding the drug class, side effects, adverse reactions, and methods of administration

401

3. Being able to distinguish **palliative** from **curative** therapy
4. Knowledge of the normal rate of delivery for each agent
5. Knowledge of the drug properties: vesicant or **nonvesicant**
6. Understanding of the vascular system
7. Educating the patient on drug side effects
8. Explaining physical and psychologic effects of the drugs
9. Awareness of Occupational Safety and Health Administration (OSHA) standards for disposal of cytoxic agents
10. Awareness of personal risks and safety precautions (INS, 1990, S63)

Cell Cycle

Antineoplastic agents are classified into two groups based on common actions on the cell cycle—the cell-cycle specific and the cell-cycle nonspecific. The cell-cycle specific agents refer to antineoplastic agents that can destroy only actively dividing cells starting at the G_0 phase. Specific agents include:

Antimetabolites
Plant alkaloids

Cell-cycle nonspecific drugs are those that can destroy cells in all five phases (Fig. 11–7). The specific agents in the grouping include:

Alkalating agents
Antitumor antibiotics
Steroids
Nitrosureas

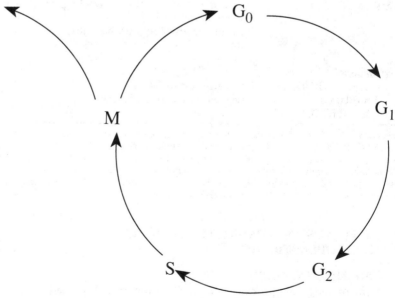

Figure 11–7 □ Five phases of the cell cycle.

General System Side Effects of Chemotherapy

The major side effects of chemotherapy involve the integumentary, gastrointestinal, and immune systems. Skin and gastrointestinal cells replicate rapidly; therefore, the adverse effects caused by chemotherapy occur within these two systems. The first step in preventing and managing adverse reactions of chemotherapy is collection of an accurate baseline assessment (Camp-Sorrell, 1991).

Alopecia (hair loss) is the most common damage to the integumentary system. Hair loss, although reversible, may affect self-esteem.

Although not an adverse effect, extravasation is a threat when infusions of vesicant drugs must be delivered. The danger of extravasation of chemotherapy vesicant drugs is of key importance for the practitioner. A small amount of a vesicant drug can damage or destroy cells if they come in contact with the tissues surrounding the vein. Damage is dependent on the amount of toxicity or irritation of the drug absorbed by the tissues. If extravasation should include tendons, nerves, or joint spaces the damage will be greater. (Chapter 8 provides treatment alternatives for extravasated drugs.)

Effects on the immune system include neutropenia, thrombocytopenia, and anemia. A decrease in white blood cell (WBC) count typically occurs 8 to 12 days after chemotherapy. The WBC count usually returns to normal levels between treatments. Generally chemotherapy is not given when the WBC count is less than $3000/mm^3$ or if neutrophils are less than $1000\ mm^3$ (Hughes, 1986). Thrombocytopenia can occur 8 to 12 days after chemotherapy. Patients with platelet counts less than 50,000 cells/mm^3 need to be taught the dangers of bleeding. Platelets are usually administered to patients whose platelet count falls below 20,000 cells/mm^3. Low hemoglobin and hematocrit levels do not prevent the patient from receiving chemotherapy. However, anemia signs and symptoms such as fatigue, shortness of breath, tachycardia, and pallor may be indicators for transfusion of packed red blood cells (PRBCs). Refer to Appendix C for normal laboratory values.

✎ **Note:** Patients with low WBC counts need to be protected against exposure to infections.

Gastrointestinal adverse effects include nausea and vomiting, which can be distressing, and stomatitis. Chemotherapy agents stimulate the brain's vomiting center and chemoreceptor trigger zone (CTZ), along with irritating the gastrointestinal mucosa. Drugs to manage nausea and vomiting include metoclopramide (Reglan), diphenhydramine (Benadryl), and lorazepam (Ativan). Oral stomatitis occurs most frequently with doxorubicine, 5-FU, cyclophosphamide, and methotrexate. Stomatitis can lead to compromised nutritional status (Walters, 1990).

✎ **PROCEDURE FOR ADMINISTRATION OF ANTINEOPLASTIC AGENTS**
1. Adequately assess the patient's venous status. Examine both arms for phlebitis, bruises, and inflammation.

403

2. Discuss with patient any past problems experienced since last treatment.
3. Each chemotherapy administration should use the patient's alternate arm.
4. Use sterile technique. Be aware that the patient might have a compromised WBC count.
5. Meticulously prepare the site.
6. An extremity with compromised circulation should not be used. Such extremities may have an invading neoplasm, existing phlebitis, or varicosities; may be on the side of a previous mastectomy; may have an immobilized fracture; or may be inflamed.
7. Assess patency of vein with 10 to 20 mL of normal saline before infusing cytoxic agent.
8. Mix chemotherapy drugs according to manufacturer's recommendations.
9. Tell the patient to inform you immediately if he or she feels any burning or stinging at the infusion site.
10. Be constantly aware of a slow leak or insidious infiltration.
11. Use a final flush of normal saline once the chemotherapeutic agent is infused to clear drug from peripheral vein.
12. Follow OSHA standards for disposal of cytotoxic agents. Refer to Appendix D for guidelines for personnel dealing with cytotoxic drugs (Camp-Sorrell, 1991; Plumer & Cosentino, 1987).

NARCOTIC INFUSION CONSIDERATIONS

Pain management begins with complete assessment of the patient's pain, including location, intensity, quality, frequency, onset, duration, aggravating and alleviating factors, associated symptoms, and coping mechanisms. Pain perception and tolerance are highly individual responses. According to McCaffery and Beebe (1989), the definition of pain is "whatever the experiencing person says it is, existing whenever he says it does."

Many therapeutic approaches are available for pain, including:

Behavioral approaches
Application of heat and cold
Massage
Physical therapy
Management with narcotics and non-narcotics via oral, subcutaneous, or I.V. routes
Neurosurgery
Anesthestics (Murphy, 1990)

Morphine is the narcotic most commonly used for continuous infusion for pain management. Continuous infusions lead to a continuous level of pain control without the peaks of side effect development and the troughs of breakthrough pain. Generally less drug is needed to prevent the recurrence of the pain (Coyle et al., 1986).

The World Health Organization (WHO) and the American Pain Society (1989) have grouped analgesia into three types:

1. Opioids
2. Non-narcotic analgesics and nonsteroidal anti-inflammatory drugs (NSAIDs)
3. Adjuvants

Opioids include narcotic analgesics and narcotic agonists. Non-narcotic analgesics, nonopioids, and NSAIDs relieve mild to moderate pain. Adjuvants include drugs to treat other signs and symptoms of pain such as depression, anxiety, and nausea; often these are referred to as coanalgesics (McGuire, 1990). Intravenous administration guidelines for narcotics are presented in Table 11–10.

Patient-Controlled Analgesia

The concept of patient-controlled analgesia (PCA), which began in 1970, is a pain management strategy that allows the patient to self-administer I.V. narcotic pain medication by pressing a button that is attached to a computerized pump (Panfilli, Brunchkorts, & Dundon, 1988). The goal of PCA is to provide the patient with a serum analgesia level for comfort with minimal sedation (Ryder, 1991). Putting patients in charge of their own pain management makes sense, as only the patient knows how much he or she is suffering.

✎ **KEY POINTS IN PROVIDING SAFE, ADEQUATE PAIN RELIEF**
1. Define the types of patients to use the PCA device.
2. Develop teaching tools.
3. Select the appropriate equipment.
4. Select the medications used and establish consistency of use and dosage.
5. Define who will handle the side effects and provide an appropriate method of communication (St. Marie, 1991).

CANDIDATES FOR WHOM PCA SHOULD BE CONSIDERED
1. Patients who are anticipating pain that is severe, yet intermittent (e.g., patients suffering from kidney stones)
2. Patients who have constant pain that gets worse with activity
3. Pediatric patients who are older than 7 years of age and able to be taught to manage the PCA machine
4. Patients who have the capability to manipulate the dose button
5. Patients who are motivated to use this system (Hadaway, 1989)

✎ **KEY CONCEPTS OF PATIENT-CONTROLLED ANALGESIA**

1. In the first 24 hours after surgery, the patient has the greatest need for pain control.
2. The best results for PCA occur when the patient can bolus every 5 to 10 minutes.
3. When patients have control of their narcotic doses, they keep the narcotic within therapeutic levels.

Table 11-10 □ **INTRAVENOUS NARCOTIC ADMINISTRATION GUIDELINES**

Narcotic	Key Point in Administration
Agonist	
Demerol 10–50 mg every 2–4 h	Avoid in patients with impaired renal function *Must be diluted* Shorter acting than morphine Not recommended I.V. in children. Caution in glaucoma, head injuries, chronic obstructive pulmonary disease Cough reflex is suppressed
Morphine 2.5–15 mg every 2–6 h	Caution in impaired ventilation, bronchial asthma, increased intracranial pressure, liver failure *Should be diluted*
Dilaudid 2–4 mg every 4–6 h	*Should be diluted* Caution in head injuries, respiratory depression, and increased intracranial pressure Slightly shorter duration than morphine
Levo-Dromoran 2–3 mg every 4–6 h	Accumulates on days 2–3, long plasma half-life I.V. is usually not the route of choice SC usual route
Agonist/Antagonist Agents	
Talwin 5–10 mg every 3–4 h	May cause psychotomimetic effect Contraindicated in myocardial infarction patient *May be given undiluted* Low addictive element Contraindicated in children under 12
Nubain 10 mg every 3–6 h	*May be given undiluted* Caution in head injury, pregnancy, lactation
Stadol 1 mg every 3–4 h	*May be given undiluted* Caution in respiratory depression, head injury, and impaired liver or kidney function
Partial Agonist	
Buprenex 0.3 mg, repeat every 6 h	May produce withdrawal in narcotic-dependent patients *May be given undiluted* Caution in asthma, respiratory depression, or impaired renal or hepatic function Contraindicated in children under 12

Source: Data from *Intravenous Medications*, 7th edition (p. 313) by B.L. Gahart, 1991, Philadelphia: Mosby-Year Book, Inc. Copyright 1991 by Mosby-Year Book, Inc. and *Principles of Analgesic Use in the Treatment of Acute Pain and Chronic Cancer Pain: A Concise Guide to Medical Practice*, 2nd edition (p. 10) by the American Pain Society, 1989. Skokie, Illinois, American Pain Society. Copyright 1989 by the American Pain Society.

4. When patients are in control and know they can get more immediate pain relief by pushing a button, they are more relaxed (White, 1988).
5. Analgesia is most effective when a therapeutic serum level is consistently maintained.
6. Postoperative patients can easily titrate doses according to need and avoid peaks and troughs associated with conventional I.V. and intramuscular administration of narcotics.
7. Studies have found that orthopedic patients seemed more tolerant of repositioning when on PCA.
8. Patients with abdominal surgery ambulate sooner postoperatively.
9. PCA patients are better able to cough and deep breathe. (Kleiman, Lipman, & Hare, 1987)

INVESTIGATIONAL DRUGS

According to INS standards of practice (1990), medications not approved for general use are administered ethically and with informed patient consent. *Administration of investigational medications shall be in accordance with state and federal regulations. Signed informed patient consent is required prior to patient participation in the investigation* (S53).

Investigational drugs are defined as medications that are not approved for general use by the Food and Drug Administration (FDA). Many **clinical trials** are conducted as a form of planned experiment that evoke appropriate treatment of future patients with a given medical condition. Clinical trials are designed to discover a drug's efficacy in selected patient populations.

The role of the registered nurse in investigational drugs is to assist the investigator (physician) in conducting the study.

✎ KEY POINTS IN THE ROLE OF THE NURSE IN INVESTIGATIONAL DRUGS

1. Communications with Institutional Review Board (IRB); familiarity with their policies and federal regulations (copies of communication between the investigator and the IRB should be sent to the sponsor)
2. Writing informed consent, explaining to patient, and obtaining signature
3. Communicating with hospital's legal counsel and ethics committee to complete protocols
4. I.V. administration of the investigational drug
5. Participating in collection of data
6. When required, assisting with blood sampling
7. Assisting with final study report, which is a requirement of the US federal regulations for the sponsor (Weinstein, 1987)

General ethical requirements of clinical research worldwide are outlined in the *Declaration of Helsinki*, issued by the World Medical Association in 1960 and revised in 1975. This document has been accepted internationally as the basis for ethical research (Popock, 1983).

PHYSICAL ASSESSMENT (INTRAVENOUS MEDICATIONS)

The nurse must use a systems approach to assess for both local and systemic complications associated with the administration of I.V. medications. The nursing assessment should include infusion rate, intake and output, and an awareness of agency policy and procedure to prevent complications associated with I.V. therapy. The following body systems should be assessed at the beginning of each shift and with each administration of each medication. Symptoms listed with each system may indicate local problems or a life-threatening situation. All laboratory findings must be monitored.

NEUROMUSCULAR
Change in level of consciousness
Confusion
Complaints of pain
Tremors
Paresthesia of the extremities
Paralysis of the extremities
Muscle weakness
Seizures

CARDIOVASCULAR
Increased or decreased blood
  pressure
Increased heart rate
Extra cardiac sounds
Pain in the chest
Distended neck veins
Bleeding from the site

RESPIRATORY
Shortness of breath
Decreased respirations
Hypoxia
Cyanosis
Respiratory distress

GASTROINTESTINAL
Nausea
Vomiting
Diarrhea
Tarry stools
Constipation

RENAL
Urinary retention
Decreased urinary output
Variance between intake and
output

INTEGUMENTARY
Fever
Profuse sweating
Pruritus
Alopecia
Edema at or near the insertion site
Change in skin color
Sensation of heat at or near the insertion site
Red line visible above the venipuncture site
Tender, cordlike vein
Bruising around or near the site of the insertion
Sluggish flow rate
Back flow absent
Coolness of the skin
Taut skin around venipuncture site

BODY WEIGHT
Rapid weight gain

SPECIAL SENSES
Pain in the jaw
Numbness of the tongue

NURSING DIAGNOSES RELATED TO INTRAVENOUS MEDICATION ADMINISTRATION

1. Altered health maintenance related to limited skills of family members with I.V. medications
2. Anxiety (mild, moderate, severe) related to threat to or change in health status; misconceptions regarding therapy
3. Altered tissue perfusion (peripheral) related to infiltration of vesicant medication
4. Decreased cardiac output related to sepsis; contamination
5. Diarrhea related to side effects of medication
6. Fear related to insertion of catheter; fear of "needle"
7. Fluid volume excess related to administration of isotonic or hypertonic solutions
8. Hyperthermia related to increased metabolic rate; illness; dehydration
9. Impaired physical mobility related to pain and discomfort resulting from placement and maintenance of I.V. catheter
10. Impaired skin integrity related to I.V. catheter; irritating I.V. solution; inflammation; infection; infiltration
11. Impaired tissue integrity related to altered circulation; fluid deficit or excess; irritating solution; inflammation; infection; infiltration
12. Impaired gas exchange related to ventilation perfusion imbalance; embolism
13. Knowledge deficit (chemotherapy side effects) related to lack of exposure
14. Pain related to physical trauma (e.g., catheter insertion)
15. Risk for infection related to broken skin or traumatized tissue
16. Sleep pattern disturbance related to external sensory stimulation owing to I.V. medications

SUMMARY OF CHAPTER 11

ADMINISTRATION OF INTRAVENOUS MEDICATION

ADVANTAGES OF I.V. MEDICATION
1. Provides a direct access to the circulatory system
2. Provides a route for drugs that irritate the gastric mucosa
3. Provides a route for instant drug action
4. Provides a route to deliver high drug concentrations
5. Provides for instant drug termination if sensitivity or adverse reaction occurs
6. Provides a route of administration in patients in whom use of the gastrointestinal tract is limited

HAZARDS OF I.V. MEDICATION
1. Drug interaction due to incompatibilities
2. Adsorption of the drug impaired owing to leaching into I.V. container or administration set
3. Errors in compounding of medication
4. Speed shock
5. Extravasation of a vesicant drug
6. Chemical phlebitis

DRUG INTERACTIONS
- Adsorption
- Errors in mixing
- Incompatibilities: chemical, physical, and therapeutic

METHODS OF I.V. MEDICATION ADMINISTRATION
Continuous infusion
Intermittent infusions
I.V. push
Subcutaneous infusions
Epidural and intrathecal
Intraperitoneal
Ventricular reservoir
Arteriovenous fistula

ANTIMICROBIAL ADMINISTRATION CONSIDERATIONS
Key questions in delivery of antimicrobial agents
- Has the infecting organism been identified?
- Is the organism resistant to any antimicrobial agents?
- Is the site of the infection identified?
- What is the status of the host defenses?
- Is the nurse familiar with the antimicrobial pharmacokinetics?
- Is the patient's renal and hepatic function known?
- Is monitoring the patient's blood levels necessary?

KEY POINTS IN ADMINISTRATION OF ANTINEOPLASTIC AGENTS
Knowledge of the cell cycle
Knowledge regarding the drug class, side effects, adverse reactions, and methods of administration
Ability to differentiate between palliative or curative treatment
Knowledge of the normal rate of delivery for each agent
Knowledge of the drug properties: vesicant or nonvesicant
Understanding of the vascular system
Educating the patient on side effects of the drugs
Explaining physical and psychologic effects of the drugs
Aware of OSHA standards for disposal of cytoxic agents
Aware of personal risks and safety precautions

THREE TYPES OF WHO AND AMERICAN PAIN SOCIETY ANALGESIA
Opioids

Non-narcotic analgesics and nonsteroid anti-inflammatory drugs
Adjuvants

INVESTIGATIONAL DRUGS
Administration in accordance with state and federal regulations

Activity Journal

1. The patient requires pain medication, and the order is for 2 mg of morphine I.V. every 2 hours as needed for pain. Discuss the key points to remember in delivering this medication by the I.V. push method.

2. You are working in a small rural outpatient clinic. A patient comes in in respiratory distress with electrolyte imbalance. The physician orders a primary solution of 5% dextrose/0.45% sodium chloride, and aminophyllin. He also orders 20 mEq of KCl to be administered over 2 hours. No pharmacist is available to assist you with this admixture. How do you infuse these medications and how do you check for compatibility?

3. You are mixing two medications in one syringe for an I.V. push administration. The solution has turned a pale yellow. Can you safely administer this drug? If not, what type of incompatibility is this?

4. A patient complains to you that the antibiotic just hung burns. The antibiotic is diluted in 100 mL of 5% dextrose in water piggybacked to run 45 minutes. What alternatives do you have in dealing with this complaint?

Quality Assessment Model

Instructions: Use this quality assessment model to conduct retrospective audits of charts, establish quality control standards, or develop outcome criteria for quality assurance. Refer to Chapter 2 for details on quality assessment.

STRUCTURE

(Resource that affects outcome)
Human Resource: Nurse
↓

PROCESS

(Actual giving and receiving of care)
Therapist activities related to safe delivery of I.V. medications are:

1. Follow standards of practice in care of intraspinal catheters.
2. Identify incompatibilities and use chart for reference.
3. Deliver I.V. medications by recommendation of manufacturer.
4. Keep I.V. medication within the prescribed rate.
5. Observation of I.V. site and site assessment every 4 to 8 hours on adults.
↓

OUTCOME STANDARDS

(Effects of care)
Documentation will reflect standards of practice:

1. I.V. medications will be charted by the correct route.
2. Dressing management of intraspinal medications will be charted with correct steps.
3. I.V. medications used for pain management will be charted at the correct time intervals and corresponding relief noted.
4. Documentation of site assessment every 4 to 8 hours.

Post-test, Chapter 11

1. List three of the five advantages of I.V. medication delivery.

   A. _____

   B. _____

   C. _____

2. Which of the following are incompatibilities of I.V. therapy?
   A. Intermittent, physical, and biotransformation
   B. Drug interaction, drug synergism, and drug tolerance
   C. Physical, chemical, and therapeutic

3. Methods in which drugs can be delivered by the I.V. route would include:
   A. I.V. push, continuous drip, and piggyback
   B. Epidural, sublingual, and intrathecal
   C. Intrathecal, I.V. push, and subcutaneous
   D. Piggyback, intradermal, and epidural

4. Key points in infusion of I.V. antifungal drugs are:
   A. Most are infused as a suspension.
   B. Drugs should not be filtered.
   C. Drugs should be administered slowly.
   D. All of the above.

5. Major side effects of antineoplastic agents involve the _____ systems.
   A. Reproductive, immune, and cardiovascular
   B. Respiratory, genitourinary, and neurologic
   C. Integumentary, gastrointestinal, and immune

6. WHO and the American Pain Society have grouped analgesics into three categories, which are
   A. Opioids, non-narcotic nonsteroid, and adjuvants
   B. Anesthetics, non-narcotic, and cholinergics
   C. Adrenergics, opioids, and opiates

7. List three nursing considerations when dealing with IP catheters:

   A. _____

   B. _____

   C. _____

8. List the important steps in dressing change of an epidural catheter.

9. The Tenckhoff catheter is used for which type of therapy?
   A. Epidural
   B. Intraperitoneal
   C. Intraspinal
   D. Subcutaneous

10. I.V. push medications should be administered according to manufacturer's recommendations, but never faster than:
   A. 30 seconds
   B. 1 minute
   C. 5 minutes
   D. 10 minutes

11. The goal of patient-controlled analgesia is to provide the patient with:
   A. A serum analgesia level for comfort without sedation
   B. A serum analgesia level to achieve sedation
   C. A method of euthanasia
   D. Limited control over pain management

12. The role of the nurse in investigational drugs is to:
   A. Conduct the study
   B. Administer the investigational drug under physician direction
   C. Take the role as investigator
   D. Observe and record the results

13. Which of the following are side effects of epidural pain medication?
   A. Urinary retention, pruritus, and respiratory depression
   B. Respiratory depression, peptic ulcers, and hemiparesis
   C. Pruritus, nausea, and urinary incontinence

Match the following definition in column 2 to the correct term in column 1.

Column 1

14. _____ Distribution

15. _____ Absorption

16. _____ Compatibility

17. _____ Curative

18. _____ Intrathecal

19. _____ Therapeutic incompatibility

20. _____ Chemical incompatibility

21. _____ Physical incompatibility

22. _____ Admixture

Column 2

A. Process of movement of medication from drug administration site to vasculature

B. Capable of being mixed and administered without undergoing undesirable changes

C. Process of delivering a drug to the various tissues of the body

D. Undesirable change that is visual

E. Undesirable effect occurring within a patient as a result of two or more drugs being given concurrently

F. Change in molecular structure of a substance

G. Combination of two or more medications

H. Inside the spinal cord

I. Healing as a remedy

415

Answers to Post-test, Chapter 11

1. A. Allows for absorption of drugs unstable in gastric juices
   B. Provides a route for drug with irritating properties
   C. Provides a route for instant drug action
   D. Permits termination of infusion if sensitivity occurs
   E. Provides better control over rate of administration of drug
2. C
3. A
4. D
5. C
6. A
7. A. Maintain strict sterile technique.
   B. Scrub all connectors with povidone/iodine.
   C. Use sterile gloves.
   D. Minimize accessing the system when possible.
   E. Irrigate catheter well before and after administering therapy.
   F. Ensure the administration set and drainage tubes are free of kinks.
   G. Perform patient teaching.
   H. Assess catheter site for signs of infection.

8. A. Wash hands with antimicrobial soap.
   B. Remove old dressing.
   C. With cotton-tipped applicator in povidone iodine solution, clean area starting at catheter and work outward.
   D. Let dry.
   E. Apply new transparent dressing.
   F. Do not use alcohol on skin or dressing site.
9. B
10. B
11. A
12. B
13. A
14. C
15. A
16. B
17. I
18. H
19. E
20. F
21. D
22. G

References

Akahoshi, M.P., Furuike-McLaughlin, T., & Enriquez, N.C. (1988). Patient controlled analgesia via intrathecal catheter in outpatient oncology patient. *Journal of Intravenous Nursing, 11*(5), 289–292.

American Pain Society. (1989). *Principles of analgesic use in the treatment of acute pain and chronic cancer pain. A concise guide to medical practice* (2nd ed.). Skokie, Illinois: American Pain Society.

Bonica, J.J. (1990). *The management of pain* (2nd ed.). Philadelphia: Lea & Febiger.

Bromage, P.R. (1980). State of art: Extradural and intrathecal narcotics. *Anesthesia and Analgesia, 59*, 473–480.

Brown, J.M. (1988). Innovative antibiotic therapy at home. *Journal of Intravenous Nursing, 11*(6), 397–401.

Burman, R., & Berkowitz, H. (1986). IV bolus: Effective, but potentially hazardous. *Critical Care Nurse, 6*(1), 22–27.

Camp-Sorrell, D. (1991). Controlling adverse effects of chemotherapy. *Nursing 91, 4*, 34–37.

Coyle, N., Mauskop, A., Maggard, J., & Foley, K.M. (1986). Continuous subcutaneous infusions of opiates in cancer patients with pain. *Oncology Nursing Forum, 13*(4), 53–57.

D'Arcy, P.F. (1983). Drug interactions with medical plastics. *Drug Intelligence Clinical Pharmacy, 17,* 726–731.

Dedrick, R. (1985). Theoretical and experimental bases of intraperitoneal chemotherapy. *Seminars in Oncology, 12*(3), 75–80.

Delaney, C.W., & Lauer, M.L. (1988). *Intravenous therapy: A guide to quality care.* Philadelphia: J.B. Lippincott.

Gahart, B.L. (1991). *Intravenous medications,* 7th ed. Philadelphia: C.V. Mosby-Year Book.

Gong, H., & King, C.Y. (1983). Inadequate drug mixing: A potential hazard in continuous intravenous admixture. *Heart and Lung, 12*(5), 528–532.

Hadaway, L.C. (1989). Evaluation and use of advanced I.V. technology: Patient controlled analgesia, part 2. *Journal of Intravenous Nursing, 12*(3), 184–191.

Howell, S.B. (1990). Intraperitoneal catheters for chemotherapy. *NAVAN, 1*(1), 8–9.

Intravenous Nursing (1990). *Standards of practice.* Philadelphia: J.B. Lippincott.

Hughes, C.B. (1986). Giving cancer drugs I.V.: Some guidelines. *American Journal of Nursing, 86*(1), 34–38.

Kleiman, A.G., Lipman, B.D., & Hare, S. (1987). PCA vs. regular IM injections for severe post-op pain. *American Journal of Nursing, 11,* 1491–1492.

LaRocca, J.C., & Otto, S.E. (1989). *Pocket guide to intravenous therapy.* St. Louis: C.V. Mosby.

Lieb, R.A., & Hurtig, J.B. (1985). Epidural and intrathecal narcotics for pain management. *Heart and Lung, 14*(2), 164–171.

Lippincott Learning System. (1984). *Incompatibilities: I.V. therapy study guide and workbook.* Philadelphia: J.B. Lippincott.

Lonsway, R.A. (1988). Care of the patient with an epidural catheter: An infection control challenge. *Journal of Intravenous Nursing, 11*(1), 52–54.

Malloy, J. (1991). Administering intraperitoneal chemotherapy, a new approach. *Nursing 91, 91*(1), 58–62.

Managing I.V. Therapy Photobook. (1980). Springhouse, PA: Intermed Communications.

Mathewson-Kuhn, M. (1991). *Pharmacotherapeutics: A nursing process approach* (2nd ed.). Philadelphia, F.A. Davis.

McCaffery, M., & Beebe, A. (1989). *Pain: Clinical manual for nursing practice.* St. Louis: C.V. Mosby.

McClay, E.F., & Howell, S.B. (1990). A review: Intraperitoneal cisplatin in the management of patients with ovarian cancer. *Gynecology Oncology, 36,* 1–6.

McGuire, L. (1990). Administering analgesics: Which drugs are right for your patient? *Nursing 90, 4,* 34–41.

McLaughlin-Hagan, M. (1990). Continuous subcutaneous infusion of narcotics. *Journal of Intravenous Therapy, 13*(2), 119–124.

Murphy, D. (1990). Home pain management of continuous infusion narcotics. *Journal of Intravenous Nursing, 13*(6), 355–358.

Nieves-Cordero, A. (1985). Compatibility of narcotic analgesic solutions with various antibiotics during simulated Y-site injections. *American Journal of Hospital Pharmacy, 42,* 1108–1109.

Nurses Drug Alert. (1985). Compatibility of antibiotics and narcotics given intravenously. *American Journal of Nursing, 85*(5), 59–60.

Panfilli, R., Brunchkhorst, L., & Dundon, R. (1988). Nursing implications of patient-controlled analgesia. *Journal of Intravenous Nursing, 11*(2), 75–77.

Piccart, M.F., Speyer, J.L., & Markman, M. (1985). Intraperitoneal chemotherapy: Technical experience at five institutions. *Seminars on Oncology, 12*(3), 90–96.

Plumer, A.L., & Cosentino, F. (1987). *Principles and practices of intravenous therapy.* Boston: Little, Brown.

Popock, S.J. (1983). *Clinical trials: A practical approach.* Chichester, England: John Wiley & Sons.

Rosen, H. (1990). An epidural analgesia program: Balancing risks and benefits. *Critical Care Nurse, 10*(8), 32–41.

Ryder, E. (1991). All about patient-controlled analgesia. *Journal of Intravenous Nursing,* 14(6), 372–379.

Slater, E.M., Zeitlin, G.L., & Edwards, M.G. (1985). Experience with epidural morphine for post-surgical pain in a community setting. *Anesthesiology Review,* 12(3).

St. Marie, B. (1989). Administration of intraspinal analgesia in the home care setting. *Journal of Intravenous Nursing,* 12(3), 164–168.

St. Marie, B. (1991). Narcotic infusions a changing scene. *Journal of Intravenous Nursing,* 14(5), 334–343.

St. Marie, B., & Henrickson, K. (1988). Intraspinal narcotic infusions for terminal cancer pain. *Journal of Intravenous Nursing,* 11(3), 161–163.

Swenson, K.K., & Eriksson, J.H. (1986). Nursing management of intraperitoneal chemotherapy. *Oncology Nursing Forum,* 12(5), 112–117.

Todd, B. (1988). Intravenous drug hazards: Interactions, absorption inadequate mixing. *Geriatric Nursing,* 1, 20–22.

Vizcarra, C. (1988). Intraperitoneal chemotherapy I.V. team responsibility. *Journal of Intravenous Nursing,* 11(3), 184–187.

Walters, P. (1990). Chemo: A nurse's guide to action, administration, and side effects. *RN,* 4, 52–57.

Wang, J.K., Nauss, L.F., & Thomas, J.E. (1979). Pain relief by intrathecally applied morphine in man. *Anesthesiology,* 50(2), 149–151.

Weinstein, S.M. (1987). Use of investigational drugs. *National Intravenous Therapy Association,* 10(5), 336–347.

White, P. (1988). Patient-controlled analgesia. *Anesthesiology,* 2(3), 339–350.

Zola, E., & McLeod, D. (1983). Comparative effects and analgesic efficacy of the agonist-antagonist opioids. *Drug Intel Clinical Pharmacy,* 17, 6–8.

Zook-Enck, D. (1990). Intraperitoneal therapy via the Tenckhoff catheter. *Journal of Intravenous Nursing,* 13(6), 375–382.

Bibliography

Anderson, A.R. (1989). Are your I.V. chemo skills up-to-date? *RN,* 52(1), 40–43.

DeMonaco, H.J. (1988). I.V. drug delivery: New technologies for consideration. *Journal of Intravenous Nursing,* 11(5), 316–320.

Ferris, E.W. (1990). A neonatal home intravenous antibiotic therapy program. *Journal of Intravenous Nursing,* 13(6), 383–388.

Garabedian-Ruffalo, S.M., & Ruffalo, R.L. (1989). Compatibilities and stabilities of IV preparations. *Critical Care Nurse,* 9(2), 81–85.

Korth-Bradley, J.M. (1991). A pharmacokinetic primer for intravenous nursing. *Journal of Intravenous Nursing,* 14(1), 16–27.

Okafor, K.C. (1990). The management of chemotherapy. *Infusion,* 13(2), 3–18.

Sesin, P., & Wiggins, M. (1987). New England Deaconess guidelines for the administration of I.V. drugs. *National Intravenous Association,* 10(1), 17–25.

Testerman, E.J. (1990). I.V. drug administration guidelines: A simplified format. *Journal of Intravenous Nursing,* 11(3), 188–190.

Central Venous Access Devices

CHAPTER 12

Central Venous Access Devices

CHAPTER CONTENTS

Glossary

Broviac silicone rubber catheter: Tunneled venous catheter with one Dacron cuff with an internal diameter of 1.0 mm; useful for infusion of nutrient solutions

CVCs: Central venous catheters

CVTCs: Central venous tunneled catheters

Distal: Farthest from the heart; farthest from the point of attachment; below previous site of cannulation

Extravascular malpositioning: Introducer of the central venous percutaneous catheter is passed out of the vessel and into the pleural space or the mediastinum

Groshong catheter: Surgically implanted, long-term tunneled Silastic catheter; unique in that it has a two-way valve adjacent to the closed tip, which prevents backflow of blood

Hickman catheter: Long-term tunneled Silastic catheter inserted surgically

Implanted ports: Catheters surgically placed into a vessel, body cavity, or organ and attached to a reservoir, which is placed under the skin

Infraclavicular: Situated below a clavicle

Intravascular malpositioning: Catheter tip of a percutaneous tunneled catheter or implanted port coils in the vessel, advances into a venous tributary other than the superior vena cava, or does not reach the superior vena

Peripherally inserted central catheter (PICC): Long (20- to 24-in) intravenous access device made of a soft flexible material (silicone or a polymer); the PICC is usually inserted into one of the superficial veins of the peripheral vascular system and advanced into the central system

Silicone: Material containing silicone carbon bond, used as lubricants, insulating resins, waterproofing materials

Thrombogenicity: Generating or production of thrombosis

Trendelenburg position: Position in which the head is lower than the feet; used to increase venous distention

Tunneled catheter: Catheter designed to have a portion lie within a subcutaneous passage before exiting the body

VADs: Vascular access device

Valsalva maneuver: Increase of intrathoracic pressure by forcible exhalation against the closed glottis. The maneuver causes a trapping of blood in the great veins, preventing it from entering the chest and right atrium. When the breath is released, the intrathoracic pressure drops, and the trapped blood is quickly propelled through the heart, producing an increase in the heart rate and blood pressure. Immediately after this event, a reflex bradycardia ensues. The increased pressure, immediate tachycardia, and reflex bradycardia can bring about cardiac arrest in vulnerable heart patients.

LEARNING OBJECTIVES

Upon completion of this chapter, the reader will be able to:

☐ Define terminology related to central venous devices
☐ Discuss the hazard associated with percutaneous insertion of central lines —intravascular malpositioning and extravascular malpositioning
☐ Differentiate between short-term and long-term access devices
☐ Identify the advantages of peripherally inserted central catheters
☐ Identify candidates for peripherally inserted central catheters
☐ Discuss the procedure for placement of peripherally inserted central catheters
☐ List the steps in dressing management of peripherally inserted central catheters
☐ Identify the complications associated with peripherally inserted central catheters
☐ Identify the advantages of tunneled Silastic catheters
☐ State the advantages of the implanted port
☐ Compare tunneled Silastic catheters with implanted ports
☐ Identify the key points of care for Hickman and Groshong catheters and implanted ports
☐ Identify the potential complications with central venous tunneled catheters and implanted ports
☐ Determine nursing diagnoses appropriate for patients with central venous access devices

Pre-test, Chapter 12

Instructions: The pre-test is to review prior knowledge of the theory related to central venous access devices. Each question in the pre-test is based on the learning objectives of the chapter.

Match the definition in column 2 to the correct term in column 1.

Column 1

1. _____ CVC

2. _____ CVD

3. _____ CVTC

4. _____ VAD

5. _____ PICC

Column 2

A. Intravenous device inserted into superior vena cava via the peripheral vasculature

B. Central venous device

C. Central venous tunneled catheter

D. Central venous catheter

E. Vascular access device

6. Advantages of the peripherally inserted catheters include:
   A. Decreases risk of pneumothorax and air embolism on insertion
   B. Preserves peripheral vascular system in the upper extremity
   C. Eliminates the pain of frequent venipunctures
   D. Decreases cost and is time efficient
   E. All of the above

7. The best site selection for a peripherally inserted central catheter placement would be the _____ vein.
   A. Basilic
   B. Innominate
   C. Jugular

8. Key points in dressing management of peripherally inserted central catheters would include:
   A. Change dressing after the first 24 hours.
   B. Use sterile technique.
   C. Inspect the catheter insertion site for redness, swelling, or drainage.
   D. Use care not to dislodge the catheter during the dressing change.
   E. Transparent dressing is recommended after first 24 hours.
   F. All of the above.

9. Complications related to the *insertion* of peripherally inserted central catheters include:
   A. Bleeding, malposition of the catheter, and nerve damage
   B. Phlebitis, infection, and air embolism
   C. Bleeding, cardiac arrhythmias, and infection

10. Advantages of central venous tunneled catheters include:
   A. Can be repaired if it breaks or leaks
   B. Is useful for all I.V. therapies
   C. Eliminates multiple venipunctures
   D. All of the above

True-False

11. **T F** Luer-locking connectors should be used on all centrally placed catheters.

12. **T F** The Hickman catheter should be flushed with 10 mL of sodium chloride and 100 U of heparin after each blood drawing.

13. **T F** Groshong catheters *must* be flushed with heparinized saline.

ANSWERS TO PRE-TEST, Chapter 12

1. D   2. B   3. C   4. E   5. A   6. E   7. A   8. F   9. A
10. D   11. T   12. T   13. F

This chapter introduces the reader to short- and long-term central venous access devices. Techniques for central catheter placement, management, and complications are reviewed. This chapter also gives an overview of peripherally inserted central catheters, their maintenance, and common complications.

ANATOMY OF THE VASCULAR SYSTEM

To understand the placement of central venous catheters (CVCs), it is necessary to understand the anatomy of the upper extremity venous system, arm, and axilla. The important veins include brachiocephalic, subclavian veins, external and internal jugular, superior vena cava, and the right and left innominate veins. It is also imperative that the registered nurse be fully aware of the anatomic position and structures of the arm and axilla venous system when insertion of peripherally inserted central catheters is desired.

Cephalic and Basilic Structures

The cephalic vein ascends along the outer border of the biceps muscle to the upper third of the arm. It passes in the space between the pectoralis major and deltoid muscles. The vein decreases in size just a few inches above the antecubital fossa and may terminate in the axillary vein or pass above or through the clavicle in a descending curve. Normally, the cephalic vein turns sharply (90 degrees) as it pierces the clavipectoral fascia and passes beneath the clavicle. Near its termination, the cephalic vein may bifurcate into two small veins, one joining the external jugular and one joining the axillary vein. Valves are located along the cephalic vein's course (Gray, 1977). The basilic vein is larger than the cephalic vein. It passes upward in a smooth path along the inner side of the biceps muscle and terminates in the axillary vein. A catheter threaded in the basilic vein may have a tendency to enter the jugular vein (Bridges, Carden, & Takac, 1979). If the patient's head is turned toward the side of insertion during catheter placement, this malposition may be avoided (Fig. 12–1.)

Vein Anatomy within the Chest

The subclavian vein extends from the outer border of the first rib to the sternal end of the clavicle and measures about 4 to 5 cm in length; the right brachiocephalic vein measures about 2.5 cm, and the left brachiocephalic vein measures about 6 to 6.5 cm. The external jugular vein lies on the side of the neck. It follows a descending inward path to join the subclavian vein along the middle of the clavicle. The internal jugular vein descends first behind and then to the outer side of the internal and common carotid arteries. The internal jugular

424

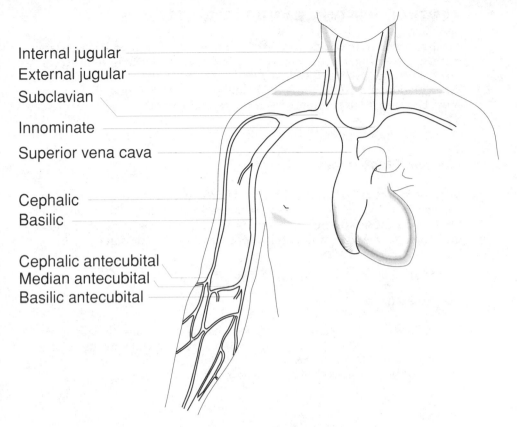

Internal jugular

External jugular

Subclavian

Innominate

Superior vena cava

Cephalic

Basilic

Cephalic antecubital

Median antecubital

Basilic antecubital

Figure 12–1 ☐ Anatomic venous structures of arm and chest. (From "Impact on Patient Care: 2652 PIC Catheter Days" by S. Markel and K. Reynan, 1990, *Journal of Intravenous Nursing, 13* (6), p. 349. Copyright 1990 by the Journal of Intravenous Nursing.)

vein joins the subclavian vein at the root of the neck. Valves are present in the venous system until approximately 1 in before the formation of the innominate vein. The right innominate vein is about 1 in long. It passes almost vertically downward and joins the left innominate just below the cartilage of the first rib. The left innominate vein is about 2.5 in long and larger than the right. It passes from left to right in a downward slant across the upper front of the chest. It joins the right innominate to form the superior vena cava. The superior vena cava receives all blood from the upper half of the body. It is composed of a short trunk 2.5 to 3 in long. It begins below the first rib close to the sternum on the right side, descends vertically slightly to the right, and empties into the right atrium of the heart (Speer, 1990). The right atrium receives blood from the upper body via the superior vena cava and from the lower body via the inferior vena cava. The venae cavae are referred to as the great veins. The right atrium is larger than the left atrium and its walls are thin (Plumer & Cosentino, 1987) (Fig. 12–1).

CENTRAL VENOUS CATHETER MATERIALS

Most vascular access devices (**VADs**) are made of biocompatible substances. Catheters are available in a variety of different materials: long-term access devices are made of silicone and polyurethane, and short-term devices of polyvinylchloride and Teflon (duPont, Wilmington, DE). Silicone, thus far, is the most biocompatible substance used for central catheters.

Silicone Elastomers

Silicone is soft and pliable and cannot be inserted by the conventional over-the-needle technique. Special insertion procedures with or without guidewires for through-the-needle insertion must be used. Silicone is less likely to damage the intima of the vein wall and is reported to be less thrombogenic.

Polyurethane

Polyurethane is stiffer and softens after insertion, making threading of the catheter easier. Polyurethane catheters have thinner walls owing to greater tensile strength than silicone catheters. Polyurethane is similar to silicone in biocompatibility and is thromboresistant and nonhemolytic.

Polyvinylchloride and Teflon

Polyvinylchloride and Teflon are used primarily for short-term venous access. Polyvinylchloride and Teflon catheters appear to have a higher tendency toward **thrombogenicity** and may damage the intima of the vessel wall, which can lead to thrombosis (McIntyre & Laidlow, 1982).

All catheters, whether used for short-term or long-term access, should have a radiopaque lateral strip or a radiopaque **distal** end for visualization on x-ray examination (Speer, 1991).

Lumens

Catheters are available in single, double, or triple lumen. Each lumen's diameter may vary from 16 to 18 gauge. The diameter of each lumen varies because of the need for larger diameters for administration of hypertonic solutions. Refer to manufacturer information to ascertain which lumen is the largest if you are administering vesicant or hypertonic solution via one lumen. Refer to Figure 12–2 for lumen sizes.

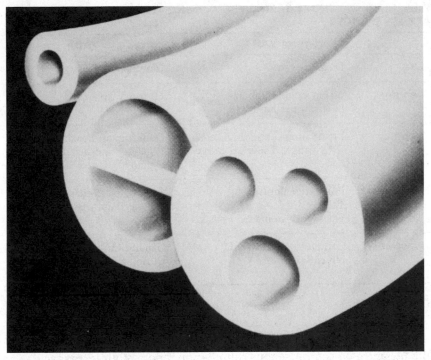

Figure 12–2 ☐ Single, double, and triple lumens. (Courtesy of Bard Access Systems, Salt Lake City, Utah.).

SHORT-TERM VERSUS LONG-TERM ACCESS DEVICES (TABLE 12–1)

Short-Term Devices

Short-term devices are intended to be used for days to weeks. These devices can be single-lumen or multiple-lumen catheters made of several materials. The short-term devices are inserted by a percutaneous venipuncture, are not tunneled under the skin, and are secured by suturing. The sites for short-term devices are infraclavicular, jugular, and femoral if performed by a physician (Hadaway, 1989). The antecubital site can be used by nurses specially trained for peripheral central venous access.

For all short-term devices with catheter tip placement in the superior vena cava, it is of utmost importance that verification by chest x-ray examination be obtained before use.

✎ **Note:** After placement of the catheter, the devices can be closed with an injection cap and heparinized while the placement is verified by x-ray examination. Do not infuse any solution except isotonic fluids without additives if the physician desires an x-ray with free-flowing solution.

427

Table 12-1 □ **SHORT-TERM VERSUS LONG-TERM ACCESS DEVICES**

	Short-Term VAD	Long-Term VAD
Use:	Days to weeks	Months to years
Length:	20-cm double lumen 30-cm triple lumen	60 to 90 cm
Gauge:	Proximal and middle lumens: 18 gauge; distal: 16 gauge	Dual lumen: Proximal (17–18 gauge) and distal (15–16 gauge)
Materials:	Polyvinylchloride Teflon Silicone elastomer	Silicone elastomer Polyurethane
Placement:	Catheter not tunneled No cuff	Usually tunneled Cuffed to fix the catheter to the subcutaneous tissue

Complications

The literature on central venous cannulation reports both **intravascular** and **extravascular malpositioning** of all types of short-term devices. Extravascular malposition can occur when the introducer slips out of the vein and the catheter is passed to the pleural space or the mediastinum. This occurs primarily during a subclavian catheterization. Intravascular malpositions are more common and can be seen with all approaches to the central vascular system (Lum & Soski, 1989). The catheter may coil in the vessel, advance into the right atrium or one of the smaller venous tributaries, or not be advanced far enough to reach the superior vena cava from the antecubital site. The catheter must be repositioned if malpositioning occurs (Vasquez, 1980; Ryan & Gough, 1984).

✎ **Note:** One way to avoid intravascular malpositioning of the catheter into the jugular is to have the patient turn the head toward the side of the venipuncture. This changes the angle of the junction between the internal jugular and subclavian veins, thus causing the catheter to move downward toward the superior vena cava.

Percutaneous Catheters

In 1961 the first intravenous catheter for accessing the central circulation was introduced (Stewart & Sanislow, 1961). The concept of subclavian catheterization was initially inserted using surgical cutdown technique such as advocated by Heimback and Ivey (1976). However, percutaneous introduction into the subclavian vein using the Seldinger through-the-needle guidewire technique is now generally preferred. The percutaneous short-term catheter is secured by suturing, and the catheter is not tunneled. This catheter may remain in place for a few days to several weeks.

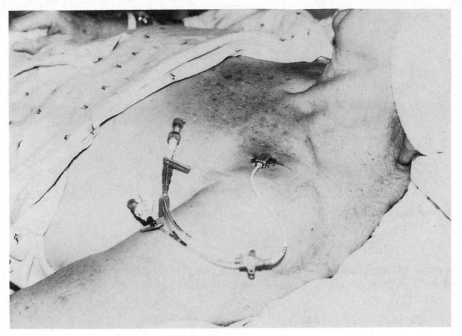

Figure 12–3 ☐ Placement of infraclavicular percutaneous catheter.

The most common site for insertion of the percutaneous catheter is the **infraclavicular** approach to the subclavian vein. The patient is placed in the **Trendelenburg position** with a rolled bath blanket or towel between the shoulders. The patient should be instructed to perform a Valsalva maneuver during the venipuncture procedure to increase the size of the veins. This exit site on the upper chest is well suited for many types of dressings, and care of the site is not complex (Fig. 12–3).

✎ **Note:** The infraclavicular approach site requires a well-hydrated patient.

The internal jugular vein is an accessible site for the physician; however, care of this site for percutaneous catheter is more difficult. The motion of the neck, a beard on men, long hair, and the proximity of respiratory secretions prevent the adequate use of transparent occlusive dressings. The femoral veins are not recommended for this type of therapy because of the difficulty in placing the catheter tip. It is also impossible to maintain an occlusive dressing on the femoral exit site (Hadaway, 1990).

Dressing Management

The percutaneous catheter can be dressed in one of two ways, depending on agency policy. An Elastoplast or a transparent semipermeable membrane dressing may be used. In today's practice the transparent semipermeable membrane dressing has gained popularity because of its occlusive nature and capability for visualization of the site. There is variability in nursing procedure, and the interpretation of various studies conflicts in support of one dressing

429

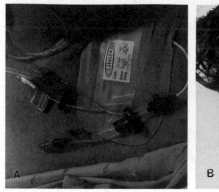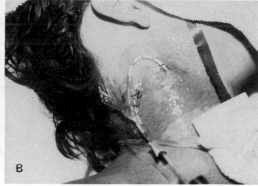

Figure 12–4 □ Elastoplast and TSM dressing for percutaneous central lines.

over another (Eisenberg, Howard, & Gianino, 1990). Therefore, both types of dressing management are presented in this text.

Elastoplast Dressings

The Elastoplast dressing (Fig. 12–4) should be changed every 48 to 72 hours, according to agency policy (Maki & Wells, 1984).

EQUIPMENT
Dressing kit
One pair gloves
Three alcohol swab sticks
Three povidone iodine swab sticks
Two 2 × 2 gauze sponges
Two 3 × 3 gauze sponges
One benzone tincture swab stick
One 4 × 7 Elastoplast dressing
One pair sterile scissors
One dressing change label
One medical tape

PROCEDURE
1. Explain procedure to patient.
2. Wash hands.
3. Prepare equipment.
4. Place patient in supine position.
5. Place mask on patient; turn patient's head away from wound site, unless this would compromise respiratory function.
6. Put mask and unsterile gloves on.
7. Remove old dressing.
8. Open dressing kit.
9. Put on sterile gloves.

10. Inspect catheter insertion site for redness, swelling, and drainage. (Culture site if needed.)
11. Cleanse area with alcohol swab sticks for full 2 minutes, beginning at the insertion site and moving in a circular motion out to the former adhesive border.
12. In same manner cleanse area with povidone iodine swab sticks and let dry for 1 to 2 minutes. (Make sure to check for iodine allergy before using povidone iodine).
13. Apply povidone iodine ointment to catheter site and cover with sterile 4 × 4 gauze.
14. Apply Elastoplast dressing, handling only the ends of the tape. Apply in one continuous motion, covering gauze sponges and creating an air-occlusive dressing.
15. Place 1-in medical tape under the exposed catheter hub and over the hub in a chevron fashion.
16. Label dressing with date and time of procedure, and initial.
17. Chart time dressing changed, condition of site, and signature.

Transparent Semipermeable Membrane Dressings

It is recommended that the transparent semipermeable membrane (TSM) dressing be changed every 4 to 7 days, and whenever the integrity of the occlusive dressing is in question (Schwartz-Fulton, Colley, & Valanis, 1981; Maki & Wells, 1984).

EQUIPMENT
Sterile gloves
Masks
Dressing kit
One pair gloves
Three acetone and alcohol swab sticks
Three povidone iodine swab sticks
Two 4 × 4 gauze sponges
One 4 × 7 transparent dressing

PROCEDURE
1–10. Use the same procedure as with the Elastoplast dressing.
    11. Cleanse the area with alcohol swab sticks, beginning at the insertion site and moving in a circular motion out to the former adhesive border. Repeat with two more swab sticks.
    12. In the same manner, cleanse area with povidone iodine swab stick three times and let air dry (Fig. 12–5).
    13. Apply transparent dressing. Fold dressing in half and remove backing to crease line. Secure half of dressing to catheter, leaving the catheter hub exposed. Peel remaining backing and secure dressing to skin.
    14. Label the dressing with date and time, along with initials.
    15. Chart dressing procedure and site assessment (refer to Fig. 12–4 for Elastoplast and TSM dressings).

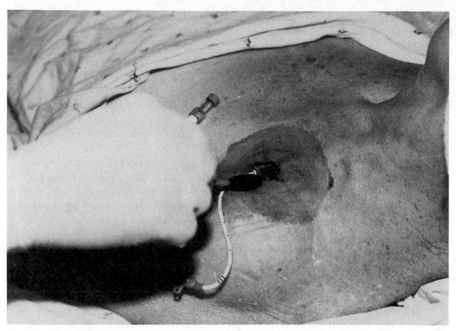

Figure 12–5 ☐ Cleansing central line site with Povidone-iodine.

Peripherally Inserted Central Catheters

The **peripherally inserted central catheter (PICC),** or long-arm catheter, is designed for short-term use. PICCs are inserted by trained intravenous (I.V.) nurses and can be inserted at the bedside. (See Table 12–2 for complete steps in insertion of the PICC.) Initially the PICC was developed for use in neonates because of the catheter's small diameter and the material's flexibility. The PICC is available as a single-lumen or a multiple-lumen device. Table 12–3 compares the PICCs currently on the market.

PICC INDICATIONS
✓ Patient who requires I.V. therapy for more than 7 days
✓ Patient with diagnosis of chest injury, radical neck dissection, radiation therapy to chest
✓ Infusion of a vesicant or irritant drug
✓ Administration of blood or blood products
✓ Patient preference
✓ Patient who is physically unstable
✓ Patient who requires hyperalimentation
✓ Patient who requires continuous narcotic infusions
✓ Difficult peripheral venous access

Table 12–2 □ **STEPS IN INSERTION OF PERIPHERALLY INSERTED CENTRAL LINE***

What to Do	Comments
• Verify the physician's request.	
• Explain the procedure to the patient and/or family.	
• Have informed consent signed.	
• Gather equipment.	
• Wash hands thoroughly.	
• Secure tourniquet around upper arm near the axilla.	
• *Examine the antecubital fossa and select a vein.*	*Preferred choices are the median basilic and the basilic veins.*
• Release the tourniquet, leaving it in place beneath the arm.	
• Position the patient for insertion — supine with the arm extended at a 90-degree angle.	
• *Measure the circumference of the upper arm.*	*To establish a baseline.*
• Measure the distance for catheter insertion.	
• Don a mask.	
• *Vigorously prep the insertion site within a 6-in radius from the midupper arm to the midlower arm. Use three alcohol swab sticks followed by six povidone iodine swab sticks. Let the area dry 2–3 min.*	*The skin prep is a key element in the prevention of infection.*
• *Reapply the tourniquet. Cover the tourniquet with a sterile 4 × 4 gauze pad.*	*To avoid contaminating the prepared arm.*
• Establish a large sterile field. Drop all supplies onto the sterile field.	
• Don a sterile gown and gloves.	
• *Draw up 10 mL 0.9% saline and 1 mL heparin (100 U/mL).*	*Have an assistant hold the vial. Using an extension set helps prevent excessive manipulation of the catheter at the site.*
• Prime the extension set and the injection cap with prepared saline.	
• *Examine the equipment for any defects. Check the patency of the introducer.*	*Trim the catheter tip at a 45-degree angle.*
• Measure the catheter with a sterile measuring tape and cut the catheter to the predetermined length.	
• Position sterile drapes under and around the insertion site.	
• *Remove gloves and don second pair.*	*Talc-free gloves are recommended.*
• Optional: Create on intradermal bleb of 0.1–0.2 mL of 1% lidocaine.	
• *Perform the venipuncture with bevel of needle facing upward.*	*Be prepared for a brisk blood return into the syringe.*

(continued)

433

Table 12–2 □ **STEPS IN INSERTION OF PERIPHERALLY INSERTED CENTRAL LINE*** — *Continued*

What to Do	Comments
• *Remove the syringe and insert the catheter through the introducer— advance the catheter 2–3 in.*	*Using forceps may help reduce the amount of particulate matter from the gloves.*
• Release the tourniquet by grasping the sterile gauze pad.	
• *Continue to advance the catheter through the introducer.*	*NEVER pull the catheter back through the needle; such motion could shear off the catheter tip.*
• Advance the catheter 4–6 in and remove the introducer carefully.	
• *When the introducer needle is clear of the skin, pinch the wings and slowly peel the introducer from around the catheter.*	*This step varies with the type of catheter used.*
• Instruct the patient to turn the head toward the cannulated arm and drop the chin to the chest.	*To help prevent accidental cannulation of the internal jugular vein.*
• Continue to advance the catheter to its final position.	
• Remove the guidewire or stylet.	
• *Connect the extension tubing and aspirate for a blood return.*	*To verify patency.*
• *Flush with the prepared saline and heparin.*	*To prevent clot formation.*
• Clean the insertion site with alcohol and povidone iodine.	
• Secure the catheter with butterfly closures placed over the catheter's hub.	
• Apply a sterile 2 × 2 gauze pad over the site and keep it in place for 24 h.	
• *Apply a sterile transparent dressing.*	*To absorb any bloody drainage.*
• Dispose of all equipment in the appropriate containers.	
• Date, time, and initial the dressing.	
• Get a chest x-ray film to verify tip placement, if inserted beyond axillary vein.	
• Document the insertion in the progress notes.	

*Insertion technique will vary somewhat with each brand of PICC used.
Source: From "The PIC Catheter: A Different Approach" by D. Roundtree, 1991, *American Journal of Nursing, 91,* p 25. Copyright 1991 by American Journal of Nursing. Reprinted with permission.

Table 12–3 □ **COMPARISON OF PICCs**

Catheter Name (Company)	Catheter Size/ Length	Material	Introducer Size/Type	Comments
Intrasil (Baxter Healthcare Corporation)	16-gauge/50.8 mm 15-gauge/55.8 mm	Silicone elastomer	15-gauge/13-gauge breakaway needle	Suture eyelets; Baxter no insertion tray guidewire available
G-PICS C-PPC (Cook Critical Care)	20-gauge/50 mm 18-gauge/50 cm/60 mm 16-gauge/50 cm/60 mm	Polyethylene or silicone	19-gauge/17-gauge/15-gauge peelaway sheath	With or without heparin; coated catheter insertion tray with or without guidewire; suture eyelets
Groshong PIC (Davol-Cath Tech Inc.)	16-gauge/55 mm	Silicone	14-gauge cannula over-the-needle introducer	Two-way valve design; insertion tray/single or double lumen, guidewire
Per-Q-Cath (Gesco International)	23-gauge/33.5 mm 20-gauge/50 mm 16-gauge/58 mm 16-gauge/40 mm	Silicone	20-gauge/18-gauge/14-gauge breakaway needle	Not sutured; insertion tray with or without guidewire

(continued)

435

Table 12–3 □ **COMPARISON OF PICCs—**_Continued_

Catheter Name (Company)	Catheter Size/ Length	Material	Introducer Size/Type	Comments
L-Cath (Luter Medical)	20-gauge/20 mm 20-gauge/56 mm 18-gauge/56 mm 16-gauge/40 mm	Polyurethane, radiopaque	19-gauge/17-gauge/14-gauge peelaway sheath	Neonatal to adult sizes; suture wings, no insertion tray; with guidewire
Ven-A-Cath (HDC Corporation)	20-gauge/40 cm 18-gauge/60 cm	Silicone, radiopaque	19-gauge/17-gauge breakaway needle	Insertion tray; preassembled Luer connection, no-suture outlets with or without guidewire
Viggo (US Viggo, Inc.)	16-gauge/50 cm	Polyurethane	16-gauge	Insertion tray; with guidewire, introducer over-the-needle catheter

5.0cm = 50mm = 22in; 3.0cm = 30mm = 12in; 14mm = .55in; 15mm = 50in; 2.3mm = 7F; 16g = 1.7mm; 14g = 2.1mm; 18g = 1.2mm; 20g = .9mm.

Source: From "Advanced Central Venous Access: Selection, Catheters, Devices, and Nursing Management" by D. Camp-Sorrell, 1990, _Journal of Intravenous Nursing, 13_, p. 362. Copyright 1990 by the Intravenous Nurses Society. Reprinted by permission.

✎ KEY POINTS OF PICCs

ADVANTAGES
1. Because of peripheral insertion, eliminates potential complication of pneumothorax or hemothorax
2. Decreases risk of air embolism owing to the ease of maintaining the insertion site below the heart
3. Decreases in pain and discomfort associated with frequent venipuncture
4. Preserves peripheral vascular system of upper extremities
5. Cost and time efficient
6. Appropriate for home placement and home I.V. therapy
7. Reliable vascular access throughout the course of antibiotic or chemotherapy

DISADVANTAGES
1. Nurses must have special training to perform this procedure.
2. Procedure takes 45 minutes to 1 hour.
3. Daily care is required.
4. Catheter maintenance guidelines must be strictly followed to prevent clotting of catheter.
5. Because of the small lumen size, some PICCs are not recommended for obtaining blood samples because the catheter could collapse on aspiration.

PROCEDURE: VEIN SELECTION
1. Basilic vein
2. Median antecubital vein
3. Cephalic vein (Refer to Fig. 12-6)

✎ **Note:** All these sites are acceptable; however, the basilic vein and the median antecubital vein are the preferred insertion sites.

EQUIPMENT
One PICC
One introducer needle
Two pair sterile gloves
Two polylined sterile drapes (one fenestrated, one nonfenestrated)
One pair sterile forceps or tweezers (nontoothed)
Two sterile 4 × 4 gauze
One tourniquet
Three povidone iodine scrub swab sticks
Three alcohol swab sticks
One sterile 2 × 2 gauze
One 4 × 6 transparent dressing
Two 10-mL syringes with 21-gauge needles
One 4-in extension tubing
One injection cap
One 10-mL vial normal saline for injection
One package of Steri-Strips
One tape measure

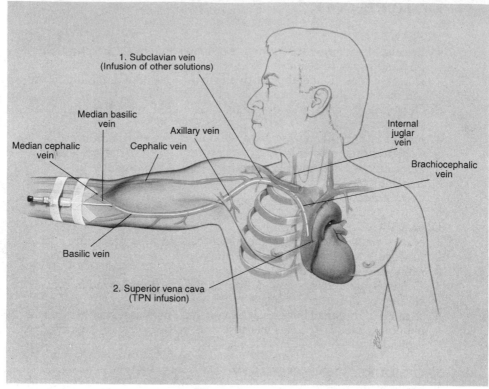

Figure 12–6 □ Anatomic placement of peripherally placed central catheter. (Courtesy of Medivisuals, Dallas, Texas.)

One face mask, goggles, and gown (according to agency policy)
One 5-mL vial of heparin, 100 U/mL

Dressing Management

After 24 hours the original dressing must be replaced with one that can remain in place up to 7 days. *This is a sterile procedure.*

✓ Wear gloves for the dressing change.
✓ Remove the transparent dressing gently, being careful not to dislodge or pull on the catheter.
✓ Assess the insertion site, the arm, and the track of the vein for redness, tenderness, edema, and drainage.
✓ Remove gloves and put on a new pair of sterile gloves to clean the skin around the insertion site.
✓ Use three alcohol swab sticks followed by three povidone iodine swab sticks.
✓ Slide a 2 × 2 split gauze pad under the catheter just below the insertion site if drainage is present.

✓ Place Steri-Strips over insertion site to prevent migration of catheter.

✓ Apply a new transparent dressing over the gauze and exposed catheter, including the hub.

✓ Initial and date your dressing (Masoorli & Angeles, 1990).

✎ **Note:** PICC dressing should be changed at intervals similar to other central line dressings. Patients who are very active or who perspire profusely will need more frequent dressing changes (Brown, 1989).

✎ **Note:** Take care to avoid stretching the catheter during dressing changes and catheter removal. Stretching or excessive pressure can cause the catheter to rupture.

Flushing Protocol

The saline–administration of medication–saline–heparin (SASH) method of flushing is recommended to eliminate problems with incompatible drugs. The amount of heparin necessary to flush the device should be equivalent to the system volume plus approximately 0.2 mL. A concentration of 10 to 100 U/mL can be used; however, 100 U/mL tends to be the recommendation (Roundtree, 1991). Flushing procedures vary from agency to agency.

Flushing Procedure

Use 2 mL of normal saline solution, followed by 1 mL of heparin (100 U/mL). If you need a heparin-free line, use 5 to 10 mL of normal saline (Roundtree, 1991).

✎ **Note:** Do not use a tuberculin syringe for flushing, as it can cause too much pressure; a 10-mL syringe may be used safely.

Declotting

The PICC line may be cleared by using urokinase according to the manufacturer's recommendation. When attempting to declot the catheter with urokinase the small volume of the PICC line must be taken into consideration, as well as catheter rupture strengths.

✎ **Note:** The drugs phenytoin (Dilantin), diazepam (Valium), and mannitol have been documented to cause problems when infused through a PICC line. When either of these drugs is given, crystals form inside the lumen, causing occlusion of the catheter. It is not known if there is an interaction between the drug and the catheter material or another drug that may have been inside the lumen (Hadaway, 1989).

Infusion Pumps

The PICC line has been used successfully with all types of infusion pumps.

Blood Sampling

If blood sampling is needed from the PICC a 2.8 F or larger catheter may be required. All companies manufacture a 3.8 F or larger catheter. Because the walls of the PICC line are soft, they collapse easily when a strong vacuum is applied. A gentle touch with a syringe rather than a Vacutainer will yield a successful sample.

Blood Administration

Blood products may be administered through a 3.8 F or larger PICC catheter. Care should be taken to flush the line thoroughly after administration of a blood product.

Repair

The PICC can be repaired in one of two ways—use of a coated blunt-end needle external repair kit or replacement of the catheter over a guidewire. PICCs can be temporarily repaired by inserting a coated blunt-end needle into the trimmed end of the broken catheter.

If the peripherally inserted central line is damaged, another catheter can be placed. An exchange-over-wire procedure can be used as a last resort to salvage the line. The guidewires used for this procedure can be extremely long; therefore, strict sterile technique with gowning is recommended. The guidewire is inserted into the catheter to be removed, and then the catheter is pulled out over the wire. A new catheter is then threaded back over the wire. Once the new catheter is in place, the guidewire can be removed. A chest x-ray examination should be done to verify placement of the new catheter tip. This procedure should be performed only by experienced I.V. nurses who are certified to insert a PICC (Intravenous Nursing Society [INS], 1990, S79). There are specific manufacturer recommendations for this procedure.

Complications

COMPLICATIONS OF PICC CATHETERS

Insertion

1. Bleeding; compartment syndrome
2. Tendon or nerve damage
3. Cardiac arrhythmias
4. Malposition of catheter
5. Catheter embolism

Postinsertion

1. Phlebitis; cellulitis
2. Infection (catheter sepsis)
3. Thrombosis; thrombophlebitis (occlusion of catheter)
4. Air embolism
5. Twiddler's syndrome

Insertion Complications

1. **Bleeding; compartment syndrome:** Bleeding is a frequent complication associated with any nontunneled catheter. Excessive bleeding beyond 24 hours after insertion is unusual. Mild pressure dressing may be required to control bleeding.
2. **Tendon or nerve damage:** Technique-related complication.
3. **Cardiac arrhythmias:** Related to placement of catheter tip. Some institutions require the patient to be monitored during placement of a PICC in the superior vena cava.
4. **Malposition of catheter:** Central venous catheter tip migration can occur while in vivo. Having patient turn head toward catheter site during insertion decreases migration into the jugular vein. However, postinsertion migration can occur with:
   - ✓ Patients who frequently experience nausea and vomiting during the course of therapy
   - ✓ Respiratory patients who may have bouts of severe coughing (causing the catheter tip to migrate)
   - ✓ Physically active patients

✎ **Note:** If the patient complains of pain in shoulder, neck, or arm on insertion side of body, catheter placement should be checked by x-ray examination at any time during the course of therapy.

5. **Catheter embolism:** Observe for pinholes, leaks, or tears in the catheter. Care should be taken to remove breakaway needle (introducer) before threading the catheter. Refer to procedure. To prevent embolism of this small-lumen catheter, avoid using larger than a 21-gauge, 1-in needle through the injection cap.

Postinsertion Complications

1. **Phlebitis; cellulitis:** Mechanical phlebitis is the most common complication seen with the PICC line. Phlebitis occurs usually in the first 48 to 72 hours after insertion. This complication occurs more frequently in women than men and with left-sided insertions more often than right-sided ones. To treat phlebitis apply warm, moist compresses to upper arm between the insertion site and the shoulder for 20 minutes four times a day. Elevation of the extremity and mild exercise can be effective in resolving or controlling the phlebitis (Brown, 1989).

   Cellulitis is usually caused by *Staphylococcus epidermis* or *Staphylococcus aureus*. Signs and symptoms are pain, tenderness, and redness at the catheter site spreading in a diffuse circular pattern into the surrounding subcutaneous tissue. Cellulitis responds well to oral antibiotics and may not require the removal of the catheter.
2. **Infection (catheter sepsis):** Infection rates of PICC lines have been extremely low when compared with those of other types of central lines. Low infection rates have been documented with studies of PICC catheters (Kyle & Meyers, 1990; Brown, 1989). Pemberton (1986) states that patients requiring multiple-lumen catheters are usually more acutely ill and therefore at higher risk for developing sepsis related to the multiple lumens.

441

3. **Thrombosis; thrombophlebitis (occlusion of catheter)**: Deep vein thrombosis of the subclavian vein is rare. The causes of deep vein thrombosis are injury to the intima of the vein wall, obstructed blood flow, and changes in the composition of the blood. The use of biocompatible catheter material has decreased this complication. Occlusions of the catheter can be avoided with routine flushing procedures, avoiding use of excess force, flushing vigorously after viscous solution, and avoiding mixing of incompatible drugs.
4. **Air embolism**: This complication is rare with PICC because the catheter exit site is below the level of the heart, which helps to maintain adequate pressure within the system.
5. **Twiddler's syndrome**: This syndrome results in dislodgment of the catheter owing to patient manipulation of the dressing and catheter. The catheter length should be assessed frequently. Inform the patient of the possible catheter dislodgment caused by fiddling with the catheter (Camp-Sorrell, 1990).

Long-Term Venous Access Devices

Devices designed for long-term use can be divided into two categories: **tunneled catheters** and **implanted ports**. These catheters require a surgical procedure for insertion, are made of Silastic material, and are available in single or double lumens. These long-term devices can remain in place up to 3 years.

Central Venous Tunneled Catheters

Central venous tunneled catheters (**CVTCs**) have been available since 1975 when Broviac catheters were introduced for long-term hyperalimentation. Inserted through a subcutaneous tunnel, these catheters are often referred to as indwelling catheters, tunneled central venous catheters, or right atrial catheters (Table 12–4). These catheters, intended for use from months to years, provide long-term venous access for obtaining blood samples and for administering drugs, blood products, and total parenteral nutrition.

Central venous tunneled catheters are composed of polymeric silicone with a Dacron polyester cuff that anchors the catheter in place subcutaneously (Fig. 12–7). This cuff is approximately 2 in from the catheter's exit site, which becomes embedded with fibroblasts within a week to 10 days after insertion, lessening the chance for accidental removal and minimizing the risk of ascending bacterial infection.

Tunneled central venous catheters are available with single, double, or triple lumens that exit midway between the nipple and sternum (Fig. 12–8). CVTCs vary in size from pediatric to adult, with most internal lumens ranging from 0.5 to 1.6 mm in diameter.

One of the general advantages of CVTCs is that a break or tear in the catheter is easy to repair without adhesive. Once repaired, the catheter is available for use within 24 hours.

✎ **Note:** CVTCs are easily maintained in the home setting.

Table 12–4 □ **COMPARISON OF CENTRAL VENOUS TUNNELED CATHETERS**

Catheter Name (Company)	Types	Internal/External Diameter	Comments
Hickman/Broviac (Bard/Davol)	Silicone; single, double, triple; 0.9–3.2 mm	0.7–1.6 mm	Permanent hub; repair kit with glue, vita cuff feature
Groshong (Bard/Cath Tech)	Silicone; single, double	0.7–1.5 mm 1.1–2.5 mm	No clamps, two-way valve design, hub not attached; repair kit with or without glue
Raaf (Quinton)	Silicone; single, double, triple; 1.5–4.5 mm	0.7–1.5 mm	Permanent hub; repair kit with glue
Hemed (Gish Biomedical)	Silicone; single, double	0.6–1.6 mm	Permanent hub; repair kit with or without glue
Chemo Cath (HDC Corporation)	Silicone; single, double	0.6–1.0 mm	Permanent hub; repair kit with glue

Source: From "Advanced Central Venous Access: Selection, Catheters, Devices, and Nursing Management" by D. Camp-Sorrell, 1990, *Journal of Intravenous Nursing*, 13, p. 363. Copyright 1990 by the Intravenous Nurses Society. Reprinted by permission.

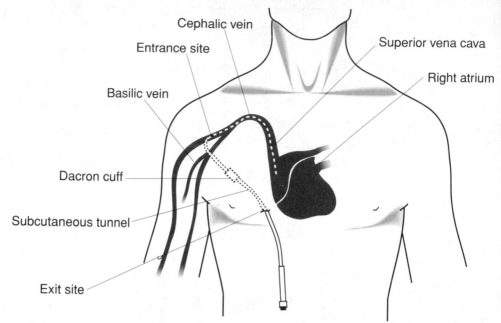

Figure 12–7 ☐ Anatomic placement of tunneled catheter. (Courtesy of Bard Access Systems, Salt Lake City, Utah.)

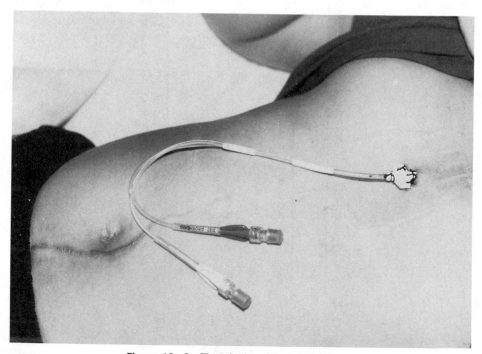

Figure 12–8 ☐ Exit site of tunneled catheter.

✎ KEY POINTS IN CENTRAL VENOUS TUNNELED DEVICES

ADVANTAGES
1. Can be repaired if it breaks or tears
2. Can be used for many purposes, including:

    Blood samples
    Monitoring central venous pressure
    Administration of hyperalimentation
    Drug administration
3. Can be used for the patient with chronic need for I.V. therapy

DISADVANTAGES
1. Daily to weekly site care
2. Cost of maintenance supplies (dressings, materials, and changes; frequency of flushing and cap changing)
3. Insertion of CVTC is a minor surgical procedure requiring postoperative care for 7 to 10 days
4. As with the PICC, can affect patient's body image (Camp-Sorrell, 1990)
5. More expensive than PICCs

Complications of Tunneled Catheters

1. **Exit site infection:** Proper dressing technique minimizes the risk of exit site infection. Temperature elevation, redness, swelling, or drainage at the site must be reported immediately to the nurse or physician.
2. **Sepsis:** All elevated temperatures need to be reported. If bacteria ascend the catheter and enter the patient's circulation, the patient may become septic. Secondary catheter sepsis may result from an infection in another body system, such as urinary tract infection or upper respiratory infection.
3. **Thrombosis:** Thrombosis can develop in the vessel in which the catheter is situated. Signs of thrombosis such as tenderness and swelling of the arms, neck, and shoulder on the catheter side of body must be reported immediately (Handy, 1989).
4. **Catheter migration:** It is good practice to infuse normal saline before and after administering medications. This clears the heparin from the catheter; also, swelling or a subcutaneous burning sensation can be detected with normal saline before injection of a medication. Dye studies can confirm catheter tip placement.
5. **Clot formation:** A clot can form in a catheter because of improper flushing technique or lack of flushing procedure with the right atrial catheter. Difficulty in flushing or total inability to flush the catheter must be reported immediately to the physician. Attempt to declot the catheter using urokinase, following agency protocol (Bjeletich, 1987).
6. **Torn or leaking catheter:** A catheter can tear or develop a leak through improper use. Always use a smooth or padded clamp on the catheter when changing the injection cap. Rotate clamping sites. Tape catheter up when not in use to prevent tugging. Never put anything sharp next

to the catheter. If a tear or leak is detected, the nurse or patient must immediately place the clamp between the tear or leak and the entry site. Call the physician.

7. **Air embolism:** If the cap is removed when the catheter is not clamped or a tear develops, air embolism can enter the system. Use only Luer-locking devices. Never allow the catheter to be open to the air. Secure all connections during an infusion.

✎ **Note:** If an air embolism occurs at home, treatment consists of closing off the open end of the catheter, placing the patient in the Trendelenburg position on his or her left side, and obtaining immediate emergency assistance.

Dressing Change

1. Wash hands.
2. Depending on agency policy, apply a povidone iodine ointment to a split 2 × 2 gauze dressing.
3. Put mask on, if patient is neutropenic; then put sterile gloves on.
4. Remove dressing from site.
5. Inspect site for redness, swelling, and drainage.
6. Remove gloves and put on second pair of sterile gloves.
7. Using alcohol swab stick, cleanse exit site, rotating in a circular method from inside outward.
8. Using povidone iodine swab stick, cleanse site, rotating in a circular method from inside outward, let dry 1 to 2 minutes. (Check for patient allergy to iodine prior to use of povidone iodine.)
9. Use a transparent semipermeable dressing over site. Apply split 2 × 2 gauze around catheter exit site if suture is present
10. Tape the catheter to the dressing and coil remaining tubing, using a chevron technique.

Injection Cap Change

1. Wear mask and gloves.
2. Swab connection of cap with povidone iodine.
3. Remove old cap.
4. Screw on new cap.
5. Wipe off excess povidone iodine with alcohol swab.

Types of Tunneled Catheters

Hickman
Broviac
Groshong

Broviac/Hickman

Specifics

The **Broviac silicone rubber catheter** (Bard Access Systems, Salt Lake City, Utah) is 90 cm in length; the pediatric catheter is 50 cm. The extended portion of this catheter is thicker than the indwelling venous portion and has a male Luer-locking hub adaptor. A small Dacron cuff encircles the catheter approximately 30 cm from the hub. This cuff stabilizes within the tunneled sheath during the 2 to 3 weeks after insertion. The internal lumen of this catheter is 1.0 mm and volume capacity 1 mL.

The **Hickman catheter** (Bard Access Systems, Salt Lake City, Utah) is similar in design to the Broviac catheter and is available with 1 to 2 Dacron cuffs. The Hickman catheter has a larger internal diameter to facilitate blood withdrawal. The outer diameter of this catheter is 3.2 mm and the volume capacity 2 mL.

A double-lumen Hickman/Broviac catheter is available. This newer design fuses the Broviac and Hickman catheters to provide two access routes. The Broviac lumen is reserved for nutrient solutions. The Hickman is reserved for blood withdrawal and administration of antibiotics and chemotherapeutic agents along with blood products.

Insertion

These catheters are inserted under local or general anesthesia by surgical cutdown of a centrally located superficial vein — usually the external jugular or cephalic vein. A separate proximal incision is made on the chest or abdominal wall, and the catheter is directed through a subcutaneous tunnel between the two incisions. The catheter is open at distal and proximal ends and trimmed to the appropriate estimated length, threaded through the subclavian vein into the superior vena cava. The position is confirmed by fluoroscopy, adjusted if needed, and then sutured to the skin or the incision is closed with Steri-Strips. These remain in place for 10 to 14 days.

✎ KEY POINTS FOR CARE OF HICKMAN OR BROVIAC CATHETERS

1. Be sure the catheter is capped at all times. If the catheter should become uncapped, follow the steps for flushing the catheter.
2. Keep all sharp objects away from the catheter. Never use scissors or pins near the catheter, as these objects may damage the external line.
3. If the catheter leaks or breaks, clamp the catheter with a nonserrated clamp between the broken area and the "exit site." Cover the broken part with a sterile gauze bandage and tape it securely. Do not use the catheter. Notify the physician.
4. Protect the catheter when showering or bathing by covering with a clear plastic wrap.
5. If flushing after a blood withdrawal use 10 mL of 0.9% sodium chloride and the correct amount of heparin.
6. Heparin is used to maintain patency of the catheter.

Flushing Procedure

Flushing procedures vary according to the agency. Generally it is accepted practice to flush the Hickman/Broviac or other tunneled catheter (except the Groshong) with twice the catheter volume of heparinized saline. After medication administration or daily maintenance, flush the catheter with saline; then

447

follow with 2.5 mL of 100 U/mL heparinized saline. A positive pressure technique should be used to flush the catheter.

Groshong

Specifics

The **Groshong catheter** (Bard Access Systems, Salt Lake City, Utah) has been marketed since 1984. This catheter has a few unique features that set it apart from other tunneled central venous catheters. This catheter is made of soft, flexible, Silastic material. The outer diameter dimensions are small. This catheter is available in single, double, or triple lumens. This Silastic material has a recoil memory that returns it to its original configuration if accidently pulled. Another unique feature of the Groshong catheter is the two-way valve placed near the distal end, which restricts blood backflow but can be purposefully overridden to obtain venous blood samples (Fig. 12–9). This valve eliminates the need for flushing with heparin. The valve is open outward during flushing or fluid infusion. After infusion the valve automatically closes inward, minimizing the risks of blood backing up the catheter lumen.

✎ **Note:** External clamps should not be used; they are unnecessary and could damage the catheter (Camp, 1988).

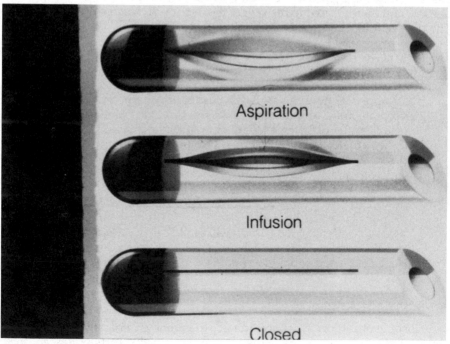

Aspiration

Infusion

Closed

Figure 12–9 ☐ Three-position Groshong valve. (Courtesy of Bard Access Systems, Salt Lake City, Utah.)

Insertion

Other catheters are tunneled up from the exit site; the Groshong catheter placement is reversed. Once the Groshong catheter is at the desired site, its length is adjusted before the connector is placed into the proximal end. The Groshong catheter distal end is closed, soft, rounded, and flexible.

Flushing Procedure

Policy and procedures for flushing vary according to the agency. The Groshong catheter should be irrigated every 7 days with 0.9% sodium chloride when not in use. Maintain aseptic technique. After administration of medication, the catheter should be flushed with 5 mL of normal saline. After the administration of viscous solutions such as lipids, flush briskly with 20 mL of normal saline to prevent crystallization of the catheter tip. Manufacturers recommend that the catheter be irrigated with a syringe attached directly to the connection hub of the Groshong catheter.

Blood Sample

To obtain a blood sample:

1. Withdraw and discard 5 mL of blood.
2. Draw sample with syringe (do not use Vacutainer).
3. Flush catheter briskly with 20 mL of normal saline.

✎ **Note:** Briskly flushing the catheter creates a swirling effect at the distal end of the catheter. If flushing is not performed briskly, a blood clot may form. Raising the patient's arms and repositioning the bed may assist in obtaining blood sample.

✎ **KEY POINTS FOR CARE OF GROSHONG CATHETERS**
1. *Do not clamp the catheter.* Clamping is not necessary because of the special valve, and clamping could cause damage such as leaking or tearing of the catheter.
2. Keep all sharp objects away from the catheter. Never use scissors or pins on or near the catheter. Never use acetone-containing products such as nail polish remover or tape remover on or near the catheter, as it can dissolve the catheter.
3. If the catheter leaks or breaks, cover the broken part with a sterile gauze bandage and tape it securely. Do not use the catheter. Notify the physician.
4. Protect the catheter when showering or bathing by covering the entire catheter with transparent dressing or clear plastic wrap.
5. Straining or heavy lifting could cause a small amount of blood to back up into the catheter. If blood is evident in the catheter line, flush.
6. After blood sample is obtained, flush briskly with 20 mL of normal saline.

✎ **Note:** Patient education—encourage patient to carry an identification card with information about the tunneled catheter.

Repair of Long-Term Central Venous Catheter

The tunneled central venous access device can tear during reinsertion of the introducer needle, during intermittent therapy when I.V. push therapy is performed, or when using scissors near the catheter site. When this happens, blood usually backs up and fluid leaks from the site. Air can enter the catheter through the tear, causing an air embolism.

Keeping current on repair methods can be difficult. Several different catheter repair kits are available. The catheters can be repaired without a kit, but this requires a certain combination of creativity and knowledge.
To repair a catheter, you will need:

Sterile gloves
Mask
Sterile drapes
Sterile scissors
Povidone iodine solution
Extension set
(Repair kit)

TYPES OF REPAIR
Blunt-end needle repair
Splicing sleeve with adhesive
Groshong repair kit
Plastic catheter method

✎ **Note:** Avoid serrated clamps on the catheter (Hadaway, 1989).

1. First, clamp the catheter immediately between the chest wall and the tear.
2. Cleanse the end of the catheter with povidone iodine if the patient is not allergic to iodine.
3. Cut off and discard the damaged portion of the catheter with sterile scissors.
4. Insert a blunt-end needle with the appropriate gauge into the end of the remaining length of catheter.

Place an injection cap in the hub of the needle and heparinize the catheter. Tie a silk suture around the needle and catheter to secure. The catheter is then ready to use until permanent repair is done. Many long-term devices come with permanent repair kits, which involve splicing a new section of catheter with an end connector to the rest of the catheter (Fig. 12–10).

OCCLUDED CENTRAL VENOUS CATHETERS: DRUG TIP

Urokinase (pH 6.0 to 7.5)

Actions

Urokinase is an enzyme, a potent direct activator of the endogenous fibrinolytic system, which converts plasminogen to the proteolytic enzyme plasmin.

Connector Instructions

1. *Transfer white sleeve (A) onto catheter from connector.*

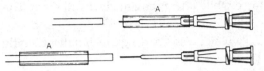

2. *Firmly push catheter onto adapter to Position B.*

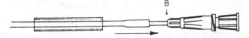

3. *Slide white sleeve onto colored hub to Position C.*

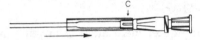

4. *Remove and discard stylet.*

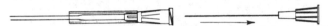

Figure 12–10 □ Example of repair kit for tunneled catheter. (Courtesy of Bard Access Systems, Salt Lake City, Utah.)

Plasmin degrades fibrin clots, as well as fibrinogen and other plasma proteins associated with clotting. The effects of fibrinolytic activity decrease within a few hours after discontinuation of drug.

Use

I.V. catheter clearance is 5000 IU (1 mL specifically diluted). The amount should be equal to the volume in the catheter.

Dilution

Sterile water for injection without preservatives is used for reconstitution of this agent.

TECHNIQUE AND RATE OF ADMINISTRATION
Confirm occlusion with 10-mL syringe.
Obtain patient consent and physician order.
Slowly and gently inject specifically diluted and premeasured urokinase into catheter.
Wait 5 minutes.
Gently aspirate to remove clot.

451

Repeat every 5 minutes until clot clears for 30 minutes.
If unsuccessful, cap catheter for 1 hour and reattempt to declot.

✎ **Note:** Residence time of urokinase ranges from 30 minutes to 3 hours before full use of the port is successfully established (Lawson, 1991).

✎ **Note:** Avoid force while attempting to clear catheters. The catheter may rupture or dislodge clot into the circulation.

✎ **Note:** Urokinase will not dissolve drug precipitate or anything other than blood products.

Contraindications

Patients who have active internal bleeding, intracranial neoplasm, hypersensitivity to urokinase, liver disease, subacute bacterial endocarditis, or visceral malignancy or who have had a cerebrovascular accident within 2 months or intracranial or intraspinal surgery should not receive urokinase.

Drug Incompatibilities

Do not mix with any other medication in any manner.

Complications

Bleeding

Bleeding may occur in two general forms: surface bleeding from invaded or disturbed sites (punctures, incision) or internal bleeding from the gastrointestinal tract, genitourinary tract, vagina, intramuscular, retroperitoneal, or intracerebral sites. *Fatalities due to cerebral or retroperitoneal hemorrhage have occurred*. The antidote to bleeding is administration of plasma volume expanders such as fresh plasma fluids, along with whole blood if hemorrhage is unresponsive to blood replacement. Aminocaproic acid can be used.

Allergic reactions

These are rare and usually in the form of rash, bronchospasm, or anaphylaxis.

Fever

Fever can occur and should be symptomatically controlled with acetaminophen rather than aspirin (Gahart, 1991, p 600).

NURSING CONSIDERATIONS
Observe patient continuously.
Do not use force when instilling urokinase into catheter.
Work with declotting the catheter every 15 minutes.
If necessary, obtain thrombin time, prothrombin time, or activated partial thromboplastin time to monitor.
Keep physician informed.

Restoring Patency of Mineral or Medication Precipitate

Hydrochloric acid (HCL) and sodium bicarbonate have been used successfully to clear a central line of precipitates caused by minerals, such as calcium and phosphate, or medications with a high pH.

HCL is indicated when there is a precipitate in the catheter of the infusate. HCL is not effective for declotting of fat globules (lipid emulsions) (Testerman, 1991). The action of HCL is to lower the pH and therefore increase the precipitation solubility, which results in dissolution and return of catheter patency.

When infusing medications with a high pH such as with phenytoin (pH 11-12) the central venous catheter can become occluded. The use of sodium bicarbonate (pH of 8) has been successfully used to restore patency (Goodwin, 1991). Check with agency for actual steps in clearing an occluded line with HCL or sodium bicarbonate.

New Development

An attachable cuff (Vita-Cuff) has been studied for tunneled central venous access devices. This cuff is made of biodegradable collagen impregnated with silver ion. The cuff is placed in the subcutaneous tissue around the central venous access device. Subcutaneous tissue grows to the cuff, providing a mechanical barrier against organism; the silver ion provides a chemical barrier. This cuff has proved to be cost effective in decreasing catheter-related septicemia (Maki, 1988).

IMPLANTED PORTS

Implanted ports have been available for venous access since 1983. Implanted ports are another form of central venous catheters. Originally, implanted ports were targeted to the oncology patient who required frequent intermittent venous access. Ports consist of a reservoir, silicone catheter, and central septum (Fig. 12–11).) The self-sealing septum can usually withstand 1000 to 2000 needle punctures. Ports have raised edges to facilitate puncture with a noncoring needle. The port is $1 \times 1.5 \times 0.5$ in and made of stainless steel or titanium. This septum is connected to a silicone catheter (Riser, 1988). Many types of implanted vascular access devices are available today, but each is the same in terms of insert site and use (Table 12–5).

✎ KEY POINTS IN THE IMPLANTED PORT

ADVANTAGES
1. Less risk of infection when used intermittently
2. Less interference with daily activities
3. Little site care
4. Needs minimal flushing
5. Easy access for fluids, blood products, or medication administration
6. Less body image disturbance owing to lack of external catheter device
7. Few limitations on patient activity

453

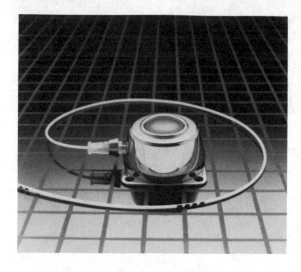

Figure 12-11 □ Implanted port. (Courtesy of Pharmacia Deltec, Inc., St. Paul, Minnesota.)

DISADVANTAGES
1. Cost of insertion (considerably higher than with other VADs)
2. Postoperative care 7 to 10 days
3. Discomfort of repeated needle sticks
4. Minor surgical procedure necessary to remove device

✎ **Note:** Placement is not recommended in the obese patient, after chest radiation, or at mastectomy sites (Camp-Sorrel, 1990).

Insertion

The port is inserted after administration of a local anesthetic, and the entire procedure takes from 30 minutes to 1 hour. An incision is made in the upper to middle chest, usually near the collarbone, to form a pocket to house the port. The Silastic catheter is inserted via cutdown into the superior vena cava; the port is then placed in the subcutaneous fascia pocket. The port contains a reservoir leading to the catheter. The incision for the port pocket is sutured closed and a sterile dressing applied.

The dressing may be removed after the first 24 hours. This area should be cleaned daily using povidone iodine solution and a sterile gauze pad until the stitches are removed and healing has taken place, approximately 10 days to 2 weeks after insertion.

SUBCUTANEOUS PORT SYSTEM CATHETER CAN BE PLACED
1. Superior vena cava
2. Hepatic artery
3. Peritoneal space (for intraperitoneal therapy)
4. Epidural space

✎ **Note:** Implanted ports are available in one- or two-septum chambers.

Table 12–5 □ **COMPARISON OF IMPLANTED PORTS**

Port Brand Name (Company)	Types	Materials	Height/ Base	Weight	Septum Diameter	Septum Depth	Internal Diameter/ Outer Diameter	Internal Volume	Catheter Attachment Style
A-Port (Therex Corporation)	Single	Titanium	14.4 mm/ 17.8 mm	9.2 g	17.8 mm	8 mm	1.5 mm/ 3.2 mm	0.5 mL	Detached or attached
Chemo-Port (HDC Corporation)	Single, peds	Stainless steel, silicone	12.1 mm/ 3.18 mm	25 g	9.1 mm	5.5 mm	1 mm/ 1.6 mm	0.8 mL	Attached
Groshong (Bard, Cath Tech)	Single, silicone	Titanium	14.4 mm/ 28.4 mm	9.2 g	13 mm	8.9 mm 2-way valve	1.5 mm/ 2.5 mm	0.5 mL	Attached, locking sleeve
Hickman (Bard/ Davol)	Single, dual 0.6 mL	Titanium, detached or stainless steel, plastic	14.0 mm/ 31.7 mm	16– 24 g	12.7 mm	10.7 mm	1–1.6 mm/ 2.5 mm		Attached
Implantolix (Burron)	Single, peds	Polyoxi-methlene	9.8 mm/ 39 mm	2.9 g	12.0 mm	9.5 mm	1.2 mm/ 1.7 mm	0.33 mL	Attached
Infus-A-Port (Shiley Corporation)	Single, dual, peds	Sulfone plastic rubber	11–15.8 mm/ 24–38 mm	2.1 g	8–14 mm	5.1 mm	1–1.6 mm/ 2.5 mm	0.2–0.7 mL	Detached or attached
Lifeport (Strato)	Single, dual	Titanium	12.2 mm/ 24 mm	16.5 g	15.9 mm	6.4 mm	1.5 mm/ 2.5 mm	0.6 mL	Bayonet lock, detached or attached
Medtronic (Medtronic Corporation)	Single, peds	Polymer, titanium, silicone	17 mm/ 50 mm	27 g	10 mm	13 mm	1 mm/ 2.2 mm	0.6 mL	Attached

(continued)

CENTRAL VENOUS ACCESS DEVICES

Table 12–5 □ **COMPARISON OF IMPLANTED PORTS—Continued**

Port Brand Name (Company)	Types	Materials	Height/Base	Weight	Septum Diameter	Septum Depth	Internal Diameter/Outer Diameter	Internal Volume	Catheter Attachment Style
Norport (Norfold Corporation)	Single, dual, peds, skin parallel	Stainless steel, silicone base	13–15 mm/ 33–38 mm	9–15 g	10.4 mm	5.5 mm	1–1.5 mm/ 2.3–4 mm	0.6 mL	Detached or attached
P.A.S. Port (Pharmacia)	Single	Titanium	7.4 mm/ 16.5 mm	5.6 g	6.6 mm	5.6 mm	1 mm/ 1.9 mm	0.2 mL	Attached, antecubital insertion/ Cath Finder System
Port-A-Cath (Pharmacia)	Single, dual	Titanium	13.5 mm/ 25 mm	16 g	1.4 mm	5.5 mm	1.5 mm/ 2.8 mm	0.5 mL	Detached
Q-Port (Quinton)	Single	Stainless steel, silicone	12.2 mm/ 31.8 mm	28.8 g	6.4 mm	6.4 mm	1.5 mm/ 3.2 mm	0.6 mL	Detached or attached, bayonet lock
Sea Port (Harbor Medical)	Single, dual, skin parallel	Titanium, catheter coated with Anthron	12 mm/ 40 mm	17 g	19.1 mm	5.1 mm	1.42 mm/ 3.0 mm	0.8 mL	Detached or attached
Vasport (Gish Corporation)	Single	Fluoropolymer titanium	14.0 mm/ 31.7 mm	9.7 mm	12.4 mm	6.7 mm	1.6 mm/ 4.6 mm	1.47 mL	Silicone anchor lock rings, detached or attached
Sea Port (Harbor Medical)	Side and top entry	Titanium	14 mm/ 32 mm	15 g	19.1 mm	6.1 mm	1.5 mm/ 2.3 mm	.55 mL	Attached

Source: From "Advanced Central Venous Access: Selection, Catheters, Devices, and Nursing Management" by D. Camp-Sorrell, 1990, *Journal of Intravenous Nursing*, 13, p 364. Copyright 1990 by the Intravenous Nurses Society. Reprinted by permission.

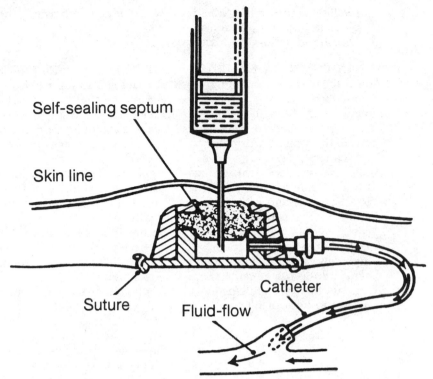

Self-sealing septum

Skin line

Suture

Fluid-flow

Catheter

Figure 12–12 ☐ Cross-section of the subcutaneous port showing fluid injection. (Courtesy of Pharmacia Deltec, Inc., St. Paul, Minnesota.)

Accessing the Port

This is a sterile procedure (Fig. 12–12).

1. Using nonsterile gloves, begin by palpating the port to find the entry septum.
2. Using povidone iodine swab, clean the injection site. Start at the center of the septum and swab outward in a circular motion until you have cleaned an area of at least 6 in in diameter. *Do not retouch site.*
3. Repeat this cleaning technique twice, using a new swab each time.
4. Put on sterile gloves.
5. Attach a 6-mL syringe of heparin solution to the stopcock at the end of the extension tubing.
6. *Connect the appropriate gauge noncoring right-angle needle* to the Luer lock at the other end and prime the tubing.
7. Palpate the port to find the center of the septum.
8. Insert a (Huber) noncoring right-angle needle into the center, pushing until the needle stops.
9. Aspirate a small amount of blood to check for patency and position.
10. Using a firm steady pressure, flush the port with approximately 10 mL of sodium chloride solution at the rate of less than 5 mL/minute. If

457

swelling occurs or the patient complains of pain or burning, the needle is improperly positioned.
11. Disconnect syringe and discard.

12A. INJECTING A BOLUS

Attach the syringe containing the prescribed drug.

Slowly inject the medication.

Disconnect the syringe to prevent any of the drug from dripping on the patient's skin.

Attach the second 10-mL syringe of saline solution and flush the injection port and catheter.

Disconnect the syringe and discard.

Attach 5-mL syringe of heparin solution and inject all 5 mL to prevent occlusion at the catheter tip.

Withdraw the needle, being careful not to twist or tilt.

Observe the injection site for signs of extravasation.

Use alcohol swabs, moving in a circular motion from the center of the port out to the povidone iodine from the skin.

12B. CONTINUOUS INFUSION

Prepare site as for a bolus.

Access the site as for a bolus.

Roll a sterile 2 × 2 gauze pad and place carefully under the needle hub and Luer lock to support the needle.

Apply tincture of benzoin to the skin on both sides of the gauze pad to help the Steri-Strips adhere.

Secure the needle and tubing by applying the Steri-Strips across the hub, using a chevron taping technique.

Apply transparent dressing over the entire system.

Attach the stopcock to the I.V. line from the infusion pump.

Tape all connections, unless using Luer-lock connections.

Note: I.V. tubing must be changed every 24 hours.

Note: Change the dressing every 4 to 7 days.

Note: Change extension tubing with needle every 4 to 7 days.

13. When infusion concluded, inject the saline and disconnect the syringe. Then attach a 10-mL syringe of heparin solution to the stopcock and flush the port.
14. Withdraw the noncoring needle without twisting or tilting.
15. Remove the tincture of benzoin with alcohol and apply a small bandage if necessary (Vialal, 1990; Pharmacia Deltec, 1989).

Flushing

Flushing procedures vary from institution to institution. Flush the system with 5 mL of heparinized saline in a 10-mL syringe. If the port is not being used, flush with heparinized saline every 4 weeks. If the port is used for medication administration or blood component therapy, the port must be flushed after every infusion (Pharmacia Deltec, 1989).

BLOOD SAMPLING

1. Insert noncoring needle attached to extension tubing and secure needle with tape.
2. Release clamp and flush with 5 mL of normal saline to confirm that fluid flows through the system.
3. Withdraw at least 3 mL of blood, clamp tubing, and discard syringe and blood.
4. Attach syringe and release clamp. Withdraw desired amount of blood for sampling.
5. Clamp tube and attach syringe with 2 mL of heparinized saline. Release clamp and flush system.
6. Clamp tube and attach syringe with 20 mL of normal saline. Release clamp and flush system.
7. Clamp tube and attach syringe with 5 mL of heparinized saline.
8. Release clamp and flush system, leaving a heparin lock (Pharmacia Deltec, 1989).

Potential Complications

The same complications associated with central venous tunneled catheters can occur with the implanted port.

1. **Site infection or breakdown:** The port site must be regularly assessed by nurse, patient, or family for redness, swelling, drainage, or breaks in skin integrity; any significant findings must be promptly reported to the physician.
2. **Sepsis:** This is a potential problem; any temperature elevations need to be reported.
3. **Thrombosis:** Any pain and tenderness in the neck, shoulder, and arm on the port side of the body must be reported, as these symptoms could indicate thrombosis.
4. **Clot formation:** The catheter portion and port of this system could be a potential site for clot formation, especially if used for blood withdrawal. Any difficulty in flushing can indicate a clot. This also must be reported to the physician or nurse as soon as it is detected.
5. **Air embolism:** When the implanted port is not in use, risk of air embolism does not exist. However, when the port has been accessed there is now a direct route from the outside to the patient's central circulation. The risks during access are the same as for other central venous catheters.
6. **Port migration:** The port is sutured in place but can move out of position if one or more sutures becomes loose. The patient and family are advised to report any difficulty in accessing the port.
7. **Extravasation:** If the special needle is not in place through the septum of the port and the position is not confirmed, fluid can extravasate and collect subcutaneously, resulting in burning or swelling around the port during infusion. Patients and nurses must always verify placement, secure needle before initiating the infusion, and observe for signs of swelling or burning.

✎ **KEY POINTS IN CARE OF THE IMPLANTED PORT**
  1. Use only *noncoring* needle for access.
  2. Change needle and extension tubing every 7 days.
  3. Flushing procedure: Flush port with normal saline and heparin every 4 weeks if port is not in use. Flush port after every infusion following procedure outlined.
  4. If continuous infusion, change dressing every 72 hours.
  5. If continuous infusion, change tubing every 24 hours.

✎ **Note:** Patient education—encourage patient to carry an identification card with information regarding implanted port.

Summary Worksheet: Central Line Management

Directions: Using this worksheet as a summary table, fill in the nursing management of each of these lines.

CENTRAL LINE	FLUSHING PROCEDURE	KEY POINTS IN MANAGEMENT
Percutaneous catheter		
Peripherally inserted central catheter		
Hickman/Broviac (tunneled) catheter		
Groshong (tunneled) catheter		
Implanted port		

PHYSICAL ASSESSMENT (CENTRAL LINES)

The nurse must use a systems approach to assess for both local and systemic complications associated with the insertion and maintenance of a central line. The nursing assessment should include infusion rate, intake and output, and an awareness of agency policy and procedure to prevent complications associated with particular lines and infusions. The following body systems should be assessed at the beginning of each shift and as needed to monitor the patient's reactions to infusions. Symptoms listed with each system may indicate local problems or life-threatening complications.

NEUROMUSCULAR
Change in level of consciousness
Confusion
Complaints of pain
Paresthesia of the neck, shoulder, or extremities
Paralysis of the neck, shoulder, or extremities

Muscle weakness

CARDIOVASCULAR
Increased or decreased blood pressure
Increased heart rate
Irregular pulse
Bleeding from the site

461

NURSING DIAGNOSES RELATED TO CENTRAL VENOUS ACCESS DEVICES

1. Anxiety (mild, moderate, severe), related to threat to or change in health status; misconceptions regarding therapy
2. Altered tissue perfusion (cardiopulmonary), related to infiltration of vesicant medication
3. Body image disturbance related to perceptions of VAD
4. Decreased cardiac output related to sepsis, contamination
5. Fear related to insertion of catheter; fear of "needles"
6. Fluid volume excess related to infusion of isotonic and hypertonic solutions
7. Hyperthermia related to increased metabolic rate, sepsis
8. Impaired gas exchange related to ventilation perfusion imbalance; dislodged VAD
9. Impaired skin integrity related to venous access device; irritating I.V. solution; inflammation; infection
10. Impaired physical mobility related to pain or discomfort resulting from placement and maintenance of VAD
11. Impaired tissue integrity related to altered circulation; leakage, extravasation, infiltration, or infection of VAD
12. Knowledge deficit (VAD and maintenance of I.V. solution) relating to lack of exposure
13. Pain related to physical trauma (e.g., catheter insertion)
14. Risk of infection related to broken skin or traumatized tissue from the VAD

RESPIRATORY
Shortness of breath
Cyanosis
Respiratory distress

RENAL
Decreased urinary output
Variance between intake and output

INTEGUMENTARY
Fever

Drainage at insertion site
Change in skin color
Sensation of heat at or near insertion site
Bruising around or near insertion site
Sluggish flow rate
Backflow absent
Coolness of the skin

SPECIAL SENSE
Burning sensation

SUMMARY OF CHAPTER 12

CENTRAL VENOUS ACCESS DEVICES

DEFINITION OF KEY TERMS
CVC = Central venous catheter
CVTC = Central venous device
VAD = Vascular access device
PICC = Peripherally inserted central catheter

Anatomy of Vascular System

Venous network for access for peripherally inserted central catheters are basilic, cephalic, and median antecubital.

ANATOMIC VEINS IN CHEST
Subclavian vein
Right and left brachiocephalic veins
External jugular vein
Internal jugular vein
Right and left innominate veins
Superior vena cava (which receives all blood from upper half of body)

CATHETER MATERIALS
Silicone elastomer
Polyurethane
Polyvinylchloride
Teflon

Lumens

These vary in gauge: Single, double, and triple.

SHORT-TERM ACCESS DEVICES
Percutaneous catheters
Peripherally inserted central catheters

LONG-TERM ACCESS DEVICES
Tunneled catheters
Implanted ports

DRESSING MANAGEMENT OF PERCUTANEOUS CATHETERS
Elastoplast dressing (change every 48 to 72 hours)
TSM dressing (change every 4 to 7 days)

PICC
Placement by certified registered nurse
Material: Silicone

Site: Peripheral, preferably basilic vein

Advantages: Decrease in risk factors associated with subclavian placements such as hemothorax, pneumothorax, and air embolism

Cost effective

Appropriate for home care

Disadvantages: Nurse must have special training, daily care is required, catheter maintenance guidelines must be followed to prevent clotting of catheter

Dressing Management

Change initial dressing after 24 hours. Thereafter, apply transparent dressing the same as any TSM central dressing.

Flushing Procedure

SASH procedure should be followed, using 100 U heparin. Use 2 mL of saline followed by 1 mL of heparinized saline. Flush after every medication administration, blood withdrawal, or blood administration. These catheters can clot easily. Maintain the integrity of the catheter.

Declotting

Use urokinase following consent from patient, physician's order, and a clear policy and procedure.

Blood Sampling

Must have a catheter larger than 3.8 F in place for blood withdrawal.

Complications of PICC

INSERTION
Bleeding at site
Tendon damage
Cardiac arrhythmias
Malposition of catheter
Catheter embolism

POSTINSERTION
Phlebitis
Infection
Thrombosis (clot formation)
Air embolism

CENTRAL VENOUS TUNNELED CATHETERS

Material: Polymeric silicone with a Dacron cuff that anchors the catheter in the subcutaneous tissue

Uses: Blood sample drawing, administering medications, blood products, and parenteral nutrition

Available: Single, double, and triple lumen

Advantages: Reparable if torn or catheter breaks, long-term therapy eliminates multiple sticks

Disadvantages: Daily, weekly care of site, cost of maintenance and supplies, surgical procedure, body image may be affected

Complications: Site infection, sepsis, thrombosis, catheter migration, clot formation, torn or leaking catheter, air embolism

Types available: Hickman, Broviac, and Groshong (refer to chart for other manufacturers of CVTCs)

KEY TIPS IN CARE OF HICKMAN/BROVIAC CATHETER

Be sure the catheter is capped at all times.

Keep all sharp objects away from the catheter.

If the catheter leaks or breaks, clamp the catheter between the broken area and exit site using a nonserrated clamp.

Protect the catheter when showering or bathing.

Flush after a blood withdrawal with 10 mL of 0.9% sodium chloride and correct amount of heparin.

Use heparin to maintain patency.

KEY TIPS IN CARE OF GROSHONG CATHETER

Do not clamp the catheter.

Keep all sharp objects away from the catheter.

If the catheter leaks or breaks, cover the broken part with a sterile gauze bandage and tape securely.

Protect the catheter when showering or bathing.

Straining or heavy lifting could cause a small amount of blood to back up into the catheter.

After blood sampling, flush with 20 mL of normal saline.

Implanted Ports

Material: Silicone catheter with a central septum made of titanium or steel

Uses: Blood sampling, medication administration, blood products, and parenteral nutrition

Available: Single or double septum

Advantages: Less risk of infection, less interference with daily activities, little site care needed, minimal flushing needed, less body image disturbance, few limitations on patient activity

Disadvantages: Cost of insertion, postoperative care 7 to 10 days, discomfort of repeated needle sticks, minor surgical procedure necessary to remove device

Complications: Site infection or breakdown, sepsis, thrombosis, clot formation, air embolism, port migration, extravasation of fluid

KEY POINTS IN CARE

Only use noncoring needle for access.

Change needle and extension tubing every 7 days.

Flush port with normal saline and heparin every 4 weeks if port is not in use. Flush port after every infusion following procedure outlined.

Tubing and dressing management only necessary with continuous use.

Drug Tip: Urokinase

Use: I.V. catheter fibrinolytic
Dose: 5000 IU in 1 mL specifically diluted solution
Technique: Insert drug into catheter; attempt every 5 minutes for 30 minutes to withdraw the clot. Reattempt after 1 hour. (Clots can usually be removed in 30 minutes to 3 hours.)

IMPLANTED PORTS
Advantages

Less risk of infection
Better self-image
No limitations on patient activity
Little site care

Disadvantages

Cost of insertion higher than other catheters
Discomfort when port accessed repeatedly through the skin
Minor surgical procedure to remove the port

Flushing: 5 mL of heparinized saline in 10-mL syringe. Flush after every use. If port not in use, flush every 4 weeks.

Activity Journal

1. As a new graduate you have been asked to change a complicated abdominal dressing on a patient postoperatively. The patient has a Hickman tunneled catheter. As you are cutting the dressing off, you accidently puncture the catheter. What do you do? How could this have been avoided?

2. Check the flushing of central lines policy and procedure at the agency where you are working. Does the procedure clearly give steps in the flushing of a Hickman catheter, Groshong catheter, and the implanted port?

3. You attempt to flush the recently inserted PICC line in order to administer the next dose of antibiotics. The line does not flush, and resistance is felt. What do you do?

4. You are the charge nurse, and a newly employed registered nurse assertively states she will insert the new PICC order on her patient because she has put in many in her former job. How do you handle this situation?

Quality Assessment Model

Instructions: Use this quality assessment model to conduct retrospective audits of charts, establish quality control standards, or develop outcome criteria for quality assurance. Refer to Chapter 2 for details on quality assessment.

STRUCTURE

(Resource that affects outcome)
Human Resource: Registered Nurse

↓

PROCESS

(Actual giving and receiving of care)
Therapist activities related to quality and integrity of central venous catheters:

1. Follow institutional policy regarding flushing the central venous access device.
2. Dressing change for the Elastoplast dressing is every 48 to 72 hours.
3. Dressing change for the transparent dressing is every 4 to 7 days.
4. Keep all sharp objects away from the central catheter.
5. Use sterile technique whenever flushing, changing dressing, or changing injection cap or accessing device.
6. Flush the catheter or port thoroughly after blood withdrawal.
7. Observe site for effects of local complications every shift.
8. Use only noncoring needles to access implanted ports.

↓

OUTCOME STANDARDS

(Effects of care)
Documentation will reflect standards of practice for delivery of safe, practical care of the patient with special needs:

1. Evidence of documented site checks every shift.
2. Evidence of documented flushing procedure, as appropriate for central venous device and institutional policy.
3. Evidence of documented dressing change in accordance with type of dressing used.
4. Evidence of signed patient consent, physician's order, and documented steps for declotting a central device with urokinase.

469

Post-test, Chapter 12

Match the following definitions in column 2 to the correct term in column 1.

Column 1

1. _____ Extravascular malpositioning
2. _____ Intravascular malpositioning
3. _____ Lymphedema
4. _____ Distal
5. _____ Cutdown

Column 2

A. Swelling of extremity caused by obstruction of lymphatic vessels

B. Farthest from heart

C. Passage of introducer into the pleural space or mediastinum instead of superior vena cava

D. Surgical procedure for exposure of a vein for cannulation

E. Advancement of catheter tip into venous tributary other than superior vena cava

True-False

6. **T F** The term central venous catheter refers to a catheter placed in the central chest vasculature, usually the superior vena cava.

7. **T F** The basilic vein is an appropriate choice for cannulation of the PICC.

8. **T F** Elastoplast dressings over percutaneous right atrial catheters should be changed every 4 to 7 days, based on agency policy.

9. **T F** The dressing over a new PICC line should be changed after 24 hours, and a TSM dressing applied.

10. **T F** Implanted ports must be accessed with noncoring needles.

11. Implanted ports, when not in use, can be flushed every:
    A. Week
    B. 2 weeks
    C. 3 weeks
    D. 4 weeks

12. A major complication of short-term central venous access devices is:
    A. Infiltration
    B. Intravascular and extravascular malpositioning
    C. Thrombosis
    D. Pulmonary edema

13. When tunneled catheters are used the advantages to the patient include:
    A. The catheter remains patent without flushing procedures.
    B. The catheter can be replaced easily.
    C. The catheter can be used for multiple purposes.
    D. The catheter causes minimal change in body image.

14. The drug of choice for declotting a clotted short-term or long-term device is:
    A. Wydase
    B. Urokinase
    C. Monoamine oxidase
    D. Acetylcholinesterase

470

15. Identify three of the seven complications of tunneled catheters:

A. _____

B. _____

C. _____

16. List the seven key points in care of the Hickman/Broviac tunneled catheter.

17. List the seven key points in care of the Groshong catheter.

18. Describe the procedure to access an implanted port for injecting a bolus.

Answers to Post-test, Chapter 12

1. C
2. E
3. A
4. B
5. D
6. T
7. T
8. T
9. T
10. T
11. D
12. B
13. C
14. B
15. A. Skin infection
    B. Sepsis
    C. Thrombosis
    D. Catheter migration
    E. Clot formation
    F. Torn or leaking catheter
    G. Air embolism
16. A. Be sure catheter is clamped at all times.
    B. Keep sharp objects away from catheter.
    C. If the catheter leaks or breaks, clamp immediately between broken area and the exit site. Cover with sterile gauze.
    D. Protect the catheter when showering or bathing.
    E. Use 10 mL of saline and heparin after blood withdrawal.
    F. Heparin must be used to keep catheter free of clots.
    G. Encourage patient to carry an identification card.
17. A. Do not clamp the catheter.
    B. Keep all sharp objects away from the catheter.
    C. If the catheter leaks or breaks, cover with sterile gauze and tape securely.
    D. Protect the catheter when showering or bathing.
    E. Straining or heavy lifting could cause a small amount of blood to back up into the catheter. If blood is evident in the catheter line, flush.
    F. After blood sample is obtained, flush briskly with 20 mL of saline.
    G. Encourage patients to carry an identification card with them.
18. A. Sterile procedure must be followed.
    B. Palpate port with sterile gloves.
    C. Use povidone iodine swabs to clean injection site: start at septum and swab outward to 6 in. Repeat three times.
    D. Attach a 6-mL syringe of heparin solution to the stopcock at the end of the extension tubing.
    E. Connect the appropriate noncoring needle to the Luer lock at the other end and prime the tubing.
    F. Put on fresh pair of sterile gloves.
    G. Palpate the port to find the center of the septum.
    H. Insert a noncoring (Huber) needle.
    I. Aspirate a small amount of blood to check for patency and position.

References

Bjeletich, J. (1987). Declotting central venous catheters with urokinase in the home by nurse clinicians. *National Intravenous Therapy Association, 10*(6), 428–430.

Bridges, B.B., Carden, E., & Takac, F.A. (1979). Introduction of central venous pressure catheters through arm veins with a high success rate. *Canadian Anaesthesia Society Journal, 26,* 128–131.

Brown, J.M. (1989). Peripherally inserted central catheter use in home care. *Journal of Intravenous Nursing, 12*(3), 144–150.

Camp, D.L. (1988). Care of the Groshong catheter. *Oncology Nursing Forum, 15*(6), 745–748.

Camp-Sorrell, D.L. (1990). Advanced central venous access selection of catheters, devices and nursing management. *Journal of Intravenous Nursing, 13*(6), 361–368.

Eisenberg, P.G., Howard, P., & Gianino, S. (1990). Improved long-term maintenance of central venous catheters with a new dressing technique. *Journal of Intravenous Nursing, 13*(5), 279–284.

Gahart, B.L. (1991). *Intravenous medications* (7th ed.). St. Louis: C.V. Mosby-Year Book.

Gray, H. (1977). *Anatomy, descriptive and surgical.* New York: Crown.

Goodwin, M.L. (1991). Using sodium bicarbonate to clear a medication precipitate from a central venous catheter. *Journal of Vascular Access Networks, 1*(2), 23.

Hadaway, L.C. (1989). Evaluation and use of advanced I.V. technology. Part I: Central venous access devices. *Journal of Intravenous Nursing, 12*(2), 73–81.

Hadaway, L.C. (1990). An overview of vascular access devices inserted via the antecubital area. *Journal of Intravenous Nursing, 13*(5), 297–306.

Handy, C.M. (1989). Vascular access devices hospital to home care. *Journal of Intravenous Nursing, 12*(1), S10–S18.

Heimbach, D.M., & Ivey, T.D. (1976). Technique for placement of a permanent home hyperalimentation catheter. *Gynecology Obstetrics, 143,* 634–646.

Intravenous Nursing Society. (1990). *Standards for practice.* Philadelphia: J.B. Lippincott.

Kyle, K.S., & Myers, J.S. (1990). PICC development of a hospital-based program. *Journal of Intravenous Nursing, 13*(5), 287–290.

Lawson, M. (1991). Partial occlusion of indwelling central venous catheters. *Journal of Intravenous Nursing, 14*(3), 157–159.

Lum, P.S., & Soski, M. (1989). Management of malpositioned central venous catheters. *Journal of Intravenous Nursing, 12*(6), 356–365.

Maki, D.G. (1988). An attachable silver-impregnated cuff for prevention of infection with central venous catheters: A prospective randomized multicenter trial. *American Journal of Medicine, 85,* 307–314.

Maki, D.G., & Wells, J. (1984). Colonization and infection associated with transparent dressings for central venous catheters: A comparison trial. Abstract paper presented at National APIC conference, Washington, DC.

Masoorli, S., & Angeles, T. (1990). PICC lines: The latest home care challenge. *RN, 1,* 44–50.

McIntyre, P.B., & Laidlow, J.M. (1982). *Lancet, 2,* 936.

Pemberton, L.B. (1986). Sepsis for triple-vs-single lumen catheters during total parenteral nutrition in surgical or critically ill patients. *Archives of Surgery, 12*(5), 591–593.

Pharmacia Deltec. (1989). *Clinician information PORT-A-CATH and P.A.S. PORT implantable access devices.* St Paul: Pharmacia Deltec.

Plumer, A.L., & Cosentino, F. (1987). *Principles and practices of intravenous therapy.* Philadelphia: J.B. Lippincott.

Riser, S. (1988). Patient care manual for implanted vascular access devices. *Journal of Intravenous Nursing, 11*(3), 166–168.

Roundtree, D. (1991). The PIC catheters: A different approach. *American Journal of Nursing, 91*(8), 22–27.

Ryan, J.A., & Gough, J. (1984). Complication of central venous catheterization for total parenteral nutrition — the role of the nurse. *National Intravenous Therapy Association, 8*(1), 29–35.

Schwartz-Fulton, J., Colley, R., & Valanis, B. (1981). Hyperalimentation dressings and skin flora. *National Intravenous Therapy Association, 4*(5), 354–357.

Speer, E.W. (1990). Central venous catheterization: Issues associated with the use of single-multiple lumen catheters. *Journal of Intravenous Nursing, 13*(1), 30–39.

Stewart, R.D., & Sanislow, G.A. (1961). Silastic intravenous catheter. *New England Journal of Medicine, 265*, 1238–1285.

Testerman, E.J. (1991). Restoring patency of central venous catheters obstructed by mineral precipitation using hydrochloric acid. *Journal of Vascular Access Networks, 1*(2), 22–23.

Vasquez, R.M. (1980). Subclavian catheterization. *American Journal of Intravenous Therapy & Clinical Nutrition, 80*(5), 11–29.

Viall, C.D. (1990a). Daily access of implanted venous ports: Implications for patient education. *Journal of Intravenous Nursing, 13*(5), 294–296.

Bibliography

Bagnall, H., & Ruccinoe, K. (1987). Experience with a totally implanted venous access device in children with malignant disease. *Oncology Nursing Forum, 14*(4), 51–56.

Goodwin, M.L. (1989). The Seldinger method for PICC insertion. *Journal of Intravenous Nursing, 12*(4), 238–243.

Holder, C., & Alexander, J. (1990). A new and improved guide to I.V. therapy. *American Journal of Nursing, 90*(2), 43–47.

I.V. Management Services. (1990). *PICC: Care, use and maintenance.* Salines: I.V. Management Services.

Markel, S., & Reynen, K. (1990). Impact on patient care 2652 PIC catheter days in the alternative setting. *Journal of Intravenous Nursing, 13*(6), 347–352.

May, G.S., & Davis, C. (1988). Percutaneous catheters and totally implantable access systems. A review of reported infection rates. *Journal of Intravenous Nursing, 11*(2), 97–103.

Perez, K. (1982). Nursing management of the Hickman Broviac catheters. *National Intravenous Therapy Association, 5*(3), 210–212.

Rutherford, C. (1989). Insertion and care of multiple lumen peripherally inserted central line catheters. *Journal of Intravenous Nursing, 11*(1), 16–20.

Schmidt, A.M., & Williams, D. (1982). The Hickman catheter: Sending your patient home safely. *RN, 2,* 57–61.

Speciale, J.L. (1985). Infuse-A-Port: New path for I.V. chemotherapy. *Nursing 85, 10,* 40–43.

Viall, C.D. (1990b). Your complete guide to central venous catheters. *Nursing 90, 2,* 34–41.

Wilson, J.M. (1983). Right atrial catheters (Broviac and Hickman): Indications, insertion, maintenances and protocol for home care. *National Intravenous Therapy Association, 6*(1), 23–26.

Nutritional Support

CHAPTER 13

Nutritional Support

CHAPTER 13 CONTENTS

Glossary

Amino acids: Chief organic component of protein

Anergy: Lack of immune response to an antigen

Anthropometry: Measurement of a part or whole of the body

BCAA: Branched chain amino acid

Central parenteral nutrition: Total nutritional support via a central venous access device, tunneled catheter, implanted port, or subclavian entry

C-TPN: Cyclic total parenteral nutrition

EFAD: Essential fatty acid deficiency

Fat emulsion: Natural product consisting of a mixture of neutral triglycerides of predominantly unsaturated fatty acids; permits inclusion of fat calories in the intravenous nutritional regimen

HTPN: Home total parenteral therapy

Kwashiorkor: Malnutrition characterized by an adequate calorie intake with inadequate amount of protein

Marasmus: Malnutrition characterized by decreased intake of calories with adequate amounts of protein intake

Peripheral parenteral nutrition: Nutritional support via a peripheral vein; glucose limited to 10 percent

Total parenteral nutrition: Nutritional support supplying glucose, protein, vitamins, electrolytes, trace elements, and sometimes fats to maintain body's growth, development, and tissue repair

LEARNING OBJECTIVES

Upon completion of this chapter, the reader will be able to:

☐ Define all terminology related to nutritional support

☐ Identify the key elements of a nutritional assessment

☐ List the six nutrients essential for total parenteral nutrition

☐ Identify the key points in administration of glucose, protein, and fat emulsions

☐ Describe the three major classifications of malnutrition

☐ Identify early candidates for total parenteral nutrition

☐ Describe the use of the additives heparin, insulin, and cimetidine to parenteral nutrition

☐ Describe three-in-one solutions

☐ List the key concepts of cyclic therapy

☐ Identify the total parenteral nutrition treatment plan for the patient with renal or liver disease

☐ Identify key concepts of peripheral parenteral nutrition

☐ State nursing considerations related to delivery of total parenteral nutrition
☐ Identify the complications related to total parenteral nutrition
☐ Determine nursing diagnoses appropriate for patients receiving nutritional support

Pre-test, Chapter 13

Instructions: The pre-test is to review prior knowledge of the theory of nutritional support. Each question in the pre-test is based on the learning objectives.

Match the definitions in column 2 to the correct term in column 1.

Column 1

1. _____ EFAD

2. _____ Anergy

3. _____ Amino acids

4. _____ Ketone bodies

5. _____ Fat emulsion

Column 2

A. Mixture of neutral triglycerides to provide fat calories

B. Lack of immune response to an antigen

C. Chief organic component of protein

D. Essential fatty acid deficiency

E. Substances formed by liver as a step in the combustion of fats

6. The most common carbohydrate used for parenteral nutrition is:
   A. Fructose
   B. Lactose
   C. Dextrose
   D. Invert sugar

7. Parenteral proteins are supplied as:
   A. Synthetic crystalline amino acids
   B. Casein amino acids
   C. Immunoglobulins

8. To treat or prevent essential fatty acid deficiency, _____ is (are) administered:
   A. Protein
   B. 10% dextrose
   C. Fat emulsion
   D. Trace elements

9. During times of stress _____ metabolism is radically altered.
   A. Protein
   B. Fat
   C. Carbohydrate
   D. Vitamin C

10. Which of the following medications may be added to total parenteral solutions?
    A. Regular insulin, heparin, and cimetidine
    B. Iron, vitamin K, and cimetidine
    C. Iron, heparin, and neutral protamine Hagedorn (NPH) insulin
    D. Regular insulin, vitamin K, and cimetidine

11. A solution of three-in-one refers to the combination of _____,
    _____, and _____ in one solution container.
    A. Fat emulsion, dextrose, amino acids
    B. Fat emulsion, vitamins, electrolytes
    C. Fat emulsion, heparin, insulin
    D. Dextrose, amino acids, trace elements

12. Components of a nutritional assessment include:
    A. Dietary history
    B. Anthropometric measurements
    C. Diagnostic tests
    D. Physical examination
    E. All of the above

13. Total parenteral nutrition includes which of the following key elements?
    A. Carbohydrates
    B. Protein
    C. Fats
    D. Electrolytes and vitamins
    E. All of the above

14. Three-in-one solutions consist of a combination of:
    A. Platelets, plasma, and white blood cells
    B. Fats, carbohydrates, and protein
    C. Fats, electrolytes, and trace elements

15. The purpose of heparin added to the total parenteral nutrition solution is to:
    A. Enhance blood glucose levels
    B. Thin the total parenteral nutrition solution, so that it infuses easily
    C. Decrease the incidence of subclavian vein thrombosis

16. The key points in delivery of cyclic therapy include:
    A. This therapy is indicated for patients receiving stabilized continuous total
       parenteral nutrition.
    B. This therapy is indicated for long-term parenteral nutrition.
    C. Cyclic total parenteral nutrition must be escalated to maintenance rate and
       tapered off gradually to avoid abrupt changes in glucose levels.
    D. All of the above.

17. Patients with liver disease have elevated levels of aromatic amino acids and
    depressed levels of branch chain amino acids. These patients require a total
    parenteral nutrition protein component that is:
    A. High in aromatic amino acids
    B. Equal in aromatic and branch chain amino acids
    C. High in branch chain amino acids

18. Criteria for peripheral parenteral nutrition include:
    A. Good venous access
    B. No fluid restrictions
    C. Ability to tolerate fat emulsion therapy
    D. Expectation that patient will resume enteral feeding within 5 to 7 days
    E. All of the above

479

ANSWERS TO PRE-TEST, Chapter 13

1. D   2. B   3. C   4. E   5. A   6. C   7. A   8. C   9. C

10. A   11. A   12. E   13. E   14. B   15. C

16. D   17. C   18. E

> Every careful observer of the sick will agree in this that thousands of
> patients are annually starved in the midst of plenty, from want of
> attention to the ways which alone make it possible for them to take food.
>
> Florence Nightingale, 1859

This chapter introduces the reader to care of the patient with **total parenteral nutritional** (TPN) support, covering nutritional assessment and concepts of peripheral and central parenteral nutrition. Nursing considerations in caring for the patient on nutritional support are strongly emphasized.

Nutritional support nursing is the care of individuals with potential or known nutritional alterations. "Nurses who specialize in nutritional support use specific expertise to enhance the maintenance and/or restoration of an individual's nutritional health" (American Society for Parenteral and Enteral Nutrition [ASPEN], 1988b).

Nutrition support nursing encompasses all nursing activities that promote optimal nutritional health. Nursing interventions are based on scientific principles. The scope of practice includes but is not limited to direct patient care; consultation with nurses and other health professionals in a variety of clinical settings; education of patients, students, colleagues, and the public; participation in research; and administrative functions (ASPEN, 1988b).

NUTRITIONAL ASSESSMENT

A nutritional assessment of high-risk patients supplies the physician and nurse with invaluable information regarding a patient's nutritional status. The nutritional assessment (Table 13–1) encompasses routine history taking with emphasis on dietary history, anthropometric measurements, diagnostic testing, and a complete physical examination (Farley, 1991).

History

The history is divided up into three major components: medical, social, and dietary. The medical history should include a specific history of weight, chronic diseases, past surgical history; presence of increased losses, such as from draining wounds and fistulas; and factors such as age and drug, alcohol, and tobacco usage. The social history affecting nutrient intake includes income, education, ethnic background, and environment during mealtime, along with re-

Table 13–1 □ **NUTRITIONAL ASSESSMENT**

1. History
      Medical
      Social
      Dietary
2. Anthropometric measurements
      Skinfolds
      Height and weight
      Midarm circumference
      Midarm muscle circumference
3. Diagnostic tests
      Anergy tests
      Total lymphocyte count
      Serum protein measurement
      Urine assays (creatinine, height index)
4. Physical examination

ligious considerations (Kennedy-Caldwell & Guenter, 1988, p 34). The dietary history often provides clues as to the cause and degree of malnutrition. The components of a dietary history include appetite, gastrointestinal (GI) disturbances, mechanical problems such as ill-fitting dentures, food allergies, medications, and food likes and dislikes (Farley, 1991).

Anthropometric Measurements

Anthropometry is the measurement of a part or whole of the body. This is a method of determining body composition. To estimate the size of the body fat mass, a skinfold test is done on the triceps of the nondominant arm using a caliper. Along with the skinfold measurement, a midarm circumference and midarm muscle circumference evaluation is performed. The height and weight are also part of this evaluation, with serial weights providing helpful information related to the protein-calorie status of the person. To calculate the current weight as a percentage of the usual weight, use the following calculation:

% usual weight = [Current weight ÷ usual weight] × 100

✎ **Note:** Mild malnutrition = 85 to 95 percent
      Moderate malnutrition = 75 to 84 percent
      Severe malnutrition = less than 75 percent (Kennedy-Caldwell & Guenter, 1988, p 37)

Diagnostic Tests

Several diagnostic tests are available to assess nutritional status. The **anergy** test, which is recommended for assessment of immunologic response, involves the intradermal injection of antigens. Proper nutrition is a key to an intact im-

481

mune system; a lack of response to antigens is considered anergic and therefore possibly indicates malnourishment. Total lymphocyte count is also measured for the body's response immunologically. Serum protein measurements, which may indicate nutritional status, include albumin, transferrin, and prealbumin tests (Farley, 1991). Radiologic findings as evidenced by osteoporosis, osteomalacia scurvy, and hypervitaminosis with widened sutures in the skull can help determine severe prolonged deficiencies or excesses (Kennedy-Caldwell & Guenter, 1988, p 39).

Physical Examination

The final phase of nutritional assessment is a complete physical examination. The findings from a physical examination can reflect protein-calorie malnutrition along with vitamin and mineral deficiencies. The physical examination should include evaluation of the hair, nails, skin, eyes, oral cavity, glands, heart, muscles, and abdomen, along with a neurologic assessment and an evaluation of delayed healing and tissue repair. Refer to Table 13–2 for the physical findings associated with deficiency states.

NUTRITIONAL REQUIREMENTS

Basic Formula Design

The basic formula must contain all essential macronutrients and micronutrients for adequate energy production, support of synthesis, replacement and repair of structural or visceral proteins, cell structure, production of hormones and enzymes, and maintenance of immune function. The basic design contains carbohydrates, protein, fat, electrolytes, vitamins, trace elements, and water (Table 13–3).

The intravenous (I.V.) source of carbohydrate is predominantly dextrose. Carbohydrate calories can also be provided by glycerol, sorbitol, or fructose. These are considered nondextrose carbohydrate sources and do not require insulin for metabolism; however, these nondextrose carbohydrates may require more energy in the metabolism process.

✎ **Note:** 1 g CHO = 4 kilocalories (kcal).

Protein hydrolysate solutions of either casein or fibrin origin were used initially for parenteral nutrition. Because of their high ammonia content and unfavorable microbial growth characteristics, these products have been replaced by synthetic amino acids. Modifications of amino acid have been recommended in situations of renal or liver disease.

✎ **Note:** Protein requirement for an adult is 0.8 g/kg per day. In disease states, this should be increased to 1 to 3 g/kg per day.

The use of I.V. fat has increased in recent years because of decreased cost and greater availability of the product. When fat is used as a calorie source in parenteral nutrition, there is less of a problem with glucose homeostasis, carbon dioxide (CO_2) production is lower, and hepatic tolerance to I.V. feedings

Table 13–2 □ **PHYSICAL FINDINGS ASSOCIATED WITH DEFICIENCY STATES**

Physical Findings	Associated Deficiencies
Hair, Nails	
Flag sign (transverse depigmentation of hair)	Protein, copper
Hair easily pluckable	Protein
Hair thin, sparse	Protein, biotin, zinc
Nails spoon-shaped	Iron
Nails lackluster, transverse riding	Protein-calorie
Skin	
Dry, scaling	Vitamin A, zinc, essential fatty acids
Flaky paint dermatosis	Protein
Follicular hyperkeratosis	Vitamins A, C; essential fatty acids
Nasolabial seborrhea	Niacin, pyridoxine, riboflavin
Petechiae, purpura	Ascorbic acid, vitamin K
Pigmentation, desquamation (sun-exposed area)	Niacin (pellagra)
Subcutaneous fat loss	Calorie
Eyes	
Angular blepharitis	Riboflavin
Corneal vascularization	Riboflavin
Dull, dry conjunctiva	Vitamin A
Fundal capillary microaneurysms	Ascorbic acid
Scleral icterus, mild	Pyridoxine
Perioral	
Angular stomatitis	Riboflavin
Cheilosis	Riboflavin
Oral Cavity	
Atrophic lingual papillae	Niacin, iron, riboflavin, folate, vitamin B_{12}
Glossitis (scarlet, raw)	Niacin, pyridoxine, riboflavin, vitamin B_{12}, folate
Hypogeusesthesia (also hyposmia)	Zinc, vitamin A
Magenta tongue	Riboflavin
Swollen, bleeding gums (if teeth present)	Ascorbic acid
Tongue fissuring, edema	Niacin
Glands	
Parotid enlargement	Protein
Sicca syndrome	Ascorbic acid
Thyroid enlargement	Iodine

(*continued*)

Table 13-2 □ **PHYSICAL FINDINGS ASSOCIATED WITH DEFICIENCY STATES — _Continued_**

Physical Findings	Associated Deficiencies
Heart	
Enlargement, tachycardia, high output failure	Thiamine ("wet" beriberi)
Small heart, decreased output	Calorie
Sudden failure, death	Ascorbic acid
Abdomen	
Hepatomegaly	Protein
Muscles, Extremities	
Calf tenderness	Thiamine, ascorbic acid (hemorrhage into muscle)
Edema	Protein, thiamine
Muscle wastage (especially temporal area, dorsum of hand, spine)	Calorie
Bones, Joints	
Bone tenderness (adult)	Vitamin D, calcium, phosphorus (osteomalacia)
Neurologic	
Confabulation, disorientation	Thiamine (Korsakoff's psychosis)
Decreased position and vibratory senses, ataxia	Vitamin B_{12}, thiamine
Decreased tendon reflexes, slowed relaxation phase	Thiamine
Ophthalmoplegia	Thiamine, phosphorus
Weakness, paresthesias, decreased fine tactile sensation	Vitamin B_{12}, pyridoxine, thiamine
Other	
Delayed healing and tissue repair (e.g., wound, infarct, abscess)	Ascorbic acid, zinc, protein

Source: From "Nutritional Assessment of Critically Ill Patients" by J. Morgan, 1984, _Focus on Critical Care, 11_, pp. 32–33. Copyright 1984 by C.V. Mosby Year Book, Inc. Reprinted by permission.

may improve. Primarily I.V. fats are supplied by safflower or soybean oil, with egg yolk phospholipids and glycerol to provide tonicity. Fat emulsions provide 1.1 and 2.0 kcal/mL for the 10% and 20% concentrations, respectively (Lang, 1987, p 120).

✎ **Note:** 1 g of fat = 9 kilocalories.

Table 13-3 □ **CHARACTERISTICS OF PARENTERAL NUTRITION**

Carbohydrates
Protein (amino acids)
Fats
Electrolytes
Vitamins
Trace elements

Carbohydrates

The major purpose of carbohydrate is to provide energy. Carbohydrates also spare body protein. Glucose, when supplied as a nutrient, is stored temporarily in the liver and muscle as glycogen. When glycogen storage capacity is reached, the carbohydrate is stored as fat. When glucose is provided parenterally it is completely bioavailable to the body without any effects of malabsorption (Table 13-4).

When dextrose is administered rapidly the solution acts as an osmotic diuretic and pulls interstitial fluid into the plasma for subsequent renal excretion. The nurse must be aware that when infusing 20 to 50% dextrose solutions the rate must be kept within 10 percent of the prescribed order. The pancreas secretes extra insulin to metabolize infused glucose. If 20 to 50% dextrose is discontinued suddenly, a temporary excess of insulin in the body may cause symptoms of hypoglycemia (Metheny, 1987, pp 151–152).

✎ **Note:** During the critical phase of illness or injury, carbohydrate metabolism is radically altered. Hyperglycemia is a hallmark of stress.

Protein

Protein is a body-building nutrient that functions to promote tissue growth, repair, and replacement of body cells. Protein is also a component in antibodies, scar tissue, and clots. Enzymes, hormones, and carrier substances also require protein for development. Protein contributes to energy needs; however, this is not its major purpose.

The amino acids are the basic unit of protein. The eight essential amino acids for adults are isoleucine, leucine, lysine, methionine, phenylalanine,

Table 13-4 □ **DEXTROSE FLUIDS FOR TOTAL PARENTERAL NUTRITION**

Solution (%)	Kcal/L	mOsm/L
10	340	505
20	680	1010
50	1700	2525
70	2380	3535

threonine, tryptophan, and valine. Parenteral proteins are elemental, providing a synthetic crystalline amino acid that does not cause an antigenic reaction. These proteins are available in concentrations of 3 to 11.4 percent and come with and without electrolytes (Metheny, 1987, p 151). Some amino acid solutions for TPN are presented in Table 13–5.

✎ **Note:** Newborn infants require another amino acid: histadine. Premature infants require cystine and tyrosine also.

Nitrogen balance is achieved when protein synthesis and breakdown are in equilibrium. During critical illness, after trauma, or in conditions of stress, protein requirements are increased. Protein is also needed for wound healing or to replace protein loss via a drain or exudate. Protein-calorie malnutrition can occur in one of three ways:

1. **Marasmus:** This type of malnutrition is caused by a decrease in the intake of calories with adequate protein-to-calorie ratio. In marasmus there is gradual wasting of body fat and skeletal muscle with preservation of visceral proteins. The individual looks emaciated and has decreased anthropometric measurements and anergy to common skin test antigens.

Table 13–5 □ **AMINO ACID FLUIDS FOR TOTAL PARENTERAL NUTRITION**

Solution	Protein Concentration (%)	Nitrogen (g/100 mL)	Osmolarity: mOsm/L
Abbott			
Aminosyn	3.5	0.55	357
Aminosyn II	3.5	0.55	308
Aminosyn	5	0.786	500
Aminosyn II	5	0.786	
Aminosyn	7	1.10	700
Aminosyn II	7	1.10	
Aminosyn	8.5	1.33	850
Aminosyn	10	1.57	873
Aminosyn II	10	1.57	1000
Baxter			
Travasol*	5.5	0.924	575
Travasol*	8.5	1.42	890
Travasol*	10	1.68	970
McGaw			
FreAmine III	3	0.46	300
FreAmine III	8.5	1.42	810
FreAmine III	10	1.57	950
FreAmine III with electrolytes	3	0.46	405

*Fluids are available with or without electrolytes.

2. **Kwashiorkor:** This malnutrition state is characterized by an adequate intake of calories but a poor protein intake. This condition causes visceral protein wasting with preservation of fat and somatic muscle. This is seen during a period of decreased protein intake as seen with liquid diets, fat diets, and long-term use of I.V. fluids containing dextrose. Loss of protein is due to depleted circulating proteins in the albumin. Individuals may appear obese and have adequate anthropometric measurements but decreased visceral proteins and depressed immune function.

3. **Mixed:** In this condition the individual has some aspects of both marasmus and kwashiorkor. The individual presents with skeletal muscle and visceral protein wasting, depleted fat stores, immune incompetence. Individuals appear cachectic and usually are in acute catabolic stress. This mixed protein-calorie disorder has the highest risk of morbidity and mortality.

✎ **Note:** Increased need for protein by the body is usually reflected in an increase in the excretion of urinary nitrogen as evidenced by laboratory values (Delaney & Lauer, 1988, p 196).

✎ **Note:** Protein sparing can be accomplished by administration of 100 to 150 g of carbohydrate daily.

Fats (Lipid Emulsions)

Fat is the primary source of heat and energy. Fat provides twice as many energy calories per gram as either protein or carbohydrate. Fat is essential for structural integrity of all cell membranes. Linoleic acid and linolenic acid are the only fatty acids essential to humans. These two acids prevent essential fatty acid deficiency **(EFAD)**. Linoleic acid is necessary as a precursor of prostaglandins and regulates cholesterol metabolism and maintains integrity of the cell wall. Signs and symptoms of EFAD include desquamating dermatitis, alopecia, brittle nails, delayed wound healing, thrombocytopenia, decreased immunity, and increased capillary fragility. Examples of lipid emulsions are presented in Table 13–6.

Complications associated with EFAD include impaired wound healing, platelet dysfunction, increased susceptibility to infection, and development of fatty liver. In patients with respiratory failure, administration of fat can help decrease CO_2 excretion. The primary purpose of fat emulsions in TPN is to prevent or treat EFAD with infusion of two to three 500-mL bottles of 10 to 20% **fat emulsion** per week (Kennedy-Caldwell & Guenter, 1988, p 70).

✎ **Note:** Use of fat can help control hyperglycemia in stress states.

Electrolytes

Electrolytes are infused either as a component already contained in the amino acid solution or as a separate additive. Electrolytes are available in several salt forms and are added based on patient's metabolic status.

The electrolytes necessary for long-term TPN include potassium, magnesium, calcium, sodium, chloride, and phosphorus. Potassium is needed for the transport of glucose and amino acids across the cell membrane. Approximately

487

Table 13–6 □ **LIPID EMULSIONS FOR TOTAL PARENTERAL NUTRITION**

Manufacturer	Emulsion	Percentages Available	Osmolarity
Abbott			
Liposyn III 10%	50/50 safflower oil, soybean oil	10% (1.1 kcal/mL)	284
Liposyn III 20%	50/50 safflower oil, soybean oil	20% (2.0 kcal/mL)	292
Baxter			
Intralipid 10%	Soybean oil	10% (1.1 kcal/mL)	280
Intralipid 20%	Soybean oil	20% (2.0 kcal/mL)	330
McGaw			
NutriLipid 10%	Soybean oil	10% (1.1 kcal/mL)	280
NutriLipid 20%	Soybean oil	20% (2.0 kcal/mL)	315

30 to 40 mEq of potassium is necessary for each 1000 calories provided by the parenteral route. Potassium may be given as potassium chloride, potassium phosphate, or potassium acetate salt. Serum potassium levels must be closely monitored during TPN.

✎ **Note:** Patients with impaired renal functions may need decreased amounts of potassium.

The other electrolytes include magnesium sulfate, at 10 to 20 mEq every 24 hours; calcium gluceptate, gluconate, or chloride at 10 to 15 mEq in 24 hours; sodium chloride, acetate, lactate, or phosphate at 60 to 100 mEq in 24 hours; and phosphorus sodium or potassium at 20 mM to 45 mM in 24 hours. Chloride is provided based on acid-base status.

Electrolytes must be individually compounded and can be highly variable in the patient receiving TPN. Choice of each of these salts depends on renal and cardiac functioning, disease-specific needs, acid-base balance, and any abnormal losses during the course of illness.

Vitamins

Vitamins are necessary for growth and maintenance, along with multiple metabolic process. The fats and water-soluble vitamins are needed for the patient requiring TPN. The Nutritional Advisory Group of the American Medical Association (AMA) has developed recommendations for the daily administration of I.V. multivitamins (AMA, 1979) (Table 13–7).

There is controversy over the exact vitamin requirements for patients receiving TPN. Certain disease states can alter vitamin requirements, and the sequelae of vitamin deficiency can be catastrophic to the very ill person. It is recommended that vitamin K, 5 mg per week, be given intramuscularly in association with C-TPN (Delaney & Lauer, 1988).

Table 13–7 □ DAILY VITAMIN RECOMMENDATIONS FROM THE AMERICAN MEDICAL ASSOCIATION (1979)

A, 3300 IU
D, 200 IU
E, 75 IU
Ascorbic acid (C), 100 mg
Folic acid, 400 μg
Niacin (B_5), 40 mg
Riboflavin (B_2), 3.6 mg
Thiamin (B_1), 3 mg
Pyridoxine (B_6), 4 mg
Cyanocobalamin (B_{12}), 5 μg
Pantothenic acid (B_3), 15 mg
Biotin (B_7), 60 μg

Trace Elements

Trace elements are found in the body in minute amounts. Basic requirements are very small, measured in milligrams. Each trace element is a single chemical, and each has an associated deficiency state.

The many functions of trace elements are often synergistic (Metheny, 1987, p 153). The AMA has also established guidelines for the daily administration of four trace elements (AMA Department of Foods and Nutrition, 1979) (Table 13–8).

Zinc contributes to wound healing by increasing the tensile strength of collagen; copper assists in iron's incorporation of hemoglobin. The other trace elements—selenium, iodine, fluorine, cobalt, nickel, and iron—all have been identified as beneficial; however, there are no guidelines established for TPN (Kennedy-Caldwell & Guenter, 1988).

Parenteral Nutrition Medication Additives

Compatibility is always an issue whenever two agents are combined. Parenteral solutions should be used immediately after mixing or else refrigerated. Stability of the admixed component dictates the appropriate length of time the solution may be refrigerated. The parenteral solutions must be infused within 24 hours or discarded (Intravenous Nursing Society [INS], 1990, S64). In addi-

Table 13–8 □ DAILY TRACE ELEMENTS RECOMMENDED BY THE AMERICAN MEDICAL ASSOCIATION

Zinc, 2.5–40 mg
Copper, 0.5–1.5 mg
Chromium, 10–15 μg
Manganese, 0.15–0.8 mg

tion to combining amino acids, dextrose, fats, electrolytes, vitamins, and trace elements, medications such as insulin, heparin, and cimetidine can be added to the TPN solution.

Hyperglycemia is the most common complication of TPN therapy, which is due to the high concentration of glucose in the TPN solutions (Johndrow, 1988). Insulin is considered to be chemically stable in parenteral nutrition. By adding regular insulin to the parenteral admixture, some patients benefit from the enhanced blood glucose levels. Insulin is responsible for adequate metabolism of carbohydrates. Insulin also has a lipolytic effect and increased muscle uptake of amino acids (Farley, 1991).

Heparin in doses of 100 to 300 U/liter has been routinely used to decrease the incidence of subclavian vein thrombosis. This is controversial because recent studies disprove this claim. It is thought that larger doses of heparin, up to 20,000 U/liter, may be needed to reduce significantly the risk of thrombosis (Brismar, 1982; Ruggiero & Aisenstein, 1983).

Cimetidine can be added to the TPN solution as a prophylactic measure against development of stress ulcers. Concentrations of 900 to 1300 mg/L are compatible with TPN solutions (Tsallas & Allen, 1982).

Other medications currently being studied to reduce the volume of fluid administration are the combination of antibiotics and corticosteroids with TPN (Farley, 1991).

THERAPEUTIC MODALITIES

Candidates for Total Parenteral Nutrition

Patients who would be good candidates for TPN are those who suffer from a multiplicity of problems and whose clinical course can be complicated by malnutrition and depletion of body protein (Fig. 13–1).

Candidates for TPN include but are not limited to:

✓ Delayed wound healing
✓ Postoperative complications
✓ Predisposition to intraoperative complications
✓ Difficulty in refeeding
✓ GI problems such as Crohn's disease, short bowel syndrome, bowel obstruction, fistulas, pancreatitis, inflammatory bowel disease, malabsorption, and radiation enteritis
✓ Ulcerative colitis
✓ Trauma
✓ Severe burns
✓ Anorexia nervosa
✓ Immunocompromised states such as in bone marrow transplants and acquired immunodeficiency syndrome (AIDS)
✓ Cancer cachexia
✓ Hyperemesis associated with pregnancy

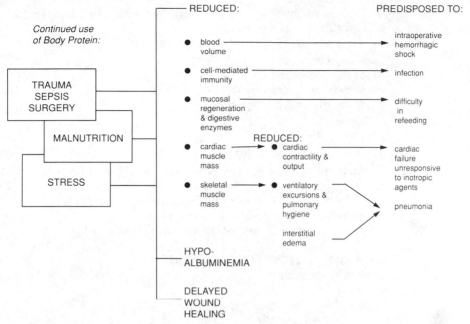

Figure 13–1 □ Body protein depletion. (From "Nutritional Support of the Surgery Patient" by R.T. Buchanan and N.S. Levine, 1983, *Annals of Plastic Surgery*, *10(2)*, pp. 159–166. Copyright 1983. Adapted by permission.)

MODALITIES FOR NUTRITIONAL SUPPORT
Enteral nutrition
Peripheral parenteral nutrition
Central parenteral nutrition
Three-in-one solutions
Cyclic therapy
Specialized parenteral formulas

Enteral Nutrition

Patients who are unable to eat regular diets have two alternatives to nutritional support: enteral or parenteral therapy. Enteral nutrition has certain advantages over parenteral nutrition: it is less expensive and more physiologic, it makes it easier to achieve a positive nitrogen balance, and it uses the GI tract. If the patient has a functioning GI tract, enteral nutrition should be used; otherwise, the parenteral route is indicated (Farley, 1991).

✎ **KEY POINTS IN DELIVERY OF ENTERAL NUTRITIONAL SUPPORT**
1. GI tract must be functioning.
2. Several approaches may be used to deliver enteral feedings.

491

3. There are three methods by which enteral nutrition can be delivered: bolus, intermittent, or continuous.
4. Six different categories of entereal formulas currently are available:

Blenderized
Meal replacement
Elemental or chemically defined
High-calorie and high-protein
Specialty
Modular

5. The patient must be monitored for:

Formula intolerance (gastric residuals every 4 to 8 hours)
Stools (frequency and consistency)
Tube tolerance (placement and maintenance checks)
Effectiveness (weight gain, nutrient intake)
Laboratory tests (Kennedy-Caldwell & Guenter, 1988, p 467)

COMPLICATIONS OF ENTERAL NUTRITION
1. Incorrect tube placement
2. Occlusion of feeding tube
3. Aspiration of feeding
4. Tracheoesopheageal fistula
5. Acute sinusitis
6. Otitis media
7. Diarrhea
8. Metabolic imbalances: hypoglycemia, hyperglycemia, hyperosmolar nonketotic dehydration, EFAD

Peripheral Parenteral Nutrition

Peripheral parenteral nutrition (PPN) was first proposed in the early 1970s as a "nitrogen-sparing" therapy. PPN is designed for mildly stressed patients who fall into the following categories:

1. Patients in whom central venous access is either impossible or contraindicated
2. Patients with no fluid restrictions
3. Patients able to tolerate fat emulsions
4. Patients expected to resume enteral feeding within 7 to 10 days (Kennedy-Caldwell & Guenter, 1988, p 487)

Generally, PPN provides dextrose in percentages below 20% with 500 mL of amino acids and fat emulsions via a peripheral line. PPN is used for therapies of less than 3 weeks. This therapy maintains the nutritional state in patients who can tolerate a relatively high fluid volume; those who usually resume bowel function and oral feeding within a few days; and those who are susceptible to catheter-related infection of central venous TPN. PPN can be delivered via an over-the-needle catheter (ONC) or by a peripherally inserted central line. Osmolarity factors of the solution must be considered when delivering PPN. It is recommended that the TPN not exceed 900 mOsm to prevent phlebitis (Hoheim et al, 1990).

Table 13–9 □ **STANDARD PERIPHERAL VEIN NUTRITION SOLUTION COMPONENTS/L**

Dextrose, 5–10%
Crystalline amino acids, 2.75–4.25%
Electrolytes, trace elements, and vitamins, as ordered
Fat emulsion, 10% or 20%
Heparin or hydrocortisone, as ordered

✎ **Note:** A commercial product designed for peripheral nutrition, Procal Amine provides 3 percent amino acids, 3 percent glycerol and electrolytes, and has an osmolarity of 735. Glycerol is used as a carbohydrate source in this product instead of dextrose (Miller, 1991). Table 13–9 gives examples of a standard PPN solution.

✎ **KEY POINTS IN DELIVERY OF PERIPHERAL PARENTERAL NUTRITION**
Advantages
1. Avoids insertion and maintenance of central catheter
2. Delivers less hypertonic solutions than central venous TPN
3. Reduces the chance of metabolic complications than central venous TPN
4. Increases calorie source, along with fat emulsion

Disadvantages
1. Cannot be used in nutritionally depleted patients
2. Cannot be used in volume-restricted patients, as higher volumes of solution are needed to provide adequate calories
3. Does not generally increase a patient's weight
4. May cause phlebitis owing to the osmolarity of the solution

Central Parenteral Nutrition

TPN by central line reverses starvation and adequately achieves tissue synthesis, repair, and growth. TPN solutions are usually administered through a central vein because of the high concentration of dextrose and the hypertonicity and hyperosmolarity of the solution. By infusing this solution into the central venous system there is a decreased incidence of phlebitis, and the highly concentrated formula can be rapidly diluted. Table 13–10 gives an example of standard **central parenteral nutrition** solution.

✎ **KEY POINTS IN DELIVERY OF CENTRAL PARENTERAL NUTRITION**
Advantages
1. Dextrose solutions of 20% to 70% administered as calorie source
2. Useful for long-term therapy (usually longer than 3 weeks)
3. Useful for patient with large caloric and nutrient needs
4. Provides calories, restores nitrogen balance; replaces essential vitamins, electrolytes, and minerals
5. Promotes tissue synthesis, wound healing, and normal metabolic function

493

Table 13–10 ☐ STANDARD CENTRAL PARENTERAL NUTRITION SOLUTION

500 mL of 8.5–10% amino acids
500 mL of 50–70% dextrose
at 3 L/d
Addition of 500 mL of 10% or 20% fat emulsion per day
Multivitamins, electrolytes, and trace elements, as needed
Heparin and insulin, as prescribed

6. Allows bowel rest and healing
7. Improves tolerance to surgery
8. Is nutritionally complete

Disadvantages
1. Requires a minor surgical procedure to insert central line
2. May cause metabolic complications: glucose intolerance, electrolyte imbalances, EFAD
3. Fat emulsions may not be used effectively in severely stressed patient (especially burn patients)
4. Risk of pneumothorax or hemothorax with central line insertion

The TPN solutions infused through a central vein are highly concentrated and range from 1800 to 2000 mOsm/kg with final additives, as compared with 300 mOsm/kg in plasma.

Three-in-One Solutions

The administration of three-in-one solutions has been found to be more efficient and cost effective than standard TPN and lipid administration. Referred to as total nutritional admixture, all-in-one, or three-in-one, this new product combines fat, amino acids, and dextrose in one container. The formula is provided in a 3-liter container that infuses over 24 hours. Lipids are mixed with dextrose and amino acid solution in the pharmacy. This solution is white and has a nonreflective surface, making precipitation difficult to observe (Larocca & Otto, 1989).

These admixtures have been shown to be stable and well tolerated by patients via central line administration (Deitel, 1987; Andrusko, 1987). Compounding of lipids, amino acids, and dextrose solutions raises the pH of the formula.

✎ **Note:** Bacterial growth may be enhanced by admixture of fat emulsions with dextrose and amino acid solutions (Green & Baptista, 1985). The solutions should be observed for pink discoloration and for separation of oils in the three-in-one admixtures (Kennedy-Caldwell, Guenter, 1988, p 408).

Cyclic Therapy

For patients requiring long-term parenteral nutritional support, cyclic TPN (C-TPN) is widely used. This therapy delivers concurrent dextrose, amino acids, and fat over a regimen of reduced time frame, usually 12 to 18 hours, versus a 24-hour continuous infusion.

✎ KEY POINTS IN DELIVERY OF CYCLIC THERAPY
1. This therapy is indicated for patients stabilized on continuous TPN.
2. This therapy is indicated for long-term parenteral nutrition.
3. The patient's cardiovascular status must be able to accommodate large fluid volume during the cyclic phase.
4. For patients without complications such as glucose intolerance or a precarious fluid balance, a 12-hour cycling regimen can be used (McClary-Bennett & Rosen, 1990).
5. To avoid abrupt changes in glucose, there must be a period of escalating to maintenance rate as well as tapering down from maintenance rate. Tapering rates vary from 1 to 2 hours.

✎ **Note:** The patient who is septic or metabolically stressed is not a good candidate for this regimen.

Advantages
1. Prevents or treats hepatotoxicity induced by continuous TPN.
2. Prevents or treats EFAD in patients on fat-free TPN (Baker & Roenberg, 1987).
3. Improves quality of life by encouraging normal daytime activities and enhances psychologic well-being

Disadvantages
1. Patients receiving C-TPN must be observed for symptoms of hypoglycemia, hyperglycemia, dehydration, excessive fluid administration, and sepsis associated with central line manipulation.
2. Patients must be carefully monitored for rebound hypoglycemia after cessation of C-TPN.
3. Hyperglycemia can develop during the peak C-TPN flow rate. Blood glucose levels should be checked anytime the patient displays symptoms of nausea, tremors, sweating, anxiety, or lethargy.

✎ **Note:** Blood glucose should be checked 1 hour after tapering off of C-TPN.

Dehydration can occur when fluid requirements are not met. Monitoring should include pulse, orthostatic blood pressures, examination of mucous membranes and skin turgor, as well as laboratory tests such as blood urea nitrogen (BUN), creatinine, hematocrit, and albumin.

Symptoms of excessive fluid administration should be monitored, such as weight gain, resulting in edema or infusion-related shortness of breath. If too much fluid is administered during the cyclic period, the time frame should be extended.

Using the C-TPN regimen requires twice the manipulations as continuous TPN; therefore, the risk of sepsis associated with central line manipulation must be considered.

Specialized Parenteral Formulas

Some parenteral formulas are designed to meet the needs of patients with specific disease states (Table 13–11). Formulas used for patients in renal failure

Table 13-11 □ **SPECIALIZED PARENTERAL FORMULAS**

Disease State	Parenteral Formulas	Treatment Plan
Renal failure	Nephramine 5.4% (McGaw) Aminosyn RF 5.2% (Abbott) RenAmin (Baxter)	Administer formulas high in essential amino acids. Administer electrolytes based on patient's clinical status. Restrict fluids based on status.
Liver disease	Hepatamine 8% (McGaw)	Administer formulas high in BCAA. Restrict total protein intake in encephalopathy.
Cardiac disease	Basic formula	Provide nutrients in as high a concentration as possible without precipitating fluid overload. Administer I.V. lipid emulsions cautiously in severe cardiac disease. Restrict fluids. Administer electrolytes based on patient's clinical status, especially potassium and magnesium.
Trauma	FreAmine HBC 6-9% (McGaw)	Administer formulas high in BCAA. Administer insulin based on patient's status.
Pulmonary disease	Basic formula	Nonprotein calories should be supplied in the following amounts: Carbohydrates 40%-50% Lipids 30%-50% Administer fluids and sodium cautiously so as not to cause fluid overload. Administer electrolytes based on patient's clinical status, especially phosphorus, magnesium, potassium, and calcium.

Table 13–11 □ **SPECIALIZED PARENTERAL FORMULAS — Continued**

Disease State	Parenteral Formulas	Treatment Plan
Burns	Basic formula	Administer higher concentrations of carbohydrates than lipids. Administer formulas high in amino acids. Administer fluid based on patient's clinical status. Administer electrolytes based on clinical status.
Sepsis	High BCAA formula 4% Branch Amin (Baxter)	Administer formulas high in BCAA. Administer lipids as 30–50% of the total nonprotein calories. Administer insulin based on patient's clinical status. Restrict the administration of iron.

Source. From *Critical Care Nursing* (p. 1147) by J.T. Dolan, 1991, Philadelphia: F.A. Davis Company. Copyright 1991 by F.A. Davis Company. Adapted by permission.

contain high amounts of essential **amino acids**. The high amounts of essential amino acids increase nephron repair in renal failure. The amino acid L-histidine enhances amino acid use in uremia (Abel, Abbott, & Fischer, 1972).

Solutions high in branched chain amino acids **(BCAA)** are designed for liver disease. Patients with chronic liver disease have elevated levels of aromatic amino acids and depressed levels of branched chain amino acids. The administration formulas high in BCAA would seem to be beneficial; however, as with formulas for renal failure, controversy exists in this area.

Formulas high in BCAA have also been recommended in the care of the trauma patient. This group of patients has a predilection to break down of BCAA in the muscles (Schmidt, Ahnefeld, & Burri, 1983). The use of formulas with high BCAA replenishes those depleted in the trauma patient.

COMPLICATIONS AND NURSING CONSIDERATIONS (TABLE 13–12)

Metabolic Complications

Hyperglycemia and Hyperosmolar Syndrome

Hyperglycemia is a common metabolic occurrence with TPN owing to the high dextrose concentrations included in the admixture. Other factors that put the

497

Table 13–12 □ **COMPLICATIONS OF TOTAL PARENTERAL NUTRITION**

Metabolic
Hyperglycemia and hyperosmolar syndrome
Postinfusion hypoglycemia
Hypomagnesemia, hypophosphatemia, and hypokalemia
Hypernatremia
EFAD
Catheter-related
Pneumothorax
Air embolus
Vein thrombosis
Catheter malposition
Infection

patient at risk for hyperglycemia are presence of overt or latent diabetes mellitus, increased age, sepsis, hypokalemia, and hypophosphatemia (Cerra, 1984, p 127).

NURSING CONSIDERATIONS
1. Begin TPN infusion at a slow rate (40 to 60 mL/hour).
2. Gradually increase the rate 25 mL/hour until maximal infusion rate is achieved.
3. Maintain a steady rate of infusion (TPN must stay within 10 percent of prescribed rate).
4. Use a rate control device to monitor the infusion.
5. Blood sugar checks should be performed every 6 hours, particularly during the first week of infusion.
6. Record fluid intake and output accurately every 8 hours.
7. Measure hourly urine output if urinary losses are above 250 mL/hour.
8. Check daily body weight using same scale. Ideally the weight gain for patients receiving TPN is approximately 2 lb/week.
9. Monitor vital signs at regular intervals. Look for signs of hypovolemia.

Postinfusion Hypoglycemia

Postinfusion hypoglycemia due to hyperinsulinism can occur if the TPN solution is abruptly discontinued.

NURSING CONSIDERATIONS
1. Wean the patient from the TPN solution gradually in decreased increments of 25 to 40 mL/hour over 24 to 48 hours.
2. If using C-TPN, gradually initiate and decrease the solution.

Electrolyte Imbalance

The complications associated with metabolic imbalances when administering TPN are either avoidable or controllable. Major electrolyte imbalances associated with TPN can occur if excessive or deficient amounts of electrolytes are supplied in the daily fluid allowance.

498

Hypophosphatemia: Adenosine triphosphate (ATP) is required for all cell energy production. Protein synthesis begins when TPN is administered and phosphate is driven into the intracellular space as a component of ATP. Therefore, a deficiency of phosphate can occur.

Hypokalemia: Potassium is also driven into the intracellular space during TPN. Serum potassium can become depleted with inadequate supply of this electrolyte along with the use of insulin in the TPN solution. Insulin administration further intensifies intracellular potassium.

Hypomagnesemia: The magnesium electrolyte also is driven into the intracellular space during TPN administration. Therefore, this electrolyte must also be included in TPN solution compounding.

Hypernatremia: To maintain homeostasis the sodium ion is driven from the intracellular space into the extracellular space. This compensatory mechanism tries to combat the extracellular anion loss (Metheny, 1987, pp 157–159). This shift could cause hypernatremia.

NURSING CONSIDERATIONS

1. Observe for signs and symptoms of hypophosphatemia, hypokalemia, hypomagnesemia, and hypernatremia. Refer to Chapter 4 for review of signs and symptoms.
2. Chemistry panel should be drawn every 3 days to check electrolyte levels.

Essential Fatty Acid Deficiency

Fat administration is important for delivery of essential fatty acids. If the regimen for nutritional support does not include a calorie source from fats, the patient is at risk for EFAD. Fats may be administered in amounts that supply 30 to 50 percent of the calories. By adding fats to the nutritional support, CO_2 production can be decreased and other metabolic complications may be avoided (Farley, 1991).

Catheter-Related Complications

Pneumothorax

This complication occurs when injury occurs during catheter placement. Blood, air, or infusion of fluid collects in the pleural cavity. Care must be taken to assess catheter placement prior to infusion of TPN. Assess for sharp chest pain, decreased breath sounds, and changes in vital signs and respiratory status. If pneumothorax has occurred, it is evident on a chest x-ray film.

Air Embolism

Passage of air into the heart can occur during insertion of the central line or during catheter maintenance. All connections should be taped and procedures strictly followed for tubing changes along with dressing management techniques. Change tubing during patient's expiratory respiratory phase. Apply an occlusive dressing over the site after the catheter has been removed.

Vein Thrombosis

Long-term central catheterization can cause vein thrombosis to occur in the superior vena cava or its tributaries. Use of a silicone catheter decreases the risk of thrombogenic factors. Pulmonary emboli can be a secondary complication of vein thrombosis. Thrombolytic therapy is beneficial when flow rates are affected owing to thrombus formation, as is the use of heparin added to the infusate to prevent thrombosis. The physician should be notified if thrombosis is suspected.

Catheter Malposition

This complication can occur during introduction of the catheter. If there is difficulty in passage of the catheter, cardiac arrhythmias during insertion along with irregularities of flow of infusate could indicate malposition of the catheter. Check dressing at least every 4 hours for signs of inadvertent displacement. Report suspected catheter malposition to the physician promptly.

Infectious Complications

When TPN is provided by a central line, concerns are related to the contamination of the central venous catheter, as discussed in Chapter 12. Catheter-related sepsis is a serious complication of central TPN therapy that is preventable with strict aseptic technique (Guthrie & Turner, 1986).

TPN patients are often immunocompromised as a result of malnutrition; these patients are highly susceptible to infection. The origin of TPN catheter-related sepsis is most often the site itself; infection related to contaminated infusates is rare (Kennedy-Caldwell & Guenter, 1988, p 523).

NURSING CONSIDERATIONS
1. Maintain aseptic technique in catheter maintenance and in administration of TPN.
2. Aseptic dressing changes should be done every 48 to 72 hours if Elastoplast dressing is used; if transparent dressing is used, aseptic dressing changes are recommended every 4 to 7 days depending on agency policy. Refer to Chapter 12 for dressing management.
3. Use of 0.22-micron inline antimicrobial filter is recommended for TPN lines, except when lipid emulsion is added to these solutions, at which time a 1.2-micron filter should be used (INS, 1990, S64).

Standards of Practice for Nutritional Support

Standards of practice related to nutritional support have been addressed by ASPEN and the INS. Presented here are the accepted standards of practice related to nutritional support.

Implementation Standards

Parenteral formulations shall be prepared according to established guidelines for safe and effective nutritional therapy.

Table 13-13 □ SUMMARY OF MONITORING OF PARENTERAL NUTRITION THERAPY

Before initiation of therapy by central line: 　Check placement of catheter tip by x-ray examination. After initiation of parenteral nutrition therapy: 　Start TPN infusion slowly. 　Check temperature and vital signs every 6 hours. 　Monitor blood sugar every 6 hours. 　Maintain strict intake and output. 　Daily weight check. 　Decrease TPN solutions gradually. 　TPN and lipid administration sets will be changed every 24 hours. Laboratory parameters to check twice weekly: 　Liver function 　Electrolyte profile 　BUN and creatinine

1. Parenteral formulations shall be sterile.
2. Parenteral formulations should be stored at 4°C.
3. Policies should be established limiting additions to the parenteral feeding formulations after they are infusing.
4. Patient and/or responsible other shall receive education and demonstrate competence in access route care in home care situations.

A summary of monitoring standards is presented in Table 13-13. Figure 13-2 is an example of a TPN order form.

Monitoring Standards

Patients should be monitored for therapeutic efficacy, adverse effects, and clinical changes that might influence specialized nutritional support.

1. Protocols shall be developed for periodic review of the patient's clinical and biochemical status.
2. Routine monitoring should include nutrient intake; review of current medications; signs of intolerance to therapy; weight changes; biochemical, hematologic, and other pertinent data, including clinical signs of nutrient deficiencies and excesses; adjustment of therapy; changes in life-style; psychosocial problems; and changes in the home environment.
3. Patient's major organ functions should be assessed periodically.

INTRAVENOUS NURSING SOCIETY STANDARDS OF PRACTICE (1990)

1. All parenteral nutrition solutions should be filtered with a 0.22-micron filter except when lipid emulsion is added to these solutions, at which time a 1.2-micron filter should be used.
2. Solutions should be compounded in the pharmacy under a horizontal laminar flow hood.
3. No medications should be added to these solutions once they are infusing.

501

TOTAL PARENTERAL NUTRITION (TPN) ORDER FORM

Date _____ Time _____

ATTENTION DOCTORS: Please order electrolyte content in **mEq/24 hours.** Pharmacy will supply a 24 hour amount. Please fill out for any ingredient or rate changes. They will be initiated with the next bag unless otherwise indicated.

Protein Source:
Aminosyn 7% (35 grams/500 ml) _____ mls/24 hours
Aminosyn 10% (50 grams/500ml) _____ mls/24 hours

Carbohydrate Caloric Source:
Dextrose 50% (850 kcal/500ml) _____ mls/24 hours
Dextrose 70% (1190 kcal/500ml) _____ mls/24 hours

Total Volume: _____ mls/24 hours,   Rate: _____ mls/hour _____

Electrolyte Additions:
Sodium Chloride _____ mEq/24 hours
Potassium Chloride _____ mEq/24 hours
Potassium Phosphate _____ mEq/24 hours
Calcium Gluconate _____ mEq/24 hours
Magnesium Sulfate _____ mEq/24 hours

Multivitamin-12 (10 ml = 1 vial/24 hours) _____ mls/24 hours
Trace Elements (1 ml = 1 vial/24 hours) _____ ml/24 hours
Regular Insulin (Humulin-R, 100 units/ml) _____ Units/24 hours

Fat Emulsion 10 % (550 kcal/500 ml unit)® Unit every _____ day(s)
Fat Emulsion 20% (1,000 kcal/500 ml unit)® Unit every _____ day(s)
Normal Serum Albumin 25% (50ml and 100ml)*

® Each unit will be piggybacked below filter and infused over 4 to 8 hours.
* All albumin shall be infused separately below final filter over no more than 4 hours as recommended by CDC and FDA since it is a blood product.

Refer to I.V. Therapy P/P for standard nursing care of TPN patients (Pol. #10-A,B,C)
☐ Blood glucose fingerstick _____ times per day.
☐ Urine S & A every _____ hours. Report 2+ or over.
☐ Baseline lab if not obtained in last 48 hours including: CBC, Chem Profile-20, Serum Magnesium, Protime & Urinalysis.
☐ Daily lab tests: Blood Sugar, Electrolytes or
☐ Ongoing lab tests including: ☐ Chem. Profile-20 & Serum Magnesium 3x weekly,
    ☐ CBC twice weekly, ☐ Protime weekly.

TO/VO_____ M.D. / _____ R.N./Pharm.D
(Circle one)   (Circle one)

(Addressograph)

Roseville Community Hospital
Roseville, California 95661
Daily TPN Order Form

Figure 13–2 ☐ Total parenteral nutrition (TPN) order form. (Courtesy of Roseville Hospital, Roseville, California.)

502

4. Except for lipid emulsions, no I.V. push or piggyback medications should be added to this line.
5. All TPN and lipid administration sets should be changed every 24 hours, coinciding with solution bag changes (INS, 1990, S55).
6. Refer to INS standards for central line tubing changes in Chapter 12 (S64).

HOME CARE

Parenteral Nutrition Therapy

Nutritional support is now well established in the home. Patients and their families can successfully be taught to administer I.V. admixtures safely, and their care can be monitored in a home setting. Hospital-to-home transition can be difficult. Keep in mind that the day of discharge is usually physically and emotionally stressful. The home care nurse should be in attendance for starting the home total parenteral nutrition (HTPN) infusion. Before home therapy for nutritional support is begun, a baseline electrolyte chemistry panel, magnesium level, and phosphorus level, along with complete blood count (CBC) within 7 days of discharge, should be obtained. Home safety must be determined before discharge from the hospital (Wiseman, 1985). Successful home therapy depends on several factors:

1. Medical stability
2. Emotional stability
3. Patient's life-style
4. Intellectual ability (patient or primary care giver)
5. Visual acuity
6. Manual dexterity
7. Home environment

    Dry storage space for supplies
    Refrigerator large enough to store admixtures
    Clean low-traffic area for procedure preparation
    Electronic outlets for any electronic equipment

Advantages

Advantages of HTPN support encompass the fact that home treatment is less expensive than treatment in the hospital. Home treatment allows the patient to remain in a familiar, comfortable surrounding, thereby decreasing the confusion associated with age-related environment changes. In many situations, home treatment allows the patient to return to normal activities. The risk of acquiring a nosocomial infection is lessened with home care. Control over one's own body and self-care responsibilities increase self-esteem (Plumer & Cosentino, 1987, p 535).

Patient Education

Home education process should include but not be limited to:

1. Verbal and written instructions of appropriate procedures
2. Demonstration and return demonstration of procedures by primary caregiver

503

3. Evaluation and documentation of competency
4. Self-monitoring instructions
5. Limitations of physical activity
6. Emergency intervention and problem-solving techniques
7. Care of infusion equipment, solutions, and supplies
8. Disposal of supplies
9. Expectations of home care and medical and nursing follow-up (Kennedy-Caldwell & Guenter, 1988, p 523)

Home care training must be individually designed according to individual capabilities. Assessment of the patient's physical and emotional status before each teaching session aids in determining goals for that session. A minimum number of people should be involved with each teaching session to limit distractions and anxiety.

PHYSICAL ASSESSMENT (NUTRITION)

The nurse must use a systems approach to assess for both local and systemic complications associated with the administration of parenteral nutritional support. The nursing assessment should include infusion rate, intake and output, and an awareness of agency policy and procedure to prevent complications associated with nutritional therapy. The following body systems should be assessed at the beginning of each shift and as needed to monitor the patient's reactions to the infusion. Symptoms listed with each system may indicate local problems or a life-threatening situation. All laboratory findings must be monitored.

NEUROMUSCULAR
Change in level of consciousness
Confusion
Complaints of pain
Paresthesia of the extremities
Paralysis of the extremities
Seizures
Tremors

CARDIOVASCULAR
Increased or decreased blood
  pressure
Increased heart rate
Distended neck veins
Bleeding from the site
Serum blood sugar level

RESPIRATORY
Shortness of breath
Wheezing

GASTROINTESTINAL
Oral intake

Nausea
Vomiting
Diarrhea

RENAL
Decreased urinary output
Variance between intake and
  output

INTEGUMENTARY
Fever
Edema at or near insertion site
Sensation of heat at or near
  insertion site
Red line visible above the
  venipuncture site
Tender, cordlike vein
Bruising around or near site of
  insertion
Sluggish flow rate
Backflow absent
Coolness of the skin
Taut skin around venipuncture site

WEIGHT
Rapid weight gain
No weight gain

SPECIAL SENSES
Taste
Appearance of oral mucous
  membranes

NURSING DIAGNOSES RELATED TO NUTRITIONAL SUPPORT

1. Altered health maintenance related to poor dietary habits, with perceptual or cognitive impairment
2. Altered nutrition (less than body requirements) related to chewing or swallowing difficulties; anorexia; nausea; vomiting; difficulty or inability to procure foods
3. Altered nutrition (greater than body requirements) related to imbalance of intake versus activity expenditure
4. Altered tissue perfusion (peripheral) related to infusion of irritating solution
5. Altered oral mucous membrane related to dehydration
6. Feeding deficit; bathing or hygiene deficit; dressing or grooming deficit; and toileting deficit — related to limited mobility because of placement of I.V. catheter and infusion of nutritional support
7. Fluid volume excess related to infusion of isotonic saline
8. Knowledge deficit (new skills) related to maintaining nutritional support
9. Ineffective family coping related to inadequate financial resources, family role changes, and stressors associated with parenteral nutrition management
10. Risk for infection related to high dextrose content of parenteral solution or break in sterile technique
11. Risk for injury related to confusion associated with altered blood sugar levels
12. Self-esteem disturbance related to negative feeling about placement of visible tunneled central line for long-term nutritional support

---

SUMMARY OF CHAPTER 13

NUTRITONAL SUPPORT

NUTRITIONAL ASSESSMENT
Dietary history
Anthropometric measurements
Diagnostic tests
Physical examination

NUTRITIONAL REQUIREMENTS
Protein (amino acids): Includes the eight essential amino acids provided

505

in 3.5% to 10% solutions; protein-calorie malnutrition: marasmus, kwashiorkor, or mixed

Carbohydrates: Dextrose in 5%, 10%, 20%, 50%, and 70%

Fats: Provided as soy or safflower oil solutions; prevents EFAD; use of fat emulsions can help control hyperglycemia

Electrolytes: Included in parenteral therapy:

Potassium 30 to 40 mEq per 1000 mL

Magnesium sulfate 10 to 20 mEq every 24 hours

Calcium glucepatate, calcium gluconate, or calcium chloride 10 to 15 mEq in 24 hours

Sodium chloride 60 to 100 mEq in 24 hours

Phosphorus sodium or phosphorus potassium 20 to 45 mEq in 24 hours

Chloride provided related to acid-base balance .

Vitamins: A, D, E, C, B_1, B_5, B_6, B_{12}, B_3, and B_7, as well as K 5 mg given intramuscularly weekly.

Trace elements: Zinc, copper, chromium, manganese

PARENTERAL NUTRITION MEDICATION ADDITIVES
Insulin

Heparin

Cimetidine (antibiotics and corticosteroids being studied)

Therapeutic Modalities

Peripheral Parenteral Nutrition

This therapy provides nutritional support in patients with mild stress. A combination of 5 to 10% dextrose, with amino acids ranging from 2.75 to 4.25 percent, along with electrolytes, trace elements, and vitamins, are administered by peripheral vein. This therapy is used for short-term duration, usually less than 3 weeks. Maximum osmolarity of this solution is 900 mOsm/L.

Central Total Parenteral Therapy

Nutritional support that provides calories for weight gain, growth, and development and wound healing usually must be administered by central line. This therapy generally has an osmolarity of 1800 to 2000 mOsm.

Three-in-One Solutions

Combination of carbohydrate, protein, and fats in one 3-liter solution bag infuses over 24 hours.

Cyclic Therapy

Cyclic therapy is indicated for patients receiving long-term nutritional support. This type of TPN is administered over 12 to 18 hours, usually at night. This leaves the patient free to lead an active life-style. The key point is that the solution must be escalated and tapered gradually so as not to cause dramatic changes in blood glucose levels.

Specialized Parenteral Formulas

Special amino acid formulas for patients with renal failure contain high amounts of essential amino acids, which helps nephron repair. Solutions high in BCAA are designed for patients with liver disease. Trauma patients benefit from formulas in BCAA.

COMPLICATIONS
Metabolic
> Hyperglycemia and hyperosmolar syndrome
> Postinfusion hypoglycemia
> Electrolyte imbalance: hypokalemia, hypomagnesemia, and hypo-
> > phosphatemia
> Hypernatremia

CATHETER-RELATED COMPLICATIONS
Infection
Catheter-related sepsis
Pneumothorax
Air embolism
Subclavian vein thrombosis
Catheter position displacement
Catheter occlusion

Activity Journal

1. Check your agency policy and procedure manual for guidelines for monitoring the patient on TPN. Is there a set policy, and how are these procedures documented?

2. You check your patient receiving TPN at the beginning of the shift and find that the fat emulsion has a 0.22-micron filter attached in the line in which it is infusing. What do you do?

3. A patient has had a blood glucose level of 100 mg/dL during the course of his first 48 hours of TPN. The next time you check the blood sugar, it is 240 mg/dL. How do you handle this situation? What could be the reason for this sudden increase in blood sugar? How would you begin to check for the problem?

4. The physician has ordered C-TPN for 12 hours on your patient who has been stabilized on nutritional support for 2 weeks. How would you explain this therapy to the patient? Upon discharge, what kind of patient guidelines would you provide?

Quality Assessment Model

Instructions: Use this quality assessment model to conduct retrospective audits of charts, establish quality control standards, or develop outcome criteria for quality assurance. Refer to Chapter 2 for details on quality assessment.

STRUCTURE

(Resource that affects outcome)
Human Resource: Nutritional Support Nurse

↓

PROCESS

(Actual giving and receiving of care)
Therapist activities related to assessment and monitoring of patient receiving TPN are:

1. Confirm catheter tip placement by x-ray film before starting TPN.
2. Begin TPN slowly by increasing the rate by 25 mL/hour until desired rate is achieved.
3. Use Luer-locking connections or tape all connections securely.
4. Maintain sterile technique during tubing, solution, and dressing changes.
5. Monitor blood sugar every 6 hours.
6. Monitor vital signs every 4 hours—especially temperature.
7. Measure daily weights.
8. Monitor accurate intake and output.
9. Use rate control device on all TPN solutions.
10. Use 0.22-micron inline filter with TPN solutions that do not contain fats.
11. Wean patient from TPN over 24 to 48 hours.
12. Change central line tubing for TPN and lipids every 24 hours.

↓

OUTCOME STANDARDS

(Effects of care)
Documentation will reflect standards of care for the practice of safe TPN delivery:

1. The catheter tip placement will be documented in the chart by x-ray examination.
2. The nursing graphics will reflect the daily weight, vital signs every 4 hours, and intake and output every 8 hours.

3. The chart will reflect the documentation of blood sugar level every 6 hours.
4. The total 8-hour parenteral fluid intake will be documented on the chart.
5. The nursing notes will reflect a review of the pertinent laboratory values.
6. The tubing and solution changes will be done concurrently and documented every 24 hours.

Post-test, Chapter 13

Match the definition in column 2 to the correct term in column 1.

Column 1

1. _____ BCAA

2. _____ Kwashiorkor

3. _____ HTPN

4. _____ Marasmus

5. _____ EFAD

Column 2

A. Essential fatty acid deficiency

B. Branched chain amino acid

C. Malnutrition caused by decreased intake of calories with adequate amount of protein

D. Malnutrition caused by adequate intake of calories with inadequate amount of protein

E. Home total parenteral nutrition

6–10. List five high-risk patient conditions that could require TPN.

11–16. Identify the six nutrients essential for TPN.

17. In addition to vitamins B and C, it is recommended that _____ intramuscularly be given weekly.
    A. Heparin 1000 U
    B. Vitamin K 5 mg
    C. Zinc 2.5 mg
    D. Biotin 60 μg

18. Cimetidine is added to parenteral nutrition for what purpose?
    A. To decrease incidence of vein thrombosis
    B. As a prophylactic measure against development of stress ulcers
    C. To increase muscle uptake of amino acids
    D. To increase tensile strength of the collagen

19. Insulin is added to parenteral nutrition for:
    A. Enhancing blood glucose levels
    B. Metabolism of carbohydrates
    C. Lipolytic effect
    D. All of the above

20. A disadvantage of three-in-one solutions is:
    A. Solution must be changed every 8 hours.
    B. Precipitation may be difficult to observe.
    C. Fats coagulate when mixed with dextrose.
    D. Risk of contamination increases owing to multiple additions to the mixture.

21. Nurses must be aware of which of the following when using C-TPN?
    A. Blood sugar can drop 1 hour after tapering off C-TPN.
    B. The patient who is metabolically stressed is not a good candidate for this therapy.
    C. Dehydration can occur if the fluid requirements are not met in 24 hours.
    D. All of the above.

22. Metabolic complications associated with TPN include:
    A. Hyperglycemia
    B. Hyperosmolar syndrome
    C. EFAD
    D. Electrolyte imbalances
    E. All of the above

True-False

23. T F An advantage of home care nutritional support is that the patient can continue with a normal routine.

24. T F A key point in delivery of PPN is that the patient should resume enteral feeding within 24 hours.

25. Identify the nursing considerations needed when responsible for TPN administration.

Answers to Post-test, Chapter 13

1. B
2. D
3. E
4. C
5. A
6–10. Patients with delayed wound healing, postoperative complications, predisposition to intraoperative hemorrhage, GI problems, trauma, severe burns, anorexia nervosa, or cancer cachexia. Also any patient with difficulty in refeeding.
11–16. Carbohydrates, protein, fats, electrolytes, trace elements, vitamins.
17. B
18. B
19. D
20. B
21. D
22. E
23. T
24. F
25. Check catheter tip placement before starting TPN.

Begin TPN slowly.
Gradually increase TPN at the rate of 25 mL/hour until maximal infusion rate is achieved.
Use rate control device to monitor the infusion.
Accucheck must be done every 6 hours.
Chart intake and output accurately every 8 hours.
Monitor daily body weights using the same scale.
Monitor vital signs every 4 hours —especially temperature.
Wean patient off TPN gradually.
Observe for signs and symptoms of electrolyte imbalances.
Check chemistry panel every 3 days.
Maintain aseptic technique in catheter maintenance and in the administration of TPN.
Use Luer-lock connector or tape all connections.
Use 0.22-micron inline filter for TPN solutions without fats added.

References

Abel, R., Abbott, W., & Fischer, J. (1972). Intravenous essential L-amino acids and hypertonic dextrose in patients with acute renal failure. *American Journal of Surgery, 123*, 632–638.

American Medical Association. (1979). Guidelines for essential trace element preparations for parenteral use: A statement by the Nutrition Advisory Group. *Journal of Parenteral and Enteral Nutrition, 3*, 263.

American Medical Association Department of Foods and Nutrition. (1979). Multivitamin preparations for parenteral use: A statement by the nutrition advisory group. *Journal of Parenteral and Enteral Nutrition, 3*, 259.

American Society for Parenteral and Enteral Nutrition (ASPEN). (1988a). Standards for home nutritional support. *Nutrition in Clinical Practice, 3*(5), 202–205.

ASPEN. (1988b). Standards of practice—nutrition support nurse. *Nutrition in Clinical Practice, 3*(2), 78–83.

Andrusko, K. (1987). Advantages and disadvantages of total nutrient admixtures in the home care patient. *Hospital Pharmacy, 22*, 4–7.

Baker, A.L., & Rosenberg, I.H. (1987). Hepatic complications of total parenteral nutrition. *American Journal of Medicine, 82*, 489–497.

Brismar, B. (1982). Reduction of catheter associated thrombosis in parenteral nutrition by intravenous heparin therapy. *Archives of Surgery* 117–1196.

Cerra, F. (1984). *Pocket manual of surgical nutrition.* St Louis: C.V. Mosby.

Delaney, C.W., & Lauer, M.L. (1988). *Intravenous therapy: A guide to quality care.* Philadelphia: J.B. Lippincott.

Deitel, M. (1987). Total nutrient admixtures. An NSS symposium in three parts. *Nutrition Support Services, 7*(13).

Farley, J.M. (1991). Nutritional support of the critically ill patient. In J.T. Dolan: *Critical care nursing,* pp 1125–1149. Philadelphia: F.A. Davis.

Guthrie, P., & Turner, W.W. (1986). Peripheral and central nutritional support. *National Intravenous Therapy Association, 9*(5), 393–398.

Green, B.A., & Baptista, R.J. (1985). Nursing assessment of 3 in 1 TPN admixture. *National Intravenous Therapy Association, 8,* 530–532.

Hoheim, D.F., O'Callaghan, T.A., Joswiak, B.J., Boysen, D.A., & Bommarito, A.A. (1990). Clinical experience with three in one admixtures administered peripherally. *Nutrition in Clinical Practice, 5*(3), 118–122.

Intravenous Nursing Society. (1990). *Standards of practice.* Philadelphia: J.B. Lippincott.

Johndrow, P.D. (1988). Making your patient and his family feel at home with T.P.N. *Nursing 88, 10,* 65–69.

Kennedy-Caldwell, C., & Guenter, P. (1988). *Nutrition support nursing core curriculum.* Maryland: American Society for Parenteral and Enteral Nutrition.

Lang, C.E. (1987). *Nutritional support in critical care.* Maryland: Aspen Publishers.

Larocca, J.C., & Otto, S.E. (1989). *Pocket guide to intravenous therapy.* St. Louis: C.V. Mosby.

Martin, D., & Jastram, C.W. (1988). Part III: Parenteral nutrition, clinical monitoring and assessment. *Nutritional Support Services, 8*(1), 12–16.

McClary-Bennett, K., & Rosen, G.H. (1990). Cyclic total parenteral nutrition. *Nutrition in Clinical Practice, 5*(4), 163–165.

Metheny, N.M. (1987). *Fluid and electrolyte balance: Nursing considerations.* Philadelphia: J.B. Lippincott.

Miller, S.J. (1991). Peripheral parenteral nutrition: Theory and practice. *Hospital Pharmacy, 26*(9), 796–801.

Plumer, A., & Cosentino, F. (1987). *Principles and practices of intravenous therapy.* Boston: Little, Brown Company.

Ruggiero, R., & Aisenstein, T. (1983). Central catheter fibrin sleeve-heparin effect. *Journal Parenteral Enteral Nutrition, 7,* 270.

Schmidt, J.E., Ahnefeld, F.W., & Burri, C. (1983). Nutritional support of the multiple trauma patient. *World Journal of Surgery, 7,* 132–142.

Tsallas, G., & Allen, L. (1982). Stability of cimetidine hydrochloride in parenteral nutrition solutions. *American Journal of Hospital Pharmacy, 39,* 484.

Wiseman, M. (1985). Setting standards for home I.V. therapy. *American Journal of Nursing, 85* 4, 421–423.

Bibliography

ASPEN. (1989). Standards for nutritional support for residents of long-term care facilities. *Nutrition in Clinical Practice, 4*(4), 148–152.

Grant, J.P. (1986). Nutritional assessment in clinical practice. *Nutrition in Clinical Practice.*

Page, C.P., & Clibon, U. (1980). Man the meal-eater and his interaction with parenteral nutrition. *JAMA, 244,* 1950–1953.

APPENDICES

Nomogram of Body Surface Areas

OLDER CHILDREN AND ADULTS

HEIGHT		SURFACE AREA	WEIGHT	
feet	centimeters	in square meters	pounds	kilograms

Figure UN–A1 ☐ Nomogram of older children and adults (Courtesy of Abbott Laboratories, Hospital Products Division, Abbott Park, Illinois.)

INFANTS AND YOUNG CHILDREN

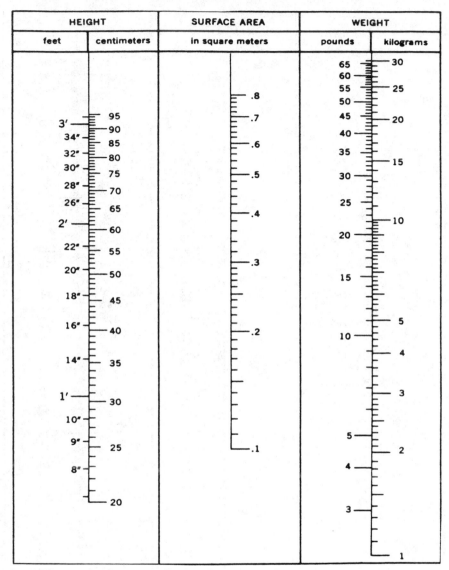

Figure UN−A2 ☐ Nomogram of body surface areas in infants and young children (From Talbot, MB, Sobel, EH, McArthur, JW, et al: Functional Endocrinology from Birth through Adolescence. Harvard University Press, Cambridge, 1980, with permission.)

Physical and Chemical Compatibility Chart*

*Source: From *Pharmacotherapeutics: A Nursing Process Approach*, second edition by M. M. Kuhn (1991), Philadelphia: F. A. Davis Company. Copyright 1991 by F. A. Davis Company. Reprinted with permission.

	Aminophylline	Ampicillin	Atropine sulfate	Bretylium	Calcium chloride	Calcium gluconate	Cefazolin	Cimetidine	Diazepam	Diazoxide	Digoxin	Dobutamine	Dopamine	Epinephrine HCl	Furosemide	Gentamicin	Heparin	Hydralazine
Aminophylline		P	N	D	N	P	S	I	N	N	P	B	P	I	B	P	P	I
Ampicillin	P		N	N	N	I	S	A	N	N	N	N	I	I	N	I	H	I
Atropine sulfate	N	N		N	N	N	N	P	N	N	N	P	N	D	N	N	P	N
Bretylium	D	N	N		C	D	N	N	N	N	D	I	C	N	N	M	N	N
Calcium chloride	N	N	N	C		N	N	N	N	N	P	I	D	I	N	N	N	N
Calcium gluconate	P	I	N	D	N		I	N	N	N	N	I	P	I	N	N	P	N
Cefazolin	S	S	N	N	N	I		P	N	N	N	N	N	N	N	I	S	N
Cimetidine	I	A	P	N	N	N	P		N	N	M	P	P	P	P	P	P	N
Diazepam	N	N	N	N	N	N	N	N		N	N	N	N	N	N	N	N	N
Diazoxide	N	N	N	N	N	N	N	N	N		N	N	N	N	N	N	N	I
Digoxin	P	N	N	D	P	N	N	M	N	N		N	N	N	N	N	N	H
Dobutamine	B	N	P	I	I	I	N	P	N	N	N		S	D	I	B	D	S
Dopamine	P	I	N	C	D	P	N	P	N	N	N	S		P	N	A	P	N
Epinephrine HCl	I	I	D	N	I	I	N	P	N	N	N	D	P		I	P	D	N
Furosemide	B	N	N	N	N	N	N	P	N	N	N	I	N	I		N	P	I
Gentamicin	P	I	N	M	N	N	I	P	N	N	N	B	A	P	N		I	N
Heparin	P	H	P	N	N	P	S	P	N	N	N	D	P	D	P	I		P
Hydralazine	I	I	N	N	N	N	N	N	N	I	H	S	N	N	I	N	P	
Insulin reg	I	N	N	P	N	N	N	A	N	N	I	I	N	N	N	N	P	P
Isoproterenol	I	P	N	I	P	P	N	P	N	N	N	P	P	N	N	P	P	P

Insulin reg	Isoproterenol	Lidocaine	Morphine sulfate	Netilmicin	Nitroglycerin	Nitroprusside	Norepinephrine	Phenytoin	Phytonadione	Potassium chloride	Procainamide	Propranolol	Quinidine	Sodium bicarbonate	Streptokinase	Tobramycin	Verapamil
I	I	P	I	N	G	N	I	N	N	P	N	N	N	B	N	N	P
N	P	P	N	N	N	N	P	N	I	P	N	N	N	N	N	N	P
N	N	N	P	P	N	N	N	N	N	P	P	N	N	I	N	N	P
P	I	C	N	N	G	N	N	N	N	P	I	N	P	C	N	N	P
N	P	P	I	N	N	N	P	N	N	P	N	N	N	I	N	I	P
N	P	D	N	N	N	N	P	N	P	P	N	N	N	I	N	I	P
N	N	I	N	P	N	N	N	N	N	S	N	N	N	N	N	N	P
A	P	D	N	N	N	D	N	P	D	N	N	P	P	P	N	N	P
N	N	N	N	N	N	N	N	N	N	N	N	I	N	N	N	N	N
N	N	N	N	N	N	N	N	N	N	N	N	I	N	N	N	N	N
I	N	P	N	N	N	N	N	N	N	Y	N	N	N	N	N	N	P
I	P	P	N	N	N	N	P	N	I	I	P	N	N	I	N	N	I
N	P	P	N	N	G	N	H	N	P	P	N	N	N	I	N	N	P
N	N	I	N	N	N	N	P	N	I	P	N	N	N	I	N	N	P
N	N	N	N	N	G	N	N	N	N	P	N	N	I	N	N	N	P
N	P	P	H	N	N	N	P	N	N	N	N	N	N	N	N	N	P
P	P	P	I	N	N	N	P	N	P	P	P	N	I	P	N	I	P
P	P	P	N	N	G	N	N	N	N	Y	N	N	N	N	N	N	S
	N	L	N	N	N	N	N	N	N	N	N	N	N	I	N	N	P
N		I	N	P	N	P	N	N	P	N	N	N	I	N	N	N	P

	Aminophylline	Ampicillin	Atropine sulfate	Bretylium	Calcium chloride	Calcium gluconate	Cefazolin	Cimetidine	Diazepam	Diazoxide	Digoxin	Dobutamine	Dopamine	Epinephrine HCl	Furosemide	Gentamicin	Heparin	Hydralazine
Lidocaine	P	P	N	C	P	D	I	D	N	N	P	P	P	I	N	P	P	P
Morphine sulfate	I	N	P	N	I	N	N	N	N	N	N	N	N	N	N	H	I	N
Netilmicin	N	N	P	N	N	N	P	N	N	N	N	N	N	N	N	N	N	N
Nitroglycerin	G	N	N	G	N	N	N	N	N	N	N	N	N	G	N	G	N	N	G
Nitroprusside	N	N	N	N	N	N	N	N	N	N	N	N	N	N	N	N	N	N
Norepinephrine	I	P	N	N	P	P	N	D	N	N	N	P	H	P	N	P	P	N
Phenytoin	N	N	N	N	N	N	N	N	N	N	N	N	N	N	N	N	N	N
Phytonadione	N	I	N	N	N	P	N	P	N	N	N	I	P	I	N	N	P	N
Potassium chloride	P	P	P	P	P	P	S	D	N	N	Y	I	P	P	P	N	P	Y
Procainamide	N	N	P	I	N	N	N	N	N	N	N	P	N	N	N	N	P	N
Propranolol	N	N	N	N	N	N	N	N	N	I	N	N	N	N	N	N	N	N
Quinidine	N	N	N	P	N	N	N	P	I	N	N	N	N	N	I	N	I	N
Sodium bicarbonate	B	N	I	C	I	I	N	P	N	N	N	I	I	I	N	N	P	N
Streptokinase	N	N	N	N	N	N	N	N	N	N	N	N	N	N	N	N	N	N
Tobramycin	N	N	N	N	I	I	N	N	N	N	N	N	N	N	N	N	I	N
Verapamil	P	P	P	P	P	P	P	P	N	N	P	I	P	P	P	P	P	S

C = Physically and chemically compatible
P = Physically compatible
D = Physically compatible only in D5W.
S = Physically compatible only in 0.9% NaCl.
G = Physically compatible only in a glass bottle.
H = Physically compatible for 24 hours.
A = Physically compatible for 4–8 hours.
B = Physically compatible for 4–8 hours only in D5W.
Y = Physically compatible through Y-site for at least 6 hours.
L = Regular insulin compatible with preservative free lidocaine solution.
M = Manufacturer claims medication should not be mixed with other medications but some compatibility data are available.
I = Incompatible.
N = Information on compatibility is not available.
SOURCE: Zeller, FP, et al: Compatibility of IV drugs in a coronary intensive care unit. Drug Intell Clin Pharm 20(5):352, 1986, with permission.

Insulin reg	Isoproterenol	Lidocaine	Morphine sulfate	Netilmicin	Nitroglycerin	Nitroprusside	Norepinephrine	Phenytoin	Phytonadione	Potassium chloride	Procainamide	Propranolol	Quinidine	Sodium bicarbonate	Streptokinase	Tobramycin	Verapamil
L	I		N	N	G	N	I	N	N	P	P	N	N	D	N	N	P
N	N	N		N	N	N	N	N	N	P	N	N	N	I	N	N	P
N	P	N	N		N	N	P	N	P	P	P	N	N	N	N	N	N
N	N	G	N	N		N	N	N	N	N	N	N	N	N	N	N	P
N	N	N	N	N	N		N	N	N	N	N	N	N	N	N	N	N
N	P	I	N	P	N	N		N	N	P	N	N	N	I	N	N	P
N	N	N	N	N	N	N	N		N	N	N	N	N	N	N	N	N
N	N	N	N	P	N	N	N	N		P	N	N	N	N	N	N	N
N	P	P	P	P	N	N	P	N	P		P	P	N	P	N	N	P
N	N	P	N	P	N	N	N	N	N	P		N	N	N	N	N	P
N	N	N	N	N	N	N	N	N	N	P	N		N	N	N	N	P
N	N	N	N	N	N	N	N	N	N	N	N	N		N	N	N	P
I	I	D	I	N	N	N	I	N	N	P	N	N	N		N	N	P
N	N	N	N	N	N	N	N	N	N	N	N	N	N	N		N	N
N	N	N	N	N	N	N	N	N	N	N	N	N	N	N	N		P
P	P	P	P	N	P	N	P	N	N	P	P	P	P	P	N	P	

Normal Reference Laboratory Values*

SERUM BLOOD VALUES

Determination	Reference Range
Albumin	3.5–5.0 g/100 mL
Ammonia	12–55 μmol/liter
Amylase	4–25 U/mL
Bilirubin	Direct: up to 0.4 mg/100 mL
	Total: up to 1.0 mg/100 mL
Calcium	8.5–10.5 mg/100 mL
	(slightly higher in children)
Carbon dioxide content	24–30 mEq/liter
Chloride	100–106 mEq/liter
Creatinine	0.6–1.5 mg/100 mL
Globulin	2.3–3.5 g/100 mL
Glucose	70–110 mg/100 mL
Lactic acid	0.6–1.8 mEq/liter
Lipids:	
Cholesterol	120–220 mg/100 mL
Triglycerides	40–150 mg/100 mL
Magnesium	1.5–2.0 mEq/liter
Osmolality	280–296 mOsm/kg
Oxygen saturation	96–100%
P_{CO_2}	35–45 mm Hg
pH	7.35–7.45
P_{O_2}	75–100 mm Hg
Phosphorus	3.0–4.5 mg/100 mL
Potassium	3.5–5.0 mEq/liter
Protein total	6.0–8.4 g/100 mL

*Source: Adapted from information appearing in *NEJM.* "Case Records of the Massachusetts General Hospital" by R.E. Scully, 1986, The New England Journal of Medicine, *324*, pp. 39–49. Copyright 1986 by The New England Journal of Medicine, by permission.

Serum glutamic-oxaloacetic transaminase (SGOT)	7–27 U/liter
Serum glutamic-pyruvic transaminase (SGPT)	1–21 U/liter
Sodium	135–145 mEq/liter
Urea nitrogen (BUN)	8–25 mg/100 mL
Uric acid	3.0–7.0 mg/100 mL

URINE VALUES

Determination	Reference Range
Amylase	24–76 U/mL
Calcium	300 mg/day or less
Catecholamines:	
Epinephrine	$< 20\mu g$/day
Norepinephrine	$< 100 \mu g$/day
Copper	1–100 μg/day
Creatinine	15–25 mg/kg of body weight per day
Hemoglobin	0
pH	5–7
Protein	<150 mg/24 hours
Glucose	0

HEMATOLOGIC VALUES

Determination	Reference Range
Coagulation screening tests	
Bleeding time	3–9.5 minutes
Prothrombin time	< 2-second deviation from control
Partial thromboplastin time	25–38 seconds
Whole blood clot lysis	No clot lysis in 24 hours
Thrombin time	Control + 5 seconds
Complete blood count	
Hematocrit	Males: 45–52 percent
	Females: 37–48 percent
Hemoglobin	Males: 13–18 g/100 mL
	Females: 12–16 g/100 mL
Leukocyte count	4300–10,800/mm^3
Erythrocyte count	4.2–5.9 million/mm^3
Platelet count	150,000–350,000/mm^3
Reticulocyte count	0.5–2.5 percent red cells

IMMUNOLOGIC TESTS

Determination	Reference Range
Rheumatoid factor	<60 IU/mL

527

Anti-DNA antibodies	Negative at 1 : 8 dilution of serum
Complement, total hemolytic	150–250 U/mL
Cryoprecipitate proteins	None detected
Immunoglobulins:	
IgG	639–1349 mg/100 mL
IgA	70–312 mg/100 mL
IgM	86–352 mg/100 mL

Guidelines for Personnel Dealing with Cytotoxic (Antineoplastic) Drugs*

The mutagenic, teratogenic, carcinogenic, and local irritant properties of many cytotoxic agents are well established and pose a possible hazard to the health of occupationally exposed individuals. These potential hazards necessitate special attention to the procedures used in the handling, preparation, and administration of these drugs and in the proper disposal of residues and wastes. These recommendations are intended to provide information for the protection of personnel participating in the clinical process of chemotherapy. It is the responsibility of institutional and private health care providers to adopt and use appropriate procedures for protection and safety.

I. **Environmental Protection**
   1. Preparation of cytotoxic agents should be performed in a Class II biologic safety cabinet located in an area with minimal traffic and air turbulence. Class II type A cabinets are the minimal requirement. Class II cabinets that are exhausted to the outside are preferred.
   2. The biologic safety cabinet must be certified by qualified personnel at least annually or any time the cabinet is physically moved.

II. **Operator Protection**
   1. Disposable surgical latex gloves are recommended for all procedures involving cytotoxic agents.
   2. Gloves should routinely be changed approximately every 30 minutes when working steadily with cytotoxic agents. Gloves should be removed immediately after overt contamination.
   3. Protective barrier garments should be worn for all procedures involving the preparation and disposal of cytotoxic agents. These gar-

---

*Source: From Recommendations for Handling Cytotoxic Agents, National Study Commission on Cytotoxic Exposure, September 1987. For additional information, contact the Commission's Chairman.

ments should have a closed front, long sleeves, and closed cuff (either elastic or knit).

4. Protective garments must not be worn outside the work area.

III. **Techniques and Precautions for Use in the Class II Biologic Safety Cabinet**

1. Special techniques and precautions must be used because of the vertical (downward) laminar airflow.

2. Clean surfaces of the cabinet using 70% alcohol and a disposal towel before and after preparation. Discard towel into a hazardous chemical waste container.

3. Prepare the work surface of the biologic safety cabinet by covering it with a plastic-backed absorbent pad. This pad should be changed when the cabinet is cleaned or after a spill.

4. The biologic safety cabinet should be operated with the blower on, 24 hours/day — 7 days a week. Where the biologic safety cabinet is used infrequently (e.g., one or two times weekly) it may be turned off after thoroughly cleaning all interior surfaces. Turn on the blower 15 minutes before beginning work in the cabinet.

5. Drug preparations must be performed only with the view screen at the recommended access opening. Professionally accepted practices concerning the aseptic preparation of injectable products should be followed.

6. All materials needed to complete the procedure should be placed into the biologic safety cabinet before beginning work to avoid interruptions of cabinet airflow. Allow a 2- to 3-minute period before beginning work for the unit to purge itself of airborne contaminants.

7. The proper procedures for use in the biologic safety cabinet differ from those used in the horizontal laminar hood because of the nature of the airflow pattern. Clean air descends through the work zone from the top of the cabinet toward the work surface. As it descends, the air is split, with some leaving through the rear perforation and some leaving through the front perforation.

8. The least efficient area of the cabinet in terms of product and personnel protection is within 3 in of the sides near the front opening, and work should not be performed in these areas.

9. Entry into and exit from the cabinet should be in a direct manner perpendicular to the face of the cabinet. Rapid movements of the hands in the cabinet and laterally through the protective air barrier should be avoided.

IV. **Compounding Procedures and Techniques**

1. Hands must be washed thoroughly before gloving and after gloves are removed.

2. Care must be taken to avoid puncturing of gloves and possible self-innoculation.

3. Syringes and I.V. sets with Luer-lock fittings should be used whenever possible to avoid spills owing to disconnection.

4. To minimize aerosolization, vials containing cytotoxic agents should be vented with a hydrophobic filter to equalize internal pressure, or the negative-pressure technique should be used.

5. Before opening ampules, care should be taken to ensure that no liquid

remains in the tip of the ampule. A sterile disposable sponge should be wrapped around the neck of the ampule to reduce aerosolization. Ampules should be broken in a direction away from the body.

6. For sealed vials, final drug measurement should be performed prior to removing the needle from the stopper of the vial and after the pressure has been equalized.

7. A closed collection vessel should be available in the biologic safety cabinet, or the original vial may be used to hold discarded excess drug solutions.

8. Cytotoxic agents should be properly labeled to identify the need for caution in handling (e.g., "Chemotherapy: Dispose of Properly").

9. The final prepared dosage form should be protected from leakage or breakage by being sealed in a transparent plastic container labeled "Do Not Open if Contents Appear to be Broken."

V. Precautions for Administration

1. Disposable surgical latex gloves should be worn during administration of cytotoxic agents. Hands must be washed thoroughly before gloving and after gloves are removed.

2. Protective barrier garments may be worn. Such garments should have a closed front, long sleeves, and closed cuff (either elastic or knit).

3. Syringes and I.V. sets with Luer-lock fittings should be used whenever possible.

4. Special care must be taken in priming I.V. sets. The distal tip or needle cover must be removed before priming. Priming can be performed into a sterile, alcohol-dampened gauze sponge. Other acceptable methods of priming such as closed receptacles (e.g., evacuated containers) or backfilling of I.V. sets may be used. Do not prime sets or syringes into the sink or any open receptacle.

VI. Disposal Procedures

1. Place contaminated materials in a leak- and puncture-proof container appropriately marked as hazardous chemical waste. These containers should be suitable to collect bottles, vials, gloves, disposable gowns, and other materials used in the preparation and administration of cytotoxic agents.

2. Contaminated needles, syringes, sets, and tubing should be disposed of intact. In order to prevent aerosolization, needles and syringes should not be clipped.

3. Cytotoxic drug waste should be transported according to the institutional procedures for hazardous material.

4. There is insufficient information to recommend any preferred method for disposal of cytotoxic drug waste.
   a. One acceptable method for disposal of hazardous waste is by incineration in an Environmental Protection Agency (EPA) permitted hazardous water incinerator.
   b. Another acceptable method of disposal is by burial at an EPA permitted hazardous waste site.
   c. A licensed hazardous waste disposal company may be consulted for information concerning available methods of disposal in the local area.

VII. Personnel Policy Recommendations

1. Personnel involved in any aspect of the handling of cytotoxic agents must receive an orientation to the agents, including their known risks, and special training in safe handling procedures.
2. Access to the compounding area must be limited to authorized personnel.
3. Personnel working with these agents should be supervised regularly to ensure compliance with procedures.
4. Acute exposures must be documented and the exposed employee referred for medical examination.
5. Personnel should refrain from applying cosmetics in the work area. Cosmetics may provide a source of prolonged exposure if contaminated.
6. Eating, drinking, chewing gum, smoking, or storing food in areas where cytotoxic agents are handled should be prohibited. Each of these can be a source of ingestion if they are accidentally contaminated.

VIII. Monitoring Procedures

1. Policies and procedures to monitor the equipment and operating techniques of personnel handling cytotoxic agents should be implemented and performed on a regular basis with appropriate documentation. Specific methods of monitoring should be developed to meet the complexities of the function.
2. It is recommended that personnel involved in the preparation of cytotoxic agents be given periodic health examinations in accordance with institutional policy.

IX. Procedures for Acute Exposure or Spills

1. Acute exposure
   a. Overtly contaminated gloves or outer garments should be removed immediately.
   b. Hands must be washed after removing gloves. Some cytotoxic agents have been documented to penetrate gloves.
   c. In case of skin contact with a cytotoxic drug product, the affected area should be washed thoroughly with soap and water. Refer for medical attention as soon as possible.
   d. For eye exposure, flush affected eye with copious amounts of water, and refer for medical attention immediately.
2. Spills
   a. All personnel involved in the clean-up of a spill should wear protective barrier garments (e.g. gloves, gowns). These garments and other material used in the process should be disposed of properly.
   b. Double gloving is recommended for cleaning up spills.

POSITION STATEMENT

The Handling of Cytotoxic Agents by Women Who Are Pregnant, Attempting to Conceive, or Breastfeeding

There are substantial data regarding the mutagenic, teratogenic, and abortifacient properties of certain cytotoxic agents both in animals and humans who

532

have received therapeutic doses of these agents. Additionally, the scientific literature suggests a possible association of occupational exposure to certain cytotoxic agents during the first trimester of pregnancy with fetal loss or malformation. These data suggest the need for caution when women who are pregnant or are attempting to conceive handle cytotoxic agents. Incidentally, there is no evidence relating male exposure to cytotoxic agents with adverse fetal outcome. There are no studies that address the possible risk associated with the occupational exposure to cytotoxic agents and the passage of these agents into breast milk. Nevertheless, it is prudent that women who are breastfeeding exercise caution in handling cytotoxic agents.

If all procedures for safe handling, such as those recommended by the Commission, are complied with, the potential for exposure will be minimized.

Personnel should be provided with information to make an individual decision. This information should be provided in written form, and it is advisable that a statement of understanding be signed.

It is essential to refer to individual state right-to-know laws to ensure compliance.

Dilution Rates of Intravenous Drugs

Drug	Type and Amount of Diluent to Use
Adrenocorticotropic hormone (ACTH) (corticotropin for injection) (Acthar)	D₅W* or NSS† At least 250 mL for whatever diagnostic dose physician orders; dilution is often 500 mL (do not mix in Soluset)
Alteplase, recombinant (Activase)	Sterile water only *without preservatives* 50 mg in 50 mL 100-mg dose; 60 mg in 1 h, 20 mg/h for 2 h
Amikacin sulfate (Amikin)	D₅W or NSS 5 mg/mL (500 mg in 200 mL of diluent)
Aminocaproic acid (Amicar)	D₅W or NSS or Ringer's injection 1 g in 50 mL of diluent
Aminophylline (multisource)	D₅W or NSS 250 mL or more (do not mix in a Soluset)
Amphotericin B (Fungizone)	Reconstitute as follows: 1. With sterile needle and syringe, rapidly inject 10 mL sterile water for injection (without additives). 2. Shake vial well until clear. 3. Dilute with D₅W (with pH of above 4.2) 1 mg/10 mL. Do not use NSS (suspension will precipitate). Do not filter (filter may block passage of antibiotic dispersion). Wrap bottle in foil to protect from exposure to light.
Ampicillin (Omnipen, Polycillin, others)	Sterile water or NSS D₅NS, D₅W 2–30 mg/mL over 10–15 min
Anistreplase (APSAC, Eminase)	Sterile water 5 mL to 30 U over 2–5 min; do not shake
Aztreonam (Azactam)	Most solutions 1 g in 100 mL over 20–60 min 1 g in 6–10 mL bolus over 3–5 min

Drug	Type and Amount of Diluent to Use
Calcium disodium edetate (Calcium Disodium Versenate)	D₅W or NSS 1 g in 250–500 mL
Carbenicillin disodium (Geopen, Pyopen)	Most solutions 1 g in 10–20 mL of sterile water for direct I.V. administration. May be added to large volumes of most solutions, including 50–100 mL additive bottles.
Cefamandole naftate (Mandol)	D₅W or NSS 1 g in 10 mL (I.V. push) 1 or 2 g in 50 mL (infusion)
Cefotaxime sodium (Claforan)	D₅W, NSS, or other compatible solution 1 g 30 to 90 min
Cefotetan (Cefotan)	D₅W or NSS 1–2 g in 10–20 mL over 3–5 min direct or 50–100 mL intermittent
Cefoxitin sodium (Mefoxin)	D₅W, NSS, sterile water for injection, lactated Ringer's solution 1 to 2 g in 50 mL
Ceftazidime (Fortaz)	D₅W 1 g diluted in 50–100 mL
Ceftizoxime sodium (Cefizox)	D₅, D₁₀W, D/NS, invert sugar, or lactated Ringer's solution 1 g in 50–100 mL bolus over 2–3 min or 30 min intermittent
Ceftriaxone sodium (Rocephin)	D₅W, D₁₀W, NSS 250 mg diluted with 50–100 mL
Cephapirin sodium (Cefadyl)	D₅W or NSS 1 g in 50 mL; 2 g in 100 mL
Cimetidine HCl (Tagamet)	D₅W 300 mg in 100 mL
Cortisol sodium succinate (Solu-Cortef, A-hydroCort)	D₅W or NSS At least 1 mL of diluent/mg
Dexamethasone phosphate (Decadron, Hexadrol)	D₅W, NSS, D₅NS, or lactated Ringer's solution 1 mg–40 mg in 500 mL
Erythromycin gluceptate (Ilotycin Gluceptate)	D₅W or 0.9% sodium chloride injection less than 500 mg in 100 mL 500 mg in 250 mL 1 g in 1000 mL (Reconstitute with sterile water, no preservatives. Add 2.5 mL sodium bicarbonate to 100 mL of I.V. solution and 5 mL sodium bicarbonate to 250 mL. Without sodium bicarbonate, solution remains stable for only 4 h and is extremely irritating to the vein wall; solution *must* run over 1 h)
Famotidine (Pepcid)	0.9% NSS, D₅W, or lactated Ringer's solution 2 mL in 100 mL infused over 15–30 min (20 mg in 2 mL)

(continued)

Drug	Type and Amount of Diluent to Use
Heparin sodium (multisource)	Usually D_5W or NSS or lactated Ringer's injection At least 250 mL and usually 500 mL or 1000 mL depending on physician's order; heparin is given by I.V. push bolus or slow I.V. infusion (do not mix in Soluset)
Imipenem-cilastatin sodium (Primaxin)	Most solutions 250 mg in 100 mL over 20–30 min 1 g over 40–60 min
Iron dextran (Imferon, Chromagen D, Dextraron-50)	Administer undiluted (drug comes already reconstituted with NSS) by slow I.V. push bolus (1 min/mL). Drug is sometimes mixed with at least 250 mL NSS and given by slow I.V. infusion (over 1–3 h), but this is not a manufacturer's recommendation. Physician should give initial test dose to check for adverse reactions.
Methicillin sodium (Staphcillin, Celbenin)	D_5W, NSS, or sterile water for injection: 1 g in 50 mL 2 g in 100 mL
Methyldopate HCl (Aldomet Ester)	D_5W 100 mL Usual dosage is 250–500 mg, but up to 1 g can be given in 100 mL. Solution usually runs over 30–60 min.
Methylprednisolone sodium succinate (Solu-Medrol, A-Methapred)	D_5W or NSS mix-o-vial Less than 1 g in 50 mL 1 g or more in 100 mL For initial reconstitution of drug in manufacturer's vial, use *only* the diluent provided by the manufacturer.
Metronidazole HCl (Flagyl I.V.)	D_5W, NSS, or lactated Ringer's solution 1. Reconstitute with 4.4 mL of diluent. 2. Add to I.V. solution in concentration not to exceed 8 mg/mL. 3. Neutralize with 5 mEq sodium bicarbonate for each 500 mg of metronidazole.
Mezlocillin sodium (Mezlin)	0.9% NSS 10–100 mg/mL Lactated Ringer's solution 10–100 mg/mL 0.9% NSS 250 mg/mL

Drug	Type and Amount of Diluent to Use
Nafcillin sodium (Nafcil, Unipen, Nallpen)	Sterile water, NSS, Ringer's injection, D$_5$W 1 g in 15–30 mL bolus over 10–15 min
Oxacillin sodium (Prostaphlin)	NSS or sterile water 1 g in 10–20 mL bolus over 10 min
Oxytocin (Pitocin, Syntocinon)	D$_5$W or NSS 10 to 40 U in 1000 mL
Penicillin G sodium	D$_5$W or NSS 3 million U or less in 50 mL More than 3 million U in 100 mL
Piperacillin sodium (Pipracil)	Sterile water, NSS, D$_5$W 1 g in 50–100 mL over 30 min or as bolus over 3–5 min
Potassium chloride (multisource)	Any standard diluent (D$_5$W, NSS, Ringer's lactate, and so on) as ordered by physician. Do not mix in Soluset (too great a concentration can cause cardiac irritability and phlebitis).
Potassium phosphate (multisource)	Any standard diluent as ordered by physician. At least 500 mL. Use vials once only; do not store used vial (solution does not contain a bacteriostatic agent.) Do not mix in Soluset.
Ranitidine (Zantac)	0.9% NSS, D$_5$W, D$_{10}$W, lactated Ringer's solution 50 mg in 20 mL injected over 5 min
Streptokinase (Streptase)	NSS, D$_5$W 5 mL to vial. Do not shake. Withdraw and dilute with additional 45 mL. 15 mL/h over 30 min; 3 mL/h maintenance dose.
Ticarcillin disodium (Ticar)	D$_5$W, NSS, or sterile water for injection 1.0 g to 5.0 g in 100 mL
Tobramycin sulfate (Nebcin)	D$_5$W or NSS 40 mg or less in 50 mL; 41–100 mg in 100 mL; more than 100 mg: 1 mg/mL
Vancomycin HCl (Vancocin)	D$_5$W or NSS less than 500 mg in 100 mL 500 mg in 200 mL
Vitamins (Folvite, 5 mg; Betalin-5, 100 mg; Berocca C, 1 amp; Hexabetalin)	All common diluents in amounts ordered by physician Added to 500 mL or more of solution, usually 1 L.

*D$_5$W = 5% dextrose in water; D$_{10}$W = 10% dextrose in water.
†NSS = Normal saline solution; D$_5$NS = 5% dextrose in normal saline.
Source: From "When You Have to Reconstitute Meds" by R. Hickman, 1981, *RN*, *4*, pp. 40–43. Copyright 1981 by Medical Economics Co. Adapted by permission.

Nursing Diagnoses Categories, NANDA — 10th National Conference

Activity intolerance
Activity intolerance, high risk for
Adjustment, impaired
Airway clearance, ineffective
Anxiety (specify level)
Aspiration, high risk for†
Body image disturbance
Body temperature, altered, high risk for
Breastfeeding, effective†
Breastfeeding, ineffective†
Breastfeeding, interrupted*
Breathing pattern, ineffective
Cardiac output, decreased
Caregiver role strain*
Caregiver role strain, high risk for*
Communication, impaired verbal
Conflict, decisional†
Conflict, parental role
Constipation
Constipation, colonic†
Constipation, perceived†
Coping, defensive†
Denial, ineffective†
Diarrhea
Disuse syndrome, high risk for†
Diversional activity deficit
Dysreflexia†
Family coping, compromised
Family coping, disabling

Family coping, potential for growth
Family processes, altered
Fatigue†
Fear
Feeding pattern, ineffective infant*
Fluid volume deficit [active loss]
Fluid volume deficit, high risk for
Fluid volume excess
Gas exchange, impaired
Grieving, anticipatory
Grieving, dysfunctional
Growth and development, altered
Health maintenance, altered
Health seeking behaviors [specify]
Home maintenance management, impaired
Hopelessness
Hyperthermia
Hypothermia
Incontinence, bowel
Incontinence, functional
Incontinence, reflex
Incontinence, stress
Incontinence, total
Incontinence, urge
Infection, high risk for
Injury, high risk for
Knowledge deficit [learning need] (specify)

---

*New diagnoses
†Revised diagnoses

Mobility, impaired physical
Noncompliance [compliance, altered] (specify)
Nutrition, altered: less than body requirements
Nutrition, altered: more than body requirements
Nutrition, altered: more than body requirements
Oral mucous membrane, altered
Pain [acute]
Pain, chronic
Parenting, altered
Parenting, altered, high risk for
Peripheral neurovascular dysfunction, high risk for*
Personal identity disturbance
Poisoning, high risk for
Post-trauma response
Powerlessness
Protection, altered†
Rape-trauma response
Rape-trauma syndrome: compound reaction
Rape-trauma syndrome: silent reaction
Relocation stress syndrome*
Role performance, altered
Self-care deficit: feeding, bathing/hygiene, dressing/grooming, toileting
Self-esteem, chronic low†
Self-esteem disturbance
Self-esteem, situational low†
Self-mutilation, high risk for*
Sensory-perceptual alterations

(specify): (visual, auditory, kinesthetic, gustatory, tactile, olfactory)
Sexual dysfunction
Sexuality patterns, altered
Skin integrity, impaired
Skin integrity, impaired high risk for
Sleep pattern disturbance
Social interaction, impaired
Social isolation
Spiritual distress
Suffocation, high risk for
Swallowing, impaired
Therapeutic regimen (individuals), ineffective management of*
Thermoregulation, ineffective
Thought processes, altered
Tissue integrity, impaired
Tissue perfusion, altered [specify] (Cerebral, cardiopulmonary, renal, gastrointestinal, peripheral)
Trauma, high risk for
Unilateral neglect
Urinary elimination, altered patterns of
Urinary retention [acute/chronic]
Ventilation, spontaneous: inability to sustain*
Ventilatory weaning response, dysfunctional*
Violence, high risk for: directed at self/others

Source: Data from *Taber's Cyclopedic Medical Dictionary,* 17th edition by C.L. Thomas (ed), 1993, Philadelphia: F.A. Davis Company. Copyright 1993 by F.A. Davis Company; and *Nurse's Pocket Guide: Nursing Diagnoses with Interventions,* 3rd edition by M.E. Doenges and M.F. Moorhouse (1990), Philadelphia: F.A. Davis Company. Copyright 1990 by F.A. Davis Company.

NANDA-Approved Nursing Diagnoses: Definitions*

Activity intolerance: The state in which an individual has insufficient physiologic or psychologic energy to endure or complete required or desired daily activities

Activity intolerance, high risk for: The state in which an individual is at risk of experiencing insufficient physiologic or psychologic energy to endure or complete required desired daily activities

Adjustment, impaired: The state in which an individual is unable to modify his or her life-style or behavior in a manner consistent with a change in health status

Airway clearance, ineffective: The state in which an individual is unable to clear secretions or obstructions from the respiratory tract to maintain airway patency

Anxiety (specify level): A vague, uneasy feeling, the source of which is often nonspecific or unknown to the individual

Aspiration, high risk for: The state in which an individual is at risk for entry of gastric secretions, oropharyngeal secretions, or exogenous food or fluids into tracheobronchial passages owing to dysfunction or absence of normal protective mechanisms

Body image disturbance: Disruption in the perception of one's body image

Body temperature, altered, high risk for: The state in which an individual is at risk for failure to maintain body temperature within normal range

Breastfeeding, ineffective: The state in which a mother, infant, and/or family experiences dissatisfaction or difficulty with the breastfeeding process

Breastfeeding, interrupted: A break in the continuity of the breastfeeding process as a result of inability or inadvisability to put baby to breast for feeding

---

Source: Data from *Taber's Cyclopedic Medical Dictionary*, 17th edition by C.L. Thomas (ed), 1993, Philadelphia: F.A. Davis Company. Copyright 1993 by F.A. Davis Company; and *Nurse's Pocket Guide: Nursing Diagnoses*, with *Interventions*, 3rd edition by M.J. Kim, G.K. McFarland, and A.M. McLane, 1989, St. Louis, C.V. Mosby Company. Copyright 1989 by C.V. Mosby Company.

Breathing pattern, ineffective: The state in which an individual's inhalation and/or exhalation pattern does not enable adequate ventilation

Cardiac output, decreased: The state in which the blood pumped by an individual's heart is sufficiently reduced that it is inadequate to meet the needs of the body's tissues

Caregiver role strain: A caregiver's felt difficulty in performing the family caregiver role.

Caregiver role strain, high risk for: A caregiver is vulnerable for felt difficulty in performing the family caregiver role.

Comfort, altered: See Pain

Communication, impaired verbal: The state in which an individual experiences a decreased or absent ability to use or understand language in human interaction

Constipation: The state in which an individual experiences a change in normal bowel habits characterized by a decrease in frequency and/or passage of hard, dry stools

Constipation, colonic: The state in which an individual's pattern of elimination is characterized by hard, dry stool that results from a delay in passage of food residue

Constipation, perceived: The state in which an individual makes a self-diagnosis of constipation and ensures a daily bowel movement through use of laxatives, enemas, and suppositories

Coping, defensive: The state in which an individual experiences falsely positive self-evaluation based on a self-protective pattern that defends against underlying perceived threats to positive self-regard

Coping, ineffective individual: Impairment of adaptive behaviors and problem-solving abilities of a person in meeting life's demands and roles

Decisional conflict (specify): A state of uncertainty about the course of action to be taken when choice among competing actions involves risk, loss, or challenge to personal life values (specify focus of conflict, e.g., choices regarding health, family relationships, career, finances, or other life events)

Denial, ineffective: A conscious or unconscious attempt to disavow the knowledge or meaning of an event to reduce anxiety/fear to the detriment of health

Diarrhea: The state in which an individual experiences a change in normal bowel habits characterized by the frequent passage of loose, fluid, unformed stools

Disuse syndrome, high risk for: The state in which an individual is at risk for deterioration of body systems as the result of prescribed or unavoidable inactivity

Diversional activity deficit: The state in which an individual experiences a decreased stimulation from, or interest or engagement in, recreational or leisure activities

Dysreflexia: The state in which an individual with a spinal cord injury at T-7 or above experiences, or is at risk of experiencing, life-threatening uninhibited sympathetic response of the nervous system to a noxious stimulus

Family coping, compromised: Insufficient, ineffective, or compromised support, comfort, assistance, or encouragement usually by a supportive primary person (family member or close friend); patient may need it to manage or master adaptive tasks related to his or her health challenge

541

Family coping, disabling: Behavior of significant person (family members or other primary person) that disables his or her own capacities and the patient's capacities to effectively address tasks essential to either person's adaptation to the health challenge

Family coping, potential for growth: Effective managing of adaptive tasks by family member involved with the patient's health challenge, who now is exhibiting desire and readiness for enhanced health and growth in regard to self and in relation to the patient

Family processes, altered: The state in which a family that normally functions effectively experiences a dysfunction

Fatigue: An overwhelming sense of exhaustion and decreased capacity for physical and mental work, regardless of adequate sleep

Fear: Feeling of dread related to an identifiable source that the person validates

Feeding pattern, ineffective infant: A state in which an infant demonstrates an impaired ability to suck or coordinate the suck-swallow response.

Fluid volume deficit [active loss]: The state in which an individual experiences vascular, cellular, or intracellular dehydration related to active loss

Fluid volume deficit [regulatory failure]: The state in which an individual experiences vascular, cellular, or intracellular dehydration related to failure of regulatory mechanisms

Fluid volume deficit, high risk for: The state in which an individual is at risk of experiencing vascular, cellular, or intracellular dehydration

Fluid volume excess: The state in which an individual experiences increased fluid retention and edema

Gas exchange, impaired: The state in which an individual experiences an imbalance between oxygen uptake and carbon dioxide elimination at the alveolar-capillary membrane gas exchange area

Grieving, anticipatory: The state in which an individual grieves before an actual loss

Grieving, dysfunctional: The state in which actual or perceived object loss (object loss is used in the broadest sense) exists; objects include people, possessions, a job, status, home, ideals, parts and processes of the body, and so on

Growth and development, altered: The state in which an individual demonstrates deviations in norms from his or her age group

Health maintenance, altered: Inability to identify, manage, and/or seek out help to maintain health

Health-seeking behaviors (specify): The state in which a patient in stable health is actively seeking ways to alter personal health habits and/or the environment in order to move toward optimal health (*stable health status* is defined as age-appropriate illness prevention measures achieved; the patient reports good or excellent health, and signs and symptoms of disease, if present, are controlled)

Home maintenance management, impaired: Inability to independently maintain a safe growth-promoting immediate environment

Hopelessness: The subjective state in which an individual sees limited or no alternatives or personal choices available and is unable to mobilize energy on own behalf

Hyperthermia: The state in which an individual's body temperature is elevated above his or her normal range

Hypothermia: The state in which an individual's body temperature is reduced below his or her normal range but not below 35.6°C (rectal)

Incontinence, bowel: The state in which an individual experiences a change in normal bowel habits characterized by involuntary passage of stool

Incontinence, functional: The state in which an individual experiences an involuntary, unpredictable passage of urine

Incontinence, reflex: The state in which an individual experiences an involuntary loss of urine occurring at somewhat predictable intervals when a specific bladder volume is reached

Incontinence, stress: The state in which an individual experiences a loss of urine of less than 50 mL occurring with increased abdominal pressure

Incontinence, total: The state in which an individual experiences a continuous and unpredictable loss of urine

Incontinence, urge: The state in which an individual experiences involuntary passage of urine occurring soon after a strong sense of urgency to void

Infection, high risk for: The state in which an individual is at increased risk for being invaded by pathogenic organisms

Injury, high risk for: The state in which an individual is at risk of injury as a result of environmental conditions interacting with the individual's adaptive and defensive resources (see also Poisoning, potential for; Suffocation, potential for; Trauma, potential for)

Knowledge deficit [Learning need] (specify): The state in which specific information is lacking

Mobility, impaired physical: The state in which an individual experiences a limitation of ability for independent physical movement

Noncompliance [compliance, altered] (specify): A person's informed decision not to adhere to a therapeutic recommendation

Nutrition, altered: less than body requirements: The state in which an individual experiences an intake of nutrients insufficient to meet metabolic needs

Nutrition, altered: more than body requirements: The state in which an individual is experiencing an intake of nutrients that exceeds metabolic needs

Nutrition, high risk for more than body requirements: The state in which an individual is at risk of experiencing an intake of nutrients that exceeds metabolic needs

Oral mucous membranes, altered: The state in which an individual experiences disruptions in the tissue layers of the oral cavity

Pain [acute]: The state in which an individual experiences and reports the presence of severe discomfort or an uncomfortable sensation

Pain, chronic: The state in which an individual experiences pain that continues for more than 6 months

Parental role conflict: The state in which a parent experiences role confusion and conflict in response to a crisis

Parenting, altered, high risk for: The state in which the ability of nurturing figure(s) to create an environment that promotes the optimum growth and development of another human being is altered or at risk

Peripheral neurovascular dysfunction, high risk for: A state in which an individual is at risk of experiencing a disruption in circulation, sensation, or motion of an extremity

Personal identity disturbance: Inability to distinguish between self and noneself

Poisoning, high risk: Accentuated risk of accidental exposure to, or ingestion of, drugs or dangerous products in doses sufficient to cause poisoning

Post-trauma response: The state in which an individual experiences a sustained painful response to (an) overwhelming traumatic event(s)

Powerlessness: Perception that one's own action will not significantly affect an outcome; a perceived lack of control over a current situation or immediate happening

Rape trauma syndrome: Forced, violent sexual penetration against the victim's will and consent; the trauma syndrome that develops from this attack or attempted attack includes an acute phase or disorganization of the victim's life-style and a long-term process of reorganization of life-style

Rape-trauma syndrome: compound reaction: An acute stress reaction to a rape or attempted rape, experienced along with other major stressors, that can include reactivation of symptoms of a previous condition

Rape-trauma syndrome: silent reaction: A complex stress reaction to a rape in which an individual is unable to describe or discuss the rape

Relocation stress syndrome: Physiologic and/or psychosocial disturbances as a result of transfer from one environment to another

Role performance, altered: Disruption in the way one perceives one's role performance

Self-care deficit, bathing/hygiene: The state in which an individual experiences an impaired ability to perform or complete bathing/hygiene activities for oneself

Self-care deficit, dressing/grooming: The state in which an individual experiences an impaired ability to perform or complete dressing and grooming activities for oneself

Self-care deficit, feeding: The state in which an individual experiences an impaired ability to perform or to complete feeding activities for oneself

Self-care deficit, toileting: The state in which an individual experiences an impaired ability to perform or complete toileting activities for oneself

Self-esteem, chronic low: Long-standing negative self-evaluation/feelings about self or self-capabilities

Self-esteem, disturbance: Negative self-evaluation/feelings about self or self-capabilities, which may be directly or indirectly expressed

Self-esteem, situational low: Negative self-evaluation/feelings about self that develop in response to a loss or change in an individual who previously had a positive self-evaluation

Self-mutilation, high risk for: A state in which an individual is at high risk to perform a deliberate act upon the self with the intent to injure, not kill, which produces immediate tissue damage to the body

Sensory-perceptual alterations (specify): visual, auditory, kinesthetic, gustatory, tactile, olfactory: The state in which an individual experiences a change in the amount or patterning of incoming stimuli accompanied by a diminished, exaggerated, distorted, or impaired response to such stimuli

Sexual dysfunction: The state in which an individual experiences a change in sexual function that is viewed as unsatisfying, unrewarding, or inadequate

Sexuality patterns, altered: The state in which an individual expresses concern regarding his or her sexuality

544

Skin integrity, impaired: The state in which an individual's skin is adversely altered

Skin integrity, impaired, high risk for: The state in which an individual's skin is at risk of being adversely altered

Sleep pattern disturbance: Disruption of sleep time causes discomfort or interferes with desired life-style

Social interaction, impaired: The state in which an individual participates in an insufficient or excessive quantity or ineffective quality of social exchange

Social isolation: Aloneness experienced by an individual and perceived as imposed by others and as a negative or threatened state

Spiritual distress: Disruption in the life principle that pervades a person's entire being and that integrates and transcends one's biologic and psychosocial nature

Suffocation, high risk for: Accentuated risk of accidental suffocation (inadequate air available for inhalation)

Swallowing, impaired: The state in which an individual has decreased ability to voluntarily pass fluids and/or solids from mouth to stomach

Therapeutic regimen (individuals), ineffective manager of: A pattern of regulating and integrating into daily living a program for treatment of illness and the sequelae of illness that is unsatisfactory for meeting specific health goals

Thermoregulation, ineffective: The state in which an individual's temperature fluctuates between hypothermia and hyperthermia

Thought processes, altered: The state in which an individual experiences a disruption in cognitive operations and activities

Tissue integrity, impaired: The state in which an individual experiences damage to mucous membrane or corneal, integumentary, or subcutaneous tissue (see also Oral mucous membrane, altered)

Tissue perfusion, altered (specify): cerebral, cardiopulmonary, renal, gastrointestinal, peripheral: The state in which an individual experiences a decrease in nutrition and oxygenation at the cellular level owing to a deficit in capillary blood supply

Trauma, high risk for: Accentuated risk of accidental tissue injury (e.g., wound, burn, fracture)

Unilateral neglect: The state in which an individual is perceptually unaware of and inattentive to one side of the body

Urinary elimination, altered patterns of: The state in which an individual experiences a disturbance in urine elimination (see also Incontinence [functional, reflex, stress, total, urge]

Urinary retention [acute/chronic]: The state in which an individual experiences incomplete emptying of the bladder

Ventilation, spontaneous: inability to sustain: A state in which a patient is unable to maintain adequate breathing to support life. This is measured by deterioration of arterial blood gases, increased work of breathing, and decreasing energy

Ventilatory weaning response, dysfunctional: A state in which a patient cannot adjust to lowered levels of mechanical ventilator support, which interrupts and prolongs the weaning process

Violence, high risk for: directed at self/others: The state in which an individual experiences behaviors that can be physically harmful either to self or others

Resource List of National Organizations Related to Intravenous Therapy

AMERICAN ASSOCIATION OF
  CRITICAL CARE NURSES
One Civic Plaza
Newport Beach, CA 92660

AMERICAN HOSPITAL
  ASSOCIATION
840 N. Lake Shore Drive
Chicago, IL 60611

AMERICAN SOCIETY FOR
  PARENTERAL AND ENTERAL
  NUTRITION (ASPEN)
8605 Cameron Street, Suite 500
Silver Spring, MD 20910
(301) 587-6315

ASSOCIATION FOR
  PRACTITIONERS IN
  INFECTION CONTROL
505 E. Hawley Street
Mundelein, IL 60060

CENTERS FOR DISEASE CONTROL
1600 Clifton Road
Atlanta, GA 30333
404-639-3311

INTRAVENOUS NURSES
  SOCIETY (INS)
Two Brighton Street, Suite 200
Belmont, MA 02178
617-489-5205

NATIONAL ASSOCIATION OF
  VASCULAR ACCESS NETWORK
  (NAVAN)
800 Menlo Avenue, Suite 115
Menlo Park, CA 94025
415-327-9430

ONCOLOGY NURSING SOCIETY
311 Banksville Road
Pittsburgh, PA 15216

Survey of Scope of Practice for LPN/LVNs by State, Related to Intravenous Therapy

This author has conducted a survey, completed December 1991, of each state to identify the role of the LPN/LVN related to I.V. therapy. The results are as follows.

The role of the LPN/LVN has changed over the past 10 years. From state to state, the issue of the LPN/LVN's role in I.V. therapy is under scrutiny. Twenty states have expanded the role of the LPN/LVN with specific guidelines and recommendations for practice, along with state certification. Twenty-six states have identified that the LPN/LVN has a designated role in I.V. therapy; however, the scope of practice is left up to each individual agency. Four states clearly state that the role of the LPN/LVN is not in the maintenance or initiation of I.V. therapy.

STATES WITH EXPANDED ROLE GUIDELINES

Alabama	Maryland
Arizona	Mississippi
California	Missouri
Colorado	Nevada
Delaware	New Hampshire
District of Columbia	New York
Florida	North Carolina
Idaho	Pennsylvania
Louisiana	South Carolina
Maine	Wyoming

STATES THAT IDENTIFY THAT THE ROLE OF THE LPN/LVN INCLUDES I.V. THERAPY, BUT DELEGATE THE RESPONSIBILITY OF EDUCATION, COMPETENCY, AND ROLE DELINEATION TO EACH AGENCY

Alaska	Ohio
Arkansas	Oklahoma
Connecticut	Oregon
Georgia	Rhode Island
Illinois	South Dakota
Indiana	Tennessee
Kansas	Texas
Kentucky	Utah
Massachusetts	Vermont
Michigan	Virginia
Minnesota	Washington
Montana	West Virginia
New Mexico	Wisconsin

STATES THAT DO NOT INCLUDE I.V. THERAPY IN THE ROLE OF THE LPN/LVN

Hawaii	Nebraska
Iowa	New Jersey

Index

An "f" following a page number indicates a figure; a "t" following a page number indicates a table.